Gulf Studies

Volume 23

This book series, indexed in Scopus, serves the growing scholarly interest in the dynamic, complex, and strategically important Arab Gulf region by offering an academic publication platform to scholars in the region and beyond. The series takes an interdisciplinary approach to documenting the changes occurring in Gulf societies. It aims to advance the understanding of Gulf societies and their interactions with the rest of the world from a non-Western perspective. The series explicitly gives scholars from the Arab Gulf region more voice and visibility in academic publications. It includes studies of the member states of the Gulf Cooperation Council (GCC), namely: Bahrain, Kuwait, Oman, Qatar, Saudi Arabia, and the United Arab Emirates, as well as Iran, Iraq, and Yemen. It accepts proposals for research monographs, edited volumes, and handbooks that explain how the Gulf societies' social, economic, and political landscapes have evolved over the past few decades. The series covers a wide range of topics within four broad themes, as follows:

(1) Social and Cultural Issues in the Gulf: Demography, migration, citizenship, gender, culture and identity, urbanization, education, new media, unemployment, youth, family, women empowerment, leadership, aging, human rights, sports, Islamic ethics, and Islam and society
(2) Politics and Security in the Gulf: Gulf defence and security, the GCC integration, Gulf politics and political systems, and the GCC's foreign policy
(3) Energy and Economics in the Gulf: The political economy of the Gulf, economic diversification, international investments, international trade, knowledge economy, energy security and geopolitics of energy, renewable energy development, environmental regulations, urban planning, and Islamic finance
(4) The GCC States and the World: The GCC and Iran, the GCC and Africa, the GCC and South Asia, the GCC and China, the GCC and East Asia, the GCC and Southeast Asia, and the GCC and Western powers.

Submission and Peer Review

All proposals will undergo peer review by the editorial board members. If accepted, the final manuscript will be peer reviewed internally by the editorial board as well as externally (single/double blind) by Springer ahead of acceptance and publication. Please submit your book proposal to the Series Editor, Md Mizanur Rahman: mizan@qu.edu.qa, and to Springer Publishing Editor, Alex Westcott Campbell: alexandra.campbell@springernature.com

Khalid Al-Naama

Domestic Abuse and Mental Health in Qatar

Challenges and Policy Interventions

Springer

Khalid Al-Naama
Doha International Family Institute
Doha, Qatar

ISSN 2662-4494 ISSN 2662-4508 (electronic)
Gulf Studies
ISBN 978-981-96-7391-9 ISBN 978-981-96-7392-6 (eBook)
https://doi.org/10.1007/978-981-96-7392-6

This Springer imprint is published by the registered company Springer Nature Singapore Pte Ltd.
The registered company address is: 152 Beach Road, #21-01/04 Gateway East, Singapore 189721, Singapore

Dedicated to my father, whose wisdom has served as my guiding light, and to my mother, whose encouragement has provided me with unwavering support. To my beloved wife, for her incredible sacrifice in taking on the family burden to support me. Your love and belief in me have been the foundation of my success. This book is for you.

Preface

This book stems from my dissertation entitled 'An Examination of the Impact of Domestic Abuse on Qatari Women's Mental Health', submitted to the University of Huddersfield in partial fulfilment of the requirements for the degree of Doctor of Philosophy in Psychology in 2023. I argue that domestic abuse against women can lead to mental health problems such as PTSD, depression, or anxiety which if not addressed can lead to serious consequences such as homicide. The key objective is to assess the occurrence of various forms of domestic abuse and investigate how domestic violence impacts the mental well-being of Qatari women. This is accomplished through the evaluation of the frequency of mental health disorders such as depression, anxiety, and post-traumatic stress disorder (PTSD). To achieve study objectives, I employ an explanatory sequential mixed approach. The overreaching research question is conceptualized to be reflected in the primary and subcategory objectives to understand domestic abuse against women in Qatar. The primary research questions are: (1) What forms of domestic abuse are prevalent and are experienced by Qatari women? (2) How does experiencing domestic abuse impact the emergence of mental health issues like PTSD, depression, and anxiety? The subcategory research questions are: (3) What factors are associated with the women's likelihood of experiencing intimate partner violence? And the subcategory question included: (4) How is woman's mindset associated with their risk of experiencing Intimate Partner Violence (IPV)? (5) Are abused women at an elevated risk of homicide? (6) Why do abused women remain in an abusive relationship? To answer these research questions, a quantitative survey with several measurement items was employed. The measurement scales for the Conflict Tactical Scale-2 and Economic Abuse Scale-12 are used to measure forms of abuse. Anxiety, depression, and PTSD are evaluated using mental health scales of the PHQ-9, Tylor Manifest Anxiety Scale, and the PCL-C civilian version, respectively.

I collected quantitative survey from mental health services organisations, family counselling centres, shelters for domestic abuse victims, university students, and public domain located in Qatar. Overall, three hundred and fifty (350) victims of domestic abuse in the past year gave their consent, and 165 women fulfilled the study's requirements to assess the prevalence of domestic abuse and its effects on women's mental health; to examine factors associated with victims of domestic abuse and effects of women's mindset on the risk of Intimate Partner Violence (IPV) victimization.

Major findings in the quantitative phase suggest that psychological aggression and economic abuse are the most reported forms of abuse whereas physical assault and sexual coercion and injury are the least reported kinds of abuse among the participants. Also, exposure to different forms of abuse is associated with increased risk of acquiring PTSD, depression, and anxiety. The results from regression analysis show that Psychological Aggression and Economic Abuse are significant positive predictors of PTSD level. In contrast, other forms of abuse are not significant predictors of PTSD. Furthermore, economic abuse is having a significant impact on depression levels. Negotiation and aggression are also significant predictors of anxiety level in contrast to the other forms of abuse.

It is additionally affirmed that an age gap between the husband and wife, having a greater number of children, a husband with lower educational attainment, a history of family violence, and being married to a polygamous partner were all linked to a heightened risk of IPV victimization.

Furthermore, results show that nearly 51 percent of the victims are having traditional and conservative attitudes while around 49 percent tend towards more equal rights and hold a liberal mindset about women's rights in society. Women with a pro-feminist mindset are at increased risk of experiencing a variety of kinds of domestic abuse. The finding could help in return to understand why women tend to adhere to a more conventional mindset to have less heated conflict in their lives. The risk of homicide is relatively low among the current sample as indicated by around 79 percent. The low score represents at variable danger, and the remaining 21 percent represents the presence of increased danger. Neither severe nor extreme danger in the current sample is reported which imply a high risk of homicide

I further explore qualitatively why abused women remain inactive or passive in the abusive relationship to augment the results obtained from the quantitative phase. Twenty women participate in the qualitative phase, and all are interviewed from WAYAK Mental Health Friends Association. Eight themes emerge from the participants' narratives in the qualitative phase centre around the individual, family, and societal factors. The eight themes are hopeless and psychological abuse, physical abuse, economic abuse during marriage and post-divorce, husband and wife socioeconomic status and risk of abuse, family pressure in marriage, bureaucracy and forms of divorce, family law and victims' rights, and risk of developing PTSD, depression and anxiety. All these were established and supported by the quantitative findings. Those distinctive patterns that emerge from the participants' narratives rationalize and provide another line of thought on understanding women's decision to remain in an abusive relationship. This is due to post-divorce arrangements in the family such as change in the child custody entitlement, victims' poor financial resources, and concern about post-divorce financial and residential arrangements among divorced mothers.

Similarly to many other countries in the region, women's domestic abuse is also prevalent in Qatar, and it is a problem that affects the mental health of women.

Furthermore, the study underscores the importance of developing policies to prevent domestic violence on a national level. I hope that this research will contribute to the growing body of literature on domestic abuse victims in the Middle East—an area that has traditionally received scanty attention in academic research.

Doha, Qatar Khalid Al-Naama

Acknowledgements

My deepest thanks go out to my family, including my wife Salwa. I am grateful to my wife Salwa for the constant support she has provided me regarding my decision to seek a doctorate in psychology. You have been very generous with your time, assistance, and compassion. I will never forget the moment when you told me, “There’s no need to waste our money and time travelling the world; instead, use that time and money to make me proud”, and all the other things you sacrificed for us. I will also never forget all the other things you did for us. To my children, who endured my absence during long hours of study and writing.

To my thesis advisors, Dr. John Synnott (Associate Professor of Psychology, University of Huddersfield) and Prof. Dr. Maria Ioannou (Professor of Psychology, University of Huddersfield), who supported me throughout my studies. They deserve my heartfelt appreciation. I want to convey my gratitude to my thesis committee members, Dr. John Synnott and Prof. Maria Ioannou, for their suggestions for improving my research project. I was able to narrow down my research subjects to ones that I could do with the help of your recommendations. You have no idea how much your words meant to me as I continued to work hard on my project. I appreciate them more than you know. It serves as a constant reminder that I am getting closer and closer to achieving my goal.

To my parents especially my mum. You have been such a fantastic and have had a positive impact on my life. I know how difficult it must have been for you to hide that feeling and the tears. You told me that the most difficult experiences in my life would make me stronger than I was before, and it was something you said to me when I had just broken my arm and had a few weeks left to do my thesis. Your memorable words “Guard both us and your aspirations” gave a reason never to give up on this dream. As soon as I came to the realisation that God had equipped me with the ability to lead others, I set new goals not just for my own family but also for the children and teenagers who lived in my neighbourhood.

Contents

List of Tables

Chapter 1
An Introduction

1.1 Domestic Abuse Against Women and Mental Health

Over the last few decades, the issue of domestic violence against women has received considerable attention in western nations. In order to better understand domestic abuse among Arab populations, a deeper understanding is needed, since Arab populations throughout the Middle East have similar perspectives and attitudes about women, which can contribute to Intimate Partner Violence (IPV) victimization. The situation in GCC nations is not different from the Arab world. In Qatar, keeping one's social identity continues to be seen as the most crucial aspect in sustaining the traditional family unit and its strong relationships. Like many other GCC countries, Qatar's social identity is shaped by triple belief systems, which constitute the basis of the family (Alshawi & Gardner, 2013). It contributes to the process of creating the basis for more non-Western conceptions involving intimate life partners. The traditional culture of Qatar is typical of an Arabic community that is collectivist (Al-Haj, 1987; Barakat, 1993), There is a historical preference for communal good over individual benefit and for social stability over social change in these societies. People tend to adhere firmly to social norms and values, as well as gender segregation rules (Al-Attiyah & Nasser, 2016).

The problem of domestic abuse against women is relevant to both public health and societal concerns. No matter how socioeconomic background or literacy status are, both men and women can be victims of domestic abuse; however, women are at greater risk for IPV (Yadav et al., 2022). This is because it denies women their fundamental rights, which may have a harmful effect on their mental health. Therefore, a comprehensive approach is essential to comprehend the aetiology of violence against women. This is because critical characteristics that were previously identified as risk factors in western research may vary by culture.

Domestic violence against women in Arab societies is little recorded, where the victims suffer in silence while their abusers go free. Drawing from prior studies, it has been determined that a more comprehensive analysis of domestic violence in

K. Al-Naama, *Domestic Abuse and Mental Health in Qatar*, Gulf Studies 23,
https://doi.org/10.1007/978-981-96-7392-6_1

the Middle East and North Africa (MENA) region is imperative for driving societal transformation via research-backed policy suggestions (Boy & Kulczycki, 2008, p. 53). The most major issue associated with being a victim of Intimate Partner Violence (IPV) is the associated social shame since Arab families see it as a very private matter. In the Middle East, Scholars argue, violence against women takes the form of honour crimes due to systematic discrimination rooted in social norms; violence that takes the form of honour crimes serves as a social control mechanism for women to avoid deviating from their traditional roles (Devers & Bacon, 2010). These worries or denials cannot be substantiated without scientific proof studies measuring the potential for violence in one of the conservative Arabic civilizations, such as Qatar. Still, some individuals may be sceptical about the prevalence and reports of domestic violence in Arabic society and therefore, understanding Qatari culture is essential and social values are essential when it comes to domestic abuse.

There is an increasing scholarship that tries to explain non-western family structures. However, the literature produced tries to explain non-western families in relation to the "universal", a synonym for the western understanding of the family. Melikian and Al-Easa's (1984) work explains Qatar's family structure. The article carries out a study conducted from 1974 to 1978 among Qatari college-going men and women to understand the significant changes that have taken place in Qatari society (Melikian & Al-Easa, 1984, p. 1). The authors first explain that Qatar has three levels of family structures: "the tribe, the clan, and the extended family" (p. 1). They explain that the branches of the tribe transcend national political boundaries; Qatar's tribes extend to Saudi Arabia, Kuwait, Bahrain, and the UAE (p. 1). However, tribal loyalties have become less important due to urbanization and the increasing importance of the modern nation-state (p. 1). They also explain that Qataris depend on their livelihood from their nation's natural resources such as oil ever since independence in 1971 rather than on pastoral grazing or camel breeding as was the case before (p. 1). They also mention that Qatar has a "booming" economy due to its oil revenue. Due to this, the state provides free education, free electricity, water, healthcare, and work opportunities to its citizens (p. 2).

After explaining Qatar's current political climate, the article explains the impact urbanization has had on the Qatari family. It contends that because of the nation's profound Islamic influence, the family continues to serve as the fundamental unit in society (p. 3). The Qatari family play the most dominant role in the socialization of their children; however, the extended family helps in this role as well, as fathers take their sons to the majlis to discuss family problems and politics while other male members are present (p. 4). In Qatari society, Islam dictates all aspects of life including "marriage, divorce, custodianship, and inheritance" (p. 3). Despite changes in society due to urbanization, it remains to be "patriarchal, extended, patrilineal, patrilocal, endogamous, and occasionally polygamous" (p. 3). The roles of its members are dominated by one's age and sex (p. 3). The practice of segregation of sexes still exists (p. 3). It also describes its features such as the large extended family consisting of grandparents, uncles, aunts and their children (p. 3). The custom is that the death of the father leads to the eldest son taking charge (p. 3). However, the article notes that the nuclear family structure is becoming more common (p. 3).

Another change is that wealth is becoming a huge factor in determining one's role (p. 3). Another increasing member of the family structure is the "nanny" who is often a foreigner; she has an impact on children as she raises them (p. 5). The article also explains the concept of marriage in Qatari families. Marriage is perceived as a responsibility (p. 5). It is based on the Islamic principle of kafaa, meaning equality. Hence, spouses look for an equal partner in descent and wealth (p. 1). It is preferred within the extended family, then with the clan, and then within the tribe (p. 1). The study conducted by the authors shows that men and women expect marriage to be monogamous (p. 6). Sixty one percent of the men preferred to marry within the extended family while only 24% of women preferred this choice (p. 6). Both men and women prefer to have fewer children and women want a more egalitarian role in marriage (pp. 6–7).

Scholars such as J. E Peterson also contribute to the literature on the changing Qatari family. According to him, the biggest impact of the discovery of oil has been the transformation of the Qatari economy (Peterson, 1990, p. 288). The economy has shifted from fishing, pastoralism, pearling, and agriculture to oil companies that at first hired nationals and then eventually internationals that encouraged consumer demand and paved the way for the service sector (p. 288). The economy has also transformed the "primitive" government and expanded its role (p. 288). The more powerful government then built a social welfare state that provided free education and gave land to people to build their homes (p. 289). This resulted in the development of "vast modern" cities and urbanization (p. 289).

Peterson (1990) argues that the discovery of oil has also "challenged the nature of personal and family relationships" (p. 278). The discovery of oil has led to increasing consumerism and increasing dependency on the government, which has resulted in "tearing the fabric of society" (p. 278). However, he argues that despite the new trends in the economy, the "core institutions" remain less impacted. Due to this, contradictory forces such as traditionalism and modernization tend to co-exist in Qatar (p. 288). He explains that the government is run on Islamic principles, hence, matters such as marriage, divorce, inherence, and custodianship are "governed on Islamic principles" (p. 290). He also explains that the family oversees socialization and age and sex determine one's status in the family (p. 290). However, he notes that some things have changed due to urbanization. There are less frequent meetups with extended family and men tend to spend more time with "schoolmates, business associates, and fellow club members" rather than the extended family (p. 291). The younger Qatari generation tends to form more nuclear families, giving more room for egalitarian roles to the spouses; women have more mobility and fathers are more involved with the socialization of daughters (p. 291). He notes that another change is the importance given to imported goods. This has led to a decline in handicrafts and local industries and the importance given to European brands (p. 291). The nation has also seen a rise in the expatriate population, which has introduced their cultural influences and impacted Qatari culture and preferences (p. 291). He also notes that expatriate teachers also teach Arabic which has influenced the socialization of children (p. 291). He argues that urbanization has led to a more non-equalitarian society with a very rigid social structure; the ruling family is placed at the top and is the wealthiest, then there are secondary elite families the wealthy businessmen. Next are the middle-class expats and finally, there are the lower classes that are the workers (pp. 293–294). He also points out that this rigid hierarchy has led to a strict religious sectarian divide as well. The Shi'as in GCC have become the "largest indigenous minority" who were at one point "established merchant families" (p. 294).

Scholarship on Qatari family structure has followed the trend of analysing what the family structure looked like before and after the discovery of oil. Al-Misnad's (1984) work follows this trend. It explains how oil transformed Qatari and GCC society. She argues that the Gulf family structure was different from the family structure of the Middle East; the Gulf family is "patrilineal, patrilocal, patriarchal, and more often than not endogamous" while Middle East family structures are based on "joint ownership of land" (Al-Misnad, 1984, p. 34). She also states that age and sex determine one's role and gender segregation is strictly practised (p. 35). However, she notes that there is an emergence of the nuclear family due to better standards of living, economic independence, and the influence of mass media (p. 35). Her research delves into the transformation of education, tracing its evolution from the "Kuttabs" to contemporary educational institutions. Additionally, she explores the progress of women's education and its societal implications. She argues that the long-term aim of these educational policies is to lessen the dependence on foreign workers and expats. She contends that following the discovery of oil, modern education became accessible to all Qatari citizens, irrespective of gender, resulting in an increase in female workforce participation (p. 70). However, equality was challenged in Qatari or GCC societies (p. 37).

Recent scholarship has started taking a much more nuanced role in Qatari family structures. Caeiro (2018) contends that research on Gulf societies is grounded in the presumption that politics, religion, family, and the economy are distinct institutions. This secular lens has produced inefficient scholarship on the region.

Similarly, increasing scholarship on Gulf and Qatari family structure has focused on women and gender issues. Al-Ghanim (2019) also writes about women's progress in Qatar. She posits that women encounter obstacles in their engagement in public life due to traditional perceptions of their role (p. 52). Structural obstacles include kinship ties that perpetuate patriarchy (p. 53). A woman cannot be a legal witness in a marriage contract (p. 65). Furthermore, roles in the family have not changed much as well as marriage remains based on the father's or the family's decision (pp. 62–64). Similarly, laws remain in favour of men; there needs to be an improvement in society in all spheres not just in educational levels (p. 55). She also maintains that despite the impact of modernization and urbanization, the deep-rooted kinship ties are much more prevalent and prevent women's socio-economic development (p. 52). She states that modernization leading to increasing educational levels of women has increased their presence in leadership roles. However, "progress remains far from satisfactory" (p. 52).

In recent years, more scholarship has been produced on gender issues in family households rather than simply analysing the pre- and post-oil transformation of the family. Al-Ghanim and Badahdah (2017) state that very little scholarship is produced analysing gender in Arab societies. They argue that this is because there are hardly any internal measures on gender (Al-Ghanim & Badahdah, 2017, p. 169). They also highlight that the research that is available on gender in Arab societies comes from non-Arab countries (p. 170).

In Arab nations, there is a widespread misconception regarding the issue of domestic abuse. Qatar, like many other Arab nations, likes to keep family and personal problems private and considers it a cultural taboo to discuss being a victim of domestic abuse. Although a few studies on domestic violence and its consequences on health have been undertaken in the past, there is currently a dearth of studies on the issue in Qatar. As an instance, in a prior study carried out in Qatar, the impact of domestic violence on women's psychological well-being was explored on a surface level, without delving into the fundamental aspects such as the various forms and prevalence of domestic abuse ingrained in Qatari society. Al-Ghanim (2009) also writes about women's experience of violence in Qatari households. She uses field research as well as documentary research sources (p. 80). She also uses a sample of women at Qatar University that represent 4.4% of Qatari females between the ages of 15 and 64 (p. 80). Her research reveals that "a significant number of women" have encountered violence, primarily within their families, perpetrated by male family members, including brothers, husbands, and fathers (p. 80). In her view, the primary factors contributing to this situation are the "absence of protective legislation" and "ineffective official institutions" aimed at safeguarding women from violence (p. 80). Her work also shows that the literature on violence towards women is little and those that have been conducted hold a very small sample size (p. 80). Hence, her work is the first national survey on violence against women in Qatar (p. 81). Her work shows that there are no legal provisions that deal with such an issue; Qatari law does not criminalize domestic violence (p. 82). However, physical assault, defamation, and molestation are deemed as crimes (p. 82). Her research shows that 23% said "yes" to the question of if they have ever been subjected to violence (p. 86). Out of the 23%, 46 stated that they have been raped and 85 said they had been subjected to sexual harassment (p. 87). Most of these women expressed that they had experienced repeated violence and most of this violence started during childhood (p. 87). 39% of these women subjected to violence said their brothers "were the prime offenders" (p. 88). The author recommends raising awareness and deeming domestic violence to be criminalized (p. 91).

However, much of the research up to now has been descriptive in nature. In addition, the sample representation was biased and did not fully reflect the entire range of abuse that occurs in society. It is quite common in Qatar, as it is in many other Arab countries in the region, for cases of domestic abuse to go unreported, either due to the shame associated with disclosing personal information or fear of further retaliation from the abuser, especially when the cultural values are heavily influenced by social stigma and family reputation principles that prioritise group and family unity over the individual interest. In his discussion of how patriarchy believes affect the social system, Scott challenges the assumption that patriarchy remains entrenched in Gulf societies whether in its traditional or modern phase (Weiner, 2016, p. 13). His work argues that previous scholarship does not show how familial patriarchy is reproduced but rather assumes patriarchy has existed and continues to exist leaving a gap in the literature (p. 13). However, he states that the issue is far more complex. For example, In Kuwait, women could not vote until 2005 and could not become prosecutors till 2014. Kuwaiti women cannot pass their citizenship to their children if they are married to a non-Kuwaiti man. However, more than half of the public sector employs women and women receive full paid maternity leave for 70 days, which is far more progressive than other societies (p. 14).

This is particularly true when cultural norms are substantially influenced by social stigma and family reputation concepts that prioritise group and family cohesion above individual interests. The most reliable research undertaken in Qatar and recognised by several scholars was conducted more than 13 years ago. The findings of the relevant study indicated that when there is an inadequate social protection system and legal framework in place, women are notably influenced in their choice to terminate a relationship with an abusive partner (Al-Ghanim, 2009).

In the research carried out in the MENA region, it was shown that violence against women in the family is quite prevalent. Moreover, women have the propensity to excuse or think that violence is their fault and many circumstances in which masculinity is questioned increase the likelihood that women will be harmed (Boy & Kulczycki, 2008).

This research was initially based on the experiences of a small number of women who fled violent and oppressive familial conditions in Qatar, only to encounter mistreatment from family members upon arrival in the United Kingdom. There is a limited understanding of the extent of domestic violence in Qatar. Due to this occurrence, international human rights organisations and activists have started scrutinising current human rights law, family policy, the effectiveness of social welfare and protection systems, and local organisations that assist victims of domestic violence.

For the sake of this research, a substantial number of anecdotes, the voices of victims, and tales that have been concealed have all been investigated in depth. These elements have led to the establishment of the framework for the variable under study, which has contextualised our understanding of domestic violence in Qatar. According to the research contained in Qatar's Second National Development Strategy (2018–2022), the number of recorded incidences of domestic violence against women reduced between 2014 and 2015 was 854. However, this percentage is expected to rise soon owing to a lack of adequate parenting skills and the transfer of children's responsibilities to housemaids and domestic labour (Ministry of Development Planning and Statistics (MDPS), 2019).

The primary aim of this study is to investigate how IPV impacts the mental health of Qatari women by examining the incidence of mental health conditions, such as anxiety, depression, and Post Traumatic Stress Disorder (PTSD). The second purpose is to identify the frequency and nature of violent actions against women, as well as their chance of being killed. The inquiry will aid in elucidating the reasons why women in abusive relationships prefer to stay passive or inactive. The research will conclude with an examination of the variables related to aggressive behaviour in intimate relationships. Consequently, the collection of data occurred in Doha, the capital and biggest city of Qatar, between December 2020 and March 2021.

In the introductory section of this chapter, as part of this study, the researcher explored the various forms of domestic violence against women and the terminology that is commonly used in the field. In addition, this chapter contains background information on Qatar, family structure and policy climate, as well as its economic progress, a problem statement, policy implications and an overview, the need for the investigation, and the reason for the research strategy used in the study. The sections that follow include the research context of Qatar and definitions of essential phrases and study questions. These phrases may be used to gain knowledge of domestic violence in Qatar.

Either new research on IPV is being conducted right now, or the previous studies have become obsolete. In addition, information is scarce regarding the numerous forms of domestic violence, such as economic abuse, the negative effects that it has on the mental health of Qatari female victims of IPV, and the possibility that it may increase the likelihood of homicide. The currently conducted study in Qatar does not make use of a tried-and-true scientific method that has already been developed to identify the frequency and severity of domestic violence. This makes it more difficult to compare the sorts of abuse that are now being reported in Qatar with those that occur in other places that have similarities to Qatar in terms of the structure of families, the common norms and values, etc. In Qatar, discussions about abusive relationships within households are infrequent, primarily due to inadequate socio-economic resources and a gendered approach to women's rights, among other factors. The researcher chose to employ a mixed-method approach in the study to offer a more comprehensive insight into the topic. This decision was made because most incidents that occur in Qatar are not recorded. The researcher decided to go with a mixed-method approach since this study is completely original in Qatar and intends to not only address a knowledge gap but also provide more up-to-date insights that may be used for the creation of future research and policies.

1.2 The Qatar Research Context

The upcoming section delves into and introduces the cultural backdrop against which the present study is taking place. Furthermore, it addresses the social and cultural dimensions of domestic abuse against women in Qatar. To gain a deeper understanding of its meaning, socioeconomic systems, marriage institutions, social beliefs, and other demographic factors are discussed.

A country located in the Middle East and part of the Arab Gulf, Qatar's capital city, Doha, is home to less than 10% of the nation's population. It has a total area of 11,586 m^2 and is located on a teeny-tiny peninsula land separating Saudi Arabia and the Gulf of the Islamic Republic of Iran to the north and south, respectively. Saudi Arabia is situated in the Middle East. The inaugural celebration of Qatar's Independence Day took place in 1971; in the intervening years, the nation has gone through several political changes and witnessed developments in its social culture as well as its economy. Various social programs have played a part in nurturing a feeling of national identity among Qatar's population. As a part of these initiatives, the 18th of December was designated as a national holiday, and as part of these initiatives, national libraries and museums were founded. In 1970, it was estimated that the population of Qatar would be somewhere around 110.000 people; by the year 2020, due to the inflow of expatriates, the population was closer to 2.7 million. It is possible that the nation's flourishing oil industry is partly to blame for this staggering increase in population (Zweiri & Al Qawasmi, 2020).

The substantial oil revenues, resulting in significant socio-economic transformations and population expansion, encouraged a greater influx of people to migrate to the Gulf Cooperation Council (GCC) region. There is a rise in life expectancy and a decline in infant mortality rates. Another trend is the rise in literacy rates, especially among girls. In the year 2015, secondary school attendance was recorded for girls aged between 8 and 17, ranging between 83 and 95%, while university enrolment for women between 18 and 23 ages stood at approximately 50% (De Bel-Air et al., 2018). GCC's family structure and dynamic had evolved and changed over time, according to the author. As a result, the fertility rate has declined, the first marriage age has increased, and consanguineous marriages remain the most popular form of marriage since the 1990s. The authors' conclusion emphasizes that the delay in marriages within the region is mainly attributable to the substantial expenses associated with marriage, including wedding costs, dowries, housing, and gold. The Gulf countries remain relatively polygamous, but divorce is relatively common. High levels of marital instability are not new, but the rising divorce rates in Qatar and other GCC countries are causing concern and sparking social debate (De Bel-Air et al., 2018).

The prevalence of domestic violence in Arab society can be explained to a large extent by the social structure of the society. Arab culture places a high value on the family unit. Traditions of family ties affect a couple's marital decisions and other important decisions in life, like many other Arab societies (Doha International Family Institute (DIFI), 2022). There is a greater importance placed on family interests than on individual interests. According to (Zahidi, 2018), it becomes pivotal to recognize the importance of extended family and older members in the lives of individuals.

Both parents' family values influence the decisions of husbands and wives after marriage in Arab culture. An integral part of Arabic culture is the role of extended family members, which goes beyond normal western principles. As a result, their opinions can influence young couples' decision-making process and shape the well-being of the couple in the long run (Al-Krenawi & Graham, 2000). Elders are often entrusted with making significant choices during life transitions such as marriage and divorce, as well as times of turmoil within the family, to preserve the dignity of the tribe and the stability of the family unit. These choices can range from whether to allow a child to attend a particular school to whether to allow a child to have a pet which was discovered as a result of a study carried out in Palestine (Haj-Yahia, 2002).

Since the discovery of oil, one of the most significant obstacles that Qatari society has had to overcome is the need to re-evaluate the essentially patriarchal and traditional cultural norms that have been upheld for generations. This is one of the problems that won't go away any time soon. Abu-Lughod (2018) argued that there has been a tendency to oppose and change the generally accepted gender roles in Arab society over the years, and that more women have joined the society in recent years. Actively working on self-development has resulted in significant improvements in female education, employment (Zahidi, 2018), and overall political representation in Arab countries (IPI Global Observatory, 2021).

There is still a patriarchal belief system that rules the social structure of the nation but the constant contact of Qataris with expatriates who have stayed in Qatar encourages them to transcend their heritage-based ideas. Expats have been living in Qatar for a long time. Despite being infrequently identified as the primary cause of violence against women in past research, patriarchal ideologies persist in Qatar, as noted by Tracy (2007). Recently, the government of Qatar has been working towards the goal of diversifying the social neighbourhoods in which inhabitants of Qatar live to stimulate intertribal socialisation. Zweiri and Al Qawasmi (2020) highlight that as part of a broader effort to diversify social neighbourhoods and foster intertribal socialization, the Qatar Foundation is actively pursuing family-friendly policies to address gender pay inequality, with the ultimate aim of enhancing the quality of life for all Qatari citizens.

A variety of social initiatives, such as the adoption of an annual celebration of a national day on December 18 and the establishment of a national library and museums, contributed to the identity formation of the people of Qatar. Other examples of these types of initiatives include the establishment of a national park.

In 1995, Qataris were able to define civil rights and make political choices thanks to the nation's first democratic elections, which they participated in. In Qatar, the Consultative Council, also known as Majlis Ash-Shura, is widely recognised as a powerful representative legal body. This council served as the venue for the advancement of women's communal roles (The Shura Council, 2018). The term "Shura Council" is used to refer to this gathering of people rather often. In the Qatar Shura Council, which is scheduled to be formally constituted in 2021, there will be four women serving as key cabinet members. These women will oversee the social development plan and will take part in a significant portion of the decision-making process for the government. In addition, there are almost as many female members of Qatar's Shura Council as there are male ones. Although women hold a disproportionate number of significant government roles at the present time, efforts to empower women have continued.

In the years that followed, the organisation expanded both in terms of number and scope, with members taking part in gatherings such as conferences and other events that brought together people from a variety of different backgrounds. The purpose of hosting the Asian Games in 2006 was to show the rest of the world that Qatar has evolved into a society that is more tolerant, open-minded, and eager to learn about the traditions and cultures of other countries.

Projects were funded by the Qatar Foundation, commonly known as the education city, with the goals of increasing women's engagement in the workforce and empowering them to do so to enhance the status of women and minimise gender disparity. It is a reasonable assumption that female students at private schools who are well-educated and successful are more aware of their position in society than their male counterparts who are less educated and less successful. This presumption is grounded in the reality that male students attending private schools often exhibit reduced educational attainment and fewer accomplishments. The Qatar Foundation was formed for the sole purpose of advancing women's rights throughout all areas of society. After residents were given access to online learning materials created by members of the global community, several initiatives that were designed to improve residents' living circumstances underwent revisions. For example, residents in Qatar are exempt from taxation and utility payments while also enjoying access to a healthcare system, education, and opportunities for career training—all free of charge (Zweiri & Al Qawasmi, 2020).

In Qatar, the bride and groom's parents often initiate the practice of getting married. In this society, there is a lack of regard for individual freedom of choice, potentially leading to adverse effects on marital satisfaction and a heightened probability of divorce. Concerns about preserving outdated Arab customs by the more traditional members of the community hinder the society from striking a harmonious balance between tradition and modernity. In contemporary society, the role of women in politics and other significant decision-making venues is still generally misunderstood, and it is often believed that women should concentrate on home chores or professions in traditionally feminine sectors. On the other hand, liberated persons favour gender-neutral opportunities for equal labour regardless of their employment status. In the most recent election, which took place in 2021, it seems that female voters were hesitant to support female candidates because they considered that female candidates were less qualified to carry out their tasks as per the views of Shockley (2018). The results of Al-Ghanim's study published in 2017 proclaimed that some men in Qatar would prefer to uphold their cultural ideals by instituting coercive control methods against women. These methods try to limit the personal freedom of women and prevent them from becoming independent persons.

Qatar has recently captured the attention of the whole world since it is the smallest country to ever host the FIFA World Cup. Qatar holds around 13% of the world's oil reserves. Additionally, the country's projected GDP is 167.225 billion Qatari Riyals, placing it in the top five wealthiest nations. The tremendous increase in GDP may be linked to the acceleration of social transformation around the world. Nevertheless, between the years 2012 and 2013, fewer than 10% of Qatari families believed themselves to be slightly destitute as a consequence of poor financial management or had excessive financial debt due to a great cultural picture of the optimum social standing of the family (Treuthart & Rosenbaum, 2013). Most women who seek divorce reconceiving with their abusive husbands. As a result, questions are raised about the role of men in the family in controlling family members and wealth. As such, it can be recognized as a form of social behaviour among Arab families (Adelman, 2000).

As a direct consequence of this, a significant number of women who are victims of domestic abuse keep silent about it and do not report it.

Nevertheless, it's crucial to emphasize Qatar's demographic makeup, revealing that 74.4% of its population falls within the 25–64 age bracket. This age group represents the vast majority of the population, with a total of 89% of the population being literate (CountryReports, n.d.). There are 14,456 persons eligible for help under Qatar's social security and welfare system, out of a total population of approximately 2.5 million. According to the MDPS (2018), the marriage rate for both genders in Qatar declined dramatically between 2011 and 2017. This is due to various variables, including the rising expense of marriage, women's high educational attainment, and their engagement in the workforce. In addition, at the time of their first marriage, 68.4% of individuals fell within the age range of 20–29. Eighty-one percent of all weddings were first marriages for the bride, while 18% were second or subsequent marriages for previously married or widowed women. According to 2017 data, 43% of all weddings included consanguineous marriages, making them the most popular and prevalent kind of union. This suggests that these relationships need to be promoted. More than 69% of all divorces based on the duration of marriage occur within the first 5 years of marriage. This is because the great majority of marriages occur during this period. Moreover, approximately 50% of divorces are initiated by couples aged 20–29, with another 25% of divorces being started by couples aged 30–39. In Qatar, female labour force participation is one of the highest indices, with women holding 51% of employment. Specifically, there was a remarkable 10% rise in female labour force participation in Qatar in 2013 as a result of improvements in social policies that encourage a work-family balance and in societal conceptions of women's responsibilities (DIFI, 2022).

1.3 The Scope and Originality

Domestic violence against women has garnered significant attention from the World Health Organization (WHO, 2021), which regards it as both a public health concern and a blatant violation of fundamental human rights. While this concerning subject has been extensively researched, there remains a notable lack of academic focus on enhancing our comprehension of IPV in Qatar, including its nature, the prevalence of various forms of IPV, the adverse effects on mental health, and the factors influencing victims to endure abusive relationships. There have been very few descriptive studies carried out, and there is a study dearth of appropriate knowledge regarding the current frequency of domestic abuse types and the effects that abuse has on the mental health of women in Qatar.

In the Qatari society, current instances of domestic abuse remain largely unreported, probably because the partners thought they would change at some point. In addition to other factors, many of these women's justifications were rooted in financial difficulties, which will be discussed in depth in this study. As majority Qatari studies look at domestic abuse as the primary cause of divorce, they ignore the psychopathological consequences of long exposure or living in a stressful environment (DIFI, 2022).

Expanding our knowledge of domestic abuse within Arab culture involves considering various societal factors and individual variables. These include residence type, nationality, religious and core beliefs of both spouses, educational levels, financial status, and traditional gender roles shaped by societal hierarchy values, all of which can be seen as contributing factors (Haj-Yahia, 2000). This contributes to the existing literature on the subject. In Sudan, for instance, a study revealed that nearly half of the participants had been subjected to some form of abuse, and among those who are attending primary clinics, one in three females had experienced domestic violence; hesitance and reluctance regarding sharing the nature of the abuse was not a concern, and approximately 86% of them were willing to share their personal story. In addition, primary care clinic attendees revealed that one in three men had suffered sexual assault (Ahmed & Elmardi, 2005). In Kuwait, for example, where male ideology and the patriarchal concept that power is in the possession of males are heavily emphasised, cultural and demographic characteristics were the most influential risk factors for domestic violence against women. Seventy-one percent of the individuals claimed having been physically assaulted, 89% reported having been mentally abused, and 81% reported having been exposed to sexual compulsion, according to the findings (Alsaleh, 2022). In Oman, for instance, Al Shidhani et al. (2020) found that the danger of IPV might arise at any point throughout a marriage. For example, the risk of violence against women is more likely to rise during pregnancy among women who reported being mistreated in the 12 months before their pregnancy. This is the case with non-exceptional cultures, such as Arabic society. Domestic violence may occur at any moment, even during pregnancy.

When a man's manhood ideology is questioned, for example, masculinity and the ideology that characterises men may lead to a range of aggressive behaviours against their spouse. In the most recent research conducted in Saudi Arabia by Alquaiz et al. (2021), it was shown that the majority of types of abuse fell within coercive control methods defined by the social situation of the roles and duties of husband and wife. In addition, the most prevalent kinds of abuse reported by participants were emotional and sexual violence, whereas physical assault was the least prevalent.

Notably, cultural elements such as social standing and public image might interact negatively with individual characteristics that enable or mitigate abuse in Qatar. This includes not seeking professional assistance or trying to terminate the abuse by reporting it to law authorities, as well as not being able to secure a divorce owing to familial pressure that a divorce would bring disgrace to the family (Soliman et al., 2019) and might escalate the situation. To comprehend how domestic violence could increase, it is vital to comprehend how women in Qatari culture see their place and rights in the larger community. The patriarchal belief system and the country's rich cultural history have a substantial effect on Qatari culture. Consequently, these circumstances impact the character of the interactions that exist between spouses and family members. In previous studies conducted in Qatar, domestic abuse prevalence and its effects on mental and physical health were not measured using pre-established validated tools (Al-Ghanim, 2009; DIFI, 2022), hence, it was difficult to compare the research's indicators and conclusions to those of other research conducted in the area.

As a consequence, the present study identified key characteristics that have been studied in western and cross-cultural studies that increase the likelihood that women would be victims of IPV. These characteristics include: all types of violence against women, including economic abuse, which was omitted from all prior surveys conducted in Qatar, focus on an additional delicate and intricate matter of Qatar's marital customs which covers the kind of marriage, polygamy, and second marriage, as well as how these factors may enhance the likelihood of domestic violence. In contrast, the current study expands the scope of the probe and uncovers the truth regarding more severe kinds of abuse, such as the murder of females and the use of sexual coercion. The methodology of the research will help to bridge the gap in knowledge and offer more recent and in-depth insights about IPV in Qatar. These findings will inspire future scholars to expand their knowledge based on the Arabic context, which will help to increase the awareness level of healthcare providers, that victims can present with no physical bruises that mostly indicated as abuse, and that advancing their pre-interview knowledge about the various forms of domestic abuse will help and protect men. The research will present an overview of how victims were interpreting the existing family policy from the victim's point of view based on their experiences during and after the separation process if they voice their real experiences.

The objective of this study is to investigate how domestic abuse impacts the mental health of Qatari women. It will also explore the factors most likely to be associated with domestic abuse victims. The objective subcategory of this study addresses the reasons victims remain passive in abusive relationships, assess the risk of domestic abuse homicide, and examines women's roles and rights within society.

In certain societies and cultures, intimate partner violence often goes unreported, considered a private matter (Bartolomei, 2015). People are often reluctant to disclose their experiences, and available data may be outdated. Given these circumstances, the chosen research methodology was the most suitable approach for conducting this study. It was the best way to conduct the research effectively. The sequential mixed methods approach helps to identify the knowledge gap and provides a basic foundation for examining the underlying factors that could lead to IPV and help in understanding the social structures that affect women's decision to leave or stay in a violent relationship.

However, the findings should be interpreted with consideration for the fact that the study focused on victims who had been in a conjugal relationship. A replicated study involving different groups of participants could result in different indicators. One of the key limitations is the generalizability of the data is limited due to the small sample size that agreed to partake in the study, along with the number of gatekeepers who rejected permitting data collection due to the sensitive nature of the research. Similarly was found in a systematic review carried out on Arabic countries by Mojahed et al. (2020). Further research could be directed towards national surveys to establish causational relationships.

The covid-19 lockdown posed time constraints and a lack of opportunities to interview and speak with government officials about the current social policy and its implications. There was a limited number of participants because not all participants completed all of the questionnaires. Therefore, the missing information and half-completed surveys were excluded from the study analysis. This is in line with previous research conducted in Jordan by Clark et al. (2010). In the present research, the extent of qualitative interviews was restricted because of the conservative nature of the society being studied and the sensitive nature of the topic under investigation. In the quality assessment phase, each transcript was reviewed by the participants themselves at the conclusion of the interview to verify the reliability and accuracy of the data.

The present findings concerning the risk of homicide should be approached with caution due to limited access to data and restrictions imposed by gatekeepers when attempting to identify and investigate cases involving victims who sought shelter due to threats of spousal murder. According to the current sample, the homicide rate does not fall within the extreme range. However, homicide data is not available in Qatar, and access to data is severely restricted, so generalizations regarding homicide rates or attempts are extremely difficult. Due to limited access to data, the research terms were broadened to include literature and empirical studies that have examined domestic abuse victims' risk of murder. This was similarly addressed in a previous study (Graham et al., 2022). The last two categories, "severe danger" and "extreme danger", both indicate a substantial potential risk of causing severe harm or even homicide. Nonetheless, this did not appear to be the situation when examining the scores of the participants in the current study. Even though these data give some evidence for a low probability of murder, one must exercise extreme caution when making inferences based on such a tiny sample size. This relationship with the present findings of DA was minor; however, future research endeavours are essential, involving a larger cohort, as the findings of this study cannot be extrapolated due to the constraints imposed by the sample size employed.

Further, the study did not consider social disparities, such as ethnicity, how particular ethnic groups are treated, how society treats women, or how the justice system responds to allegations made by victims, which might provide a different perspective on understanding domestic abuse with those covariables. Further, the societal factor in this study has been limited to attitudes towards women's rights and roles in society. Previous study shows the importance of addressing domestic abuse from a family violence perspective (Anderson, 2018). This study did not explore social policies and cultural norms as they fell outside the study's scope. A future study should examine economic abuse before and after divorce considering socio-demographic and societal factors. This research also showed that the second most common form of abuse encountered by participants was economic abuse.

Despite extensive testing of the psychometric properties of the study scales in western societies, some of the study scales were not conducted in Arabic cultures. It raises the possibility that some forms of abuse may be overlooked or not captured by this proposed scale. Some of the scale subcategory items seem redundant when it was converted to the Arabic language, rephrasing a sentence or contextualising them improved the accuracy of the response. The limitation was consistent with those found in previous research conducted in Saudi Arabia (Almubaddel, 2022).

Some participants were unable to discuss sexual coercion or were hesitant to elaborate on that topic because of the topic's sensitivity and due to concerns surrounding the consequences that prevented them from sharing details of the incidents. Programs that raise awareness about revealing abuse to professionals may help victims to understand their rights and terminate abuse. In addition, they may handle victims and perpetrators in a professional manner (Bottoms et al., 2016). There was discussion about the increased risk of sexual coercion among mothers with more children, and this provided further insight into the topic of sexual coercion. However, the limitation becomes the direction for future research to develop the general population's understanding of this issue and to capture their feelings about domestic violence and sexual coercion.

Either studies on IPV are currently being undertaken or they are out of date. In addition, there is a dearth of knowledge addressing the many types of domestic violence, such as economic abuse, its detrimental impact on the mental health of Qatari female victims of IPV, and the fact that it might raise the likelihood of murder. Existing research in Qatar lacks a pre-established, verified scientific instrument for detecting the prevalence and severity of domestic violence. This lowers the capacity to compare the presently reported types of abuse with those in other locations that have parallels with Qatar in terms of family structure, prevalent norms and values, etc. Due to a lack of resources on economic and social concerns, gender viewpoints towards women's rights, And other factors, domestic abuse is seldom addressed in Qatar. Since the great majority of instances in Qatar go unreported, the researcher chose to use a mixed methods approach throughout the whole study to get a thorough grasp of the problem. The researcher adopted a mixed method approach since this study is wholly unique in Qatar and aims to fill a knowledge vacuum as well as give more current insights for future research and policy development.

Considerable research has delved into the policy implications of child custody arrangements for victims of domestic violence. These studies suggest that at times, legal authorities may not adequately address female complaints regarding the nature of Intimate Partner Violence. Such oversight can deter women from taking action to end or mitigate abuse due to concerns about the implications for new family arrangements following a divorce (Hamel et al., 2009).

Family courts are designed to safeguard child welfare and the rights of mothers, ensuring protection against any discriminatory factors that could impact children and their mothers during or following divorce; however, a lack of comprehension of the legal proceedings and the ability to furnish adequate evidence can sway the court's rulings (Abdul Hak et al., 2019). It is a joint activity that must be allowed (165–188 of the family law) by both parents after a divorce for the child's best interests, with the mother having the upper power. Child custody is a mother's right by default until this entitlement is lost (Al Meezan, 2022d). A survey conducted in Saudi Arabia indicated that 56.6% of the total 223 Saudi women are unable to continue living in their husband's house after divorce, since the majority of them are forced to leave their homes, and separate housing is not an option for all divorced moms (Pervin,

2014). As a consequence of Qatar's acknowledgement of post-divorce financial aid as a critical component of the preservation of women's dignity and rights, a provision in Qatari family law might entitle women to more than 2 years of financial support after a divorce. The family laws of Qatar protect the rights of women both before and after a divorce, such as the right to maintenance, which requires the husband to give the wife and any children an adequate quality of life (Al Meezan, 2022a).

While the marital financial support provided by the husband to his wife is determined by the husband's financial capacity and the economic circumstances of both partners, which are evaluated by the court to ensure that justice is served for both life partners, the financial support provided by the husband to his wife is based on his financial capacity (Wickrama et al., 2006). Other studies have emphasized the financial constraints frequently reported by divorced mothers and how these alterations lead to a decreased standard of living for their children. Divorce or separation does not guarantee that abuse will cease. Numerous academic studies have shown that post-divorce violence worries prompt women to rethink leaving an abusive husband. This is especially true for women who are responsible for children, since leaving with them may be difficult and costly, especially for mothers who have nowhere to reside with their children (Hardesty, 2002).

Divorced moms are under a tremendous deal of strain when it comes to property and housing following a divorce, but Qatari family law protects them by declaring and outlining the role of a husband to arrange suitable housing. Property and housing post-divorce pose some of the most formidable challenges that divorced mothers encounter (Al Meezan, 2022e). While a component of Pakistani legislation does not contain post-divorce support for women, and such action and economic uncertainty were intended to deter women from getting divorced, the divorced indicator grew for more than half of Shahid's population (Shahid, 2013).

Another research has emphasised the need of granting women property rights, which in turn necessitates that law enforcement comprehends the context of the economic circumstances that impede women from achieving their entitlements.

According to the results of another researcher (Peterman, 2011), property rights abuses against a broad category of women have grown increasingly prevalent, particularly among divorced or widowed women (Deere et al., 2014). For example, the majority of participants concurred that a woman granted child custody rights should reside in the family home. On the other hand, some stressed the necessity for a conjugal living arrangement to ensure the safety of vulnerable family members during disputes or divorces (Davis, 2010). Before initiating a divorce, women's choices are heavily influenced by their high living expenses and property rentals. In her research, Stepney (2016) finds that, in the near future, around 40% of Qatari people would be unable to purchase homes due to high rental costs that deplete their resources for constructing or purchasing a new home. Moreover, 62% of individuals who resided in rental homes are divorced or in the process of divorce. In research conducted in France by Ferrari et al. (2019), it was shown that divorced mums are more likely to relocate to a smaller house owing to financial constraints and that the custodial mother prefers to be in her husband's home if the choice is available. Both results are comparable to those of research conducted in France by Ferrari et al. (2019).

Since single parents cannot afford to buy half of the property and renting a home is costly, it is customary for them to leave the family home following a divorce (Murinkó, 2019). The housing repercussions that follow a divorce are one of the key concerns that divorced mothers face. Lack of understanding of women's rights is another reason for concern since it inhibits a woman's ability to halt violence against her or defend her own and her family's rights via the legal and welfare systems (Abu-Ras, 2007). Concerns over the policy implications of the post-divorce period are a common source of concern for divorced mothers, especially those who have been victims of domestic abuse and those with little financial means.

This book is structured in seven chapters including this one. Chapter 2, "Domestic Abuse: Global and Local", addresses domestic violence against women from local, regional, and global perspectives. It offers a summary of the body of research by examining multiple kinds of intimate partner domestic abuse and how they affect victims' mental health in terms of psychopathology. The theoretical underpinnings of violence against women and the aggravating variables that increase IPV victimisation are then succinctly discussed for further elaboration. Chapter 3, "Research Setting and Design", offers the outline of the research methodology and go over how to carry out an explanatory sequential mixed methods study. The theoretical and rational case for employing an explanatory sequential mixed method approach is presented in the first section. The research design is covered in the second section, and the justification for implementing data analysis shown in the third section. Chapter 4, "Domestic Abuse against Women: Correlates and Conundrums", looks into the relationship between several variables, and the quantitative results are presented in this chapter. Given the current state of the violet normal distribution for some scales and the constraints of the short sample size, four statistical analyses and a descriptive analysis are conducted. When the normality assumptions were violated, parametric and non-parametric procedures such as ANOVA, Pearson correlation, Kruskal-Wallis test, and Mann-Whitney U test were required to evaluate the data. The study participants' PTSD, depression, and anxiety have been examined using multiple regression analysis to see if abuse histories are predictive of these conditions. Because the independent and dependent variables in this study were continuous, the regression model was chosen based on the characteristics of the variables under investigation. This chapter expounds upon the manner in which the victims' perspective gave rise to the prevailing attitude towards women. Chapter 5, "Narratives of Domestic Abuse Against Women", elaborates the types of domestic violence experienced by women in Qatar and the reasons behind their refusal to leave abusive relationships through the use of qualitative data and explanation. It advances our understanding of whether the participants' choices to stay silent in an abusive relationship are influenced by the social setting and societal elements. Chapter 6, "The Sounds of Silence: Making Sense of the Domestic Abuse", evaluates the risk of homicide, the prevalence of intimate partner victimisation (IPV), and the detrimental consequences these factors have on the mental health of Qatari women. This chapter analyses the causes of intimate partner violence (IPV) in women and the reasons for their passivity in violent relationships. The goals and objectives of the study are reflected in the arrangement of this discussion chapter. Each point is examined, evaluated, and interpreted in order to produce a summary of the study's findings and conclusions. Chapter 7, "Conclusions and Policy Implications", concludes with policy recommendations.

References

Abdul Hak, N., Mansor, A. M., & Che Soh, R. (2019). Resolution of child custody dispute: Legislative foundation and contemporary application of Sulh in the Shariah court of Malaysia. *Journal of Islam in Asia, 53*(9), 1689–1699. https://journals.iium.edu.my/jiasia/index.php/jia/article/view/990/451

Abu-Lughod, L. (2018). Do Muslim women really need saving? Anthropological reflections on cultural relativism and its others. *American Anthropologist, 104*(3), 783–790. https://doi.org/10.1525/AA.2002.104.3.783

Abu-Ras, W. (2007). Cultural beliefs and service utilization by battered Arab immigrant women. *Violence Against Women, 13*(10), 1002–1028. https://doi.org/10.1177/1077801207306019

Adelman, M. (2000). No way out: Divorce-related domestic violence in Israel. *Violence Against Woman, 6*(11), 1223–1254. https://doi.org/10.1177/10778010022183613

Ahmed, A. M., & Elmardi, A. E. (2005). A study of domestic violence among women attending a medical centre in Sudan. *Eastern Mediterranean Health Journal, 11*(1–2), 164–174. https://pubmed.ncbi.nlm.nih.gov/16532685/

Al Meezan. (2022a). Articles 61–73. Law No. 22 of 2006 Promulgating 'The Family Law'. Date:29/06/2006, Official Gazette: Issue:8. Starting Date: 28/08/2006. https://www.almeezan.qa/LawArticles.aspx?LawTreeSectionID=8748&lawId=2558&language=en

Al Meezan. (2022d). *Article 170. Law No. 22 of 2006 Promulgating 'The Family Law'*. Date:29/06/2006, Official Gazette: Issue:8. Starting Date: 28/08/2006. https://www.almeezan.qa/LawArticles.aspx?LawArticleID=36311&LawID=2558&language=en

Al Meezan. (2022e). *Article 181. Law No. 22 of 2006 Promulgating 'The Family Law'*. Date:29/06/2006, Official Gazette: Issue:8. Starting Date: 28/08/2006. https://www.almeezan.qa/LawArticles.aspx?LawArticleID=36322&LawId=2558&language=en

Al Shidhani, N. A., Al Kendi, A. A., & Al Kiyumi, M. H. (2020). Prevalence, risk factors and effects of domestic violence before and during pregnancy on birth outcomes: An observational study of literate Omani women. *International Journal of Women's Health, 12*, 911–925. https://doi.org/10.2147/IJWH.S272419

Al-Attiyah, A., & Nasser, R. (2016). Gender and age differences in life satisfaction within a sex-segregated society: Sampling youth in Qatar. *International Journal of Adolescence and Youth, 21*(1), 84–95. https://doi.org/10.1080/02673843.2013.808158

Al-Ghanim, K. (2019). Perceptions of women's roles between traditionalism and modernity in Qatar. *Journal of Arabian Studies, 9*(1), 52–74. https://doi.org/10.1080/21534764.2019.1646502

Al-Ghanim, K. A. (2009). Violence against women in Qatari society. *Journal of Middle East Women's Studies, 5*(1), 80–93. https://doi.org/10.2979/mew.2009.5.1.80

Al-Ghanim, K. A., & Badahdah, A. M. (2017). Gender roles in the Arab world: Development and psychometric properties of the Arab adolescents' gender roles attitude scale. *Sex Roles, 77*(3–4), 169–177. https://doi.org/10.1007/s11199-016-0722-y

Al-Haj, M. (1987). *Social change and family processes*. Westview Press.

Al-Krenawi, A., & Graham, J. R. (2000). Culturally sensitive social work practice with Arab clients in mental health settings. *Health & Social Work, 25*(1), 9–22. https://doi.org/10.1093/hsw/25.1.9

Al-Misnad, S. A. (1984). *The development of modern education in Bahrain, Kuwait and Qatar with special reference to the education of women and their position in modern Gulf society* [Doctoral dissertation, Durham University]. Durham e-Theses. http://etheses.dur.ac.uk/10485/.

Almubaddel, A. (2022). Psychometric properties of a Saudi Arabian version of the Positive Mental Health (PMH) scale. *Psicologia: Reflexao e Critica, 35*(1), 29. https://doi.org/10.1186/s41155-022-00232-0

Alquaiz, A. M., Almuneef, M., Kazi, A., & Almeneessier, A. (2021). Social determinants of domestic violence among Saudi married women in Riyadh, Kingdom of Saudi Arabia. *Journal of Interpersonal Violence, 36*(3–4), NP1561–NP1585. https://doi.org/10.1177/088626051774 6128

Alsaleh, A. (2022). Violence against Kuwaiti women. *Journal of Interpersonal Violence, 37*(5–6), NP3628–NP3649. https://doi.org/10.1177/0886260520916280

Alshawi, A. H., & Gardner, A. (2013). Tribalism, identity and citizenship in contemporary Qatar. *Anthropology of the Middle East, 8*(2), 46–59. https://doi.org/10.3167/ame.2013.080204

Anderson, K. L. (2018). Gender, status, and domestic violence: An integration of feminist and family violence approaches. *Domestic Violence, 59*(3), 263–277. https://doi.org/10.4324/978 1315264905-20

Barakat, H. (1993). *The Arab world: Society, culture and state*. University of California Press.

Bartolomei, M. R. (2015). Domestic violence and human rights. An anthropological view. *Ex Aequo - Revista Da Associação Portuguesa de Estudos Sobre as Mulheres*, (31), 91–104. https://doi.org/10.22355/exaequo.2015.31.07

Bottoms, B. L., Peter-Hagene, L. C., Epstein, M. A., Wiley, T. R. A., Reynolds, C. E., & Rudnicki, A. G. (2016). Abuse characteristics and individual differences related to disclosing childhood sexual, physical, and emotional abuse and witnessed domestic violence. *Journal of Interpersonal Violence, 31*(7), 1308–1339. https://doi.org/10.1177/0886260514564155

Boy, A., & Kulczycki, A. (2008). What we know about intimate partner violence in the Middle East and North Africa. *Violence Against Women, 14*(1), 53–70. https://doi.org/10.1177/107780120 7311860

Caeiro, A. (2018). The politics of family cohesion in the Gulf: Islamic authority, new media, and the logic of the modern rentier state. *Arabian Humanities - International Journal of Archaeology and Social Sciences in the Arabian Peninsula, 10*. https://doi.org/10.4000/cy.3762

Clark, C. J., Silverman, J. G., Shahrouri, M., Everson-Rose, S., & Groce, N. (2010). The role of the extended family in women's risk of intimate partner violence in Jordan. *Social Science and Medicine, 70*(1), 144–151. https://doi.org/10.1016/j.socscimed.2009.09.024

CountryReports. (n.d.). *Qatar demographics*. Retrieved March 18, 2023, from https://www.countr yreports.org/country/Qatar/population.htm

Davis, D. (2010). Who gets the house? Renegotiating property rights in post-socialist urban China. *Modern China, 36*(5), 463–492. https://doi.org/10.1177/0097700410373265

De Bel-Air, F., Safar, J., & Destremau, B. (2018). Marriage and Family in the Gulf Today: Storms over a patriarchal institution? *Chroniques Yéménites, 10*. https://doi.org/10.4000/cy.4399

Deere, C. D., Contreras, J., & Twyman, J. (2014). Patrimonial violence: A study of women's property rights in Ecuador. *Latin American Perspectives, 41*(1), 143–165. https://doi.org/10.1177/009458 2X13492133

Devers, L. N., & Bacon, S. (2010). Interpreting honor crimes: The institutional disregard towards female victims of family violence in the Middle East. *International Journal of Criminology and Sociological Theory, 3*(1), 359–371. https://ijcst.journals.yorku.ca/index.php/ijcst/article/download/25925/24007

Doha International Family Institute (DIFI). (2022). *The state of Qatari Families: Strengths and challenges*. https://doi.org/10.5339/difi_9789927161629

Ferrari, G., Bonnet, C., & Solaz, A. (2019). "Will the one who keeps the children keep the house?" Residential mobility after divorce by parenthood status and custody arrangements in France. *Demographic Research, 40*(February), 359–394. https://doi.org/10.4054/DEMRES.2019.40.14

Graham, L. M., Macy, R. J., Rizo, C. F., & Martin, S. L. (2022). Explanatory theories of intimate partner homicide perpetration: A systematic review. *Trauma, Violence & Abuse, 23*(2), 408–427. https://doi.org/10.1177/1524838020953800

Haj-Yahia, M. M. (2000). Wife abuse and battering in the sociocultural context of Arab society. *Family Process, 39*(2), 237–255. https://doi.org/10.1111/j.1545-5300.2000.39207.x

Haj-Yahia, M. M. (2002). Attitudes of Arab women toward different patterns of coping with wife abuse. *Journal of Interpersonal Violence, 17*(7), 721–745. https://doi.org/10.1177/088626050 20170070

Hamel, J., Desmarais, S. L., Nicholls, T. L., Malley-Morrison, K., & Aaronson, J. (2009). Domestic violence and child custody: Are family court professionals' decisions based on erroneous beliefs? *Journal of Aggression, Conflict and Peace Research, 1*(2), 37–52. https://doi.org/10.1108/175 96599200900011

Hardesty, J. L. (2002). Separation assault in the context of postdivorce parenting. *Violence Against Women, 8*(5), 597–625. https://doi.org/10.1177/107780120200800505

IPI Global Observatory. (2021). *Women's political participation in the Arab world*. https://theglo balobservatory.org/2021/01/womens-political-participation-arab-world/

Melikian, L. H., & Al-Easa, J. S. (1984). Oil and social change in the Gulf. In A. Ghabra (Ed.), *Political behavior in the Arab states* (1st ed., p. 14). Routledge.

Ministry of Development Planning and Statistics (MDPS). (2018). *Marriage & divorce in the State of Qatar, 2017 (Review & analysis)*. https://www.psa.gov.qa/en/statistics/Statistical%20Releases/General/StatisticalAbstract/2017/population-chapters/marriage_divorce_qatar_2017_En.pdf

Ministry of Development Planning and Statistics (MDPS). (2019). *Qatar second national development strategy 2018~2022*. https://www.psa.gov.qa/en/knowledge/Documents/NDS2Fi nal.pdf

Mojahed, A., Alaidarous, N., Shabta, H., Hegewald, J., & Garthus-Niegel, S. (2020). Intimate partner violence against women in the Arab countries: A systematic review of risk factors. *Trauma, Violence & Abuse, 23*(2), 1–18. https://doi.org/10.1177/1524838020953099

Murinkó, L. (2019). Housing consequences of divorce and separation in a "super home ownership" regime: The case of Hungary. *Demographic Research, 40*(June), 975–1014. https://doi.org/10. 4054/DemRes.2019.40.34

Pervin, D. (2014). Post-divorce maintenance for Muslim women : Which path to follow in Bangladesh? *Society & Change, 8*(1), 7–26. https://societyandchange.com/uploads/150959 7310.pdf

Peterman, A. (2011). Women's property rights and gendered policies: Implications for women's long-term welfare in rural Tanzania. *Journal of Development Studies, 47*(1), 1–30. https://doi. org/10.1080/00220381003600366

Peterson, J. E. (1990). Change and continuity in Arab Gulf society. In C. Davies (Ed.), *After the War: Iraq, Iran and the Arab Gulf* (pp. 287–312). Carden Publications. http://jepeterson.net/sit ebuildercontent/sitebuilderfiles/Peterson_Change_and_Continuity_in_Gulf_Society_1990.pdf

Shahid, A. (2013). Post-divorce maintenance for Muslim women in Pakistan and Bangladesh: A comparative perspective. *International Journal of Law, Policy and the Family, 27*(2), 197–215. https://doi.org/10.1093/lawfam/ebt004

Shockley, B. (2018). Competence and electability: Exploring the limitations on female candidates in Qatar. *Journal of Women, Politics & Policy, 39*(4), 467–489. https://doi.org/10.1080/1554477x. 2018.1511125

Soliman, A., Alyafie, A., & Gomaa, A.-S. (2019). *Factors that influence Qatari family stability: Testing a vulnerability and resiliency model.* Doha International Family Institute (DIFI), 1–27. https://www.difi.org.qa/wp-content/uploads/2022/09/B-h-1.pdf

Stepney, E. (2016). *Housing tenure and economic inequality among Qatari citizens.* SESRI Policy Brief, 2016(3), 3–4. The Social and Economic Survey Research Institute, Qatar University. https://qspace.qu.edu.qa/bitstream/handle/10576/5116/Qatari-Renters-Eng-Final.pdf?seq uence=2&isAllowed=y

The Shura Council. (2018). *History*. https://www.shura.qa/en/Pages/About-Council/History

Tracy, S. R. (2007). Patriarchy and domestic violence: Challenging common misconceptions. *Journal of the Evangelical Theological Society, 50*(3), 573–594.

Treuthart, M. P., & Rosenbaum, S. A. (2013). Engendering a clinic: Lessons learned from a domestic violence clinical course in Qatar. *International Review of Law, 2013*(4), 1–24. https://doi.org/10.5339/irl.2013.dv.1

Weiner, S. (2016). Rethinking patriarchy and kinship in the Arab Gulf states. *Women and gender in Middle East politics workshop* (March 11, 2016). Project on Middle East Political Science. https://pomeps.org/rethinking-patriarchy-and-kinship-in-the-arab-gulf-states

Wickrama, K. A. S., Lorenz, F. O., Conger, R. D., Elder, G. H., Abraham, W. T., & Fang, S.-A. (2006). Changes in family financial circumstances and the physical health of married and recently divorced mothers. *Social Science & Medicine, 63*(1), 123–136. https://doi.org/10.1016/j.socscimed.2005.12.003

World Health Organization (WHO). (2021). *Caring for women subjected to violence: a WHO training curriculum for health care providers (Revised edition).* https://apps.who.int/iris/handle/10665/349539

Yadav, A., Kumar, P., & Kumar, J. (2022). Domestic violence: Consequences, causes and preventive measures. *Indian Journal of Psychology and Education, 12*(2), 40–43. https://www.researchgate.net/publication/362760828_Domestic_Violence_Consequences_Causes_and_Preventive_Measures

Zahidi, S. (2018). *Fifty million rising: The new generation of working women transforming the Muslim World* (1st ed.). Nation Books.

Zweiri, M., & Al Qawasmi, F. (Eds.). (2020). *Contemporary Qatar - Examining state and society* (4th ed.). Springer. https://doi.org/10.1007/978-981-16-1391-3

Chapter 2
Domestic Abuse: Global and Local

This chapter offers a synopsis of the existing literature examining the various forms of intimate partner domestic abuse and its impact on the mental health of victims with regard to psychopathology. Following this, there is a concise presentation of the theoretical framework related to violence against women and the contributing factors that elevate IPV victimization. This has helped to form the logical consideration to understand the nature of domestic abuse and its impacts that have been addressed by the study's key questions. Including them helps in setting the foundation for the research hypothesis to deep research understanding about key variables that should be considered in a cross-cultural setting. A considerable amount of literature has been published on domestic abuse in western societies and the Middle East, yet in Qatar, little attention was drawn to domestic abuse issues. As part of this chapter research about domestic abuse in Qatar will be included to support and rationalize the current study framework that has been evolved and established to become a cornerstone in drawing a new viewpoint by utilizing preestablished and tested tools to examine domestic violence which has not been considered in previous research in Qatar.

2.1 Domestic Violence Against Women

Intimate partner violence is a public health issue for which victims are deprived of their fundamental rights, which has a profound impact on the mental and physical health of women. It has been associated with long-term health issues and heightens the psychopathology symptoms among victims of domestic abuse (Alejo, 2014; Clements et al., 2019). Post Traumatic Stress Disorder (PTSD), depression, and anxiety are commonly presented mental health issues among victims of domestic abuse, some presented with minor brain injuries which go unnoticed (Karakurt et al., 2021) Umubyeyi et al. (2014) found that women who had experienced intimate partner violence were three times more likely to report major depressive disorder,

K. Al-Naama, *Domestic Abuse and Mental Health in Qatar*, Gulf Studies 23,
https://doi.org/10.1007/978-981-96-7392-6_2

suicidal thoughts, and general anxiety disorder compared to those who had not encountered any forms of such violence. The National Intimate Partner and Sexual Violence Survey (NISVS) in the United States reveal that around 22.3% of women have experienced abuse at some stage in their lives.

Extensive research has delved into the physical repercussions of IPV on women, and further investigation is warranted to examine the potential for psychopathological effects and its enduring impact (Campbell, 2002; Stöckl et al., 2013). Several studies across different cultural settings have demonstrated the impact of intimate partner violence on and the associated risk of developing a range of mental health problems and poor physical health after domestic violence incidents (Dillon et al., 2013). IPV can present and attribute to lethal and non-lethal consequences, for example; 36% of IPV victims were physically hurt and 8% of victims were at greater risk of homicide as a result of being stabbed or shot (Bureau of Justice Statistics, 2013). Even though violence has ended, the negative effects of violence may persist which have lifelong consequences (Dutton et al., 2015). These factors negatively affect their health, reproductive lives, and mental health, in addition to financial disadvantages (Breiding et al., 2015).

In addition to its destructive effects on victims, domestic abuse adversely affects the lifestyle and well-being of family members (Yadav et al., 2022). Results from a cross-sectional study in Rabat show that victims of IPV were indicating high levels of psychopathological symptomology and substance abuse among those who were subjected to a broad range of psychological violence (Bellali et al., 2019). In meta-analysis reviews, strong evidence of depressive symptoms and drug abuse was found among those who presented with IPV in the past 12 months (Bacchus et al., 2018). Results from research conducted by Stuart et al. (2006) on women victims of IPV showed that forms of domestic abuse increase the likelihood of women developing forms of psychopathology; for example, PTSD, depression, general anxiety disorder, panic disorder and some forms of personality disorder were significantly associated with women experiencing IPV. And far more detrimental effects on IPV survivors have predicted substance abuse outcomes, psychological problems, and chronic pain as consequences of IPV victimization which has been demonstrated in two independent systematic reviews (Ogden et al., 2022; Rizo et al., 2017). A growing body of literature confirmed the association between major depressive disorder, anxiety disorder, PTSD, social thoughts and IPV (Sabri, 2021; Ulloa & Hammett, 2016). Similarly, a high level of IPV exposure was associated with the somatoform disorder and anxiety disorder (Sezgin & Punamäki, 2021). In a more recent study, Other mental health issues such as eating disorder and PTSD were found among survivors of IPV who is living in shelters (Holmes et al., 2023). Despite the physical assaults' adverse outcomes on mental health, In meta-analysis reviews demonstrated that psychological and emotional aggression was found strongly associated with PTSD, depression, and anxiety among victims of IPV, and the strength of association differs across the context (Dokkedahl et al., 2022). Another study has shown that IPV was associated with poor physical and mental health issues in both genders. However, women are more likely to suffer systematic abuse and physical violence as a result of their gender (Carbone-López et al., 2006).

A more comprehensive approach is required to understand the multivariate of the complex nature that influences IPV (Flynn & Graham, 2010). Individuals who were exposed to domestic abuse during their childhood are more likely to be either victims or perpetrators, and several reported psychopathology conditions commonly include PTSD, depression and substance abuse (Rioli et al., 2017). These results seem to be consistent with other research which found that children witnessing violence in their family of origin may influence their sense of insecurity and attachment, consequently increasing their chance of IPV victimization or perpetration in their adulthood life (Levendosky et al., 2012). Likewise, Priestley and Lee (2021) claims that being physically abused after the age of 15 and undergoing family violence were also key predictors of later life chances of perpetrating a life partner.

In addition, there is very little published or outdated research on IPV in Qatar (Al-Ghanim, 2009). There is a lack of clarity regarding the risk of death among victims of IPV. According to Pinto et al. (2021), there is a significantly higher risk of death among individuals who have been exposed to a wide range of physical violence. In contrast, pregnant women appear to have a lower risk of death. Nevertheless, no research has been found in Qatar that surveyed the fatal form of abuse that could lead to the risk of death. Concordantly, homicide might occur during serious and escalated cases of disputes (Atiyat, 2015).

Long-term exposure to any kind of violence against women particularly that committed by an intimate partner or inside the household may be detrimental to mental health. It is a significant violation of human rights because it deprives women of the right to feel safe and secure in their own homes. Several studies have focused on the prevalence of domestic violence against women in western countries and its negative repercussions on their mental health. However, there is a dearth of research in Qatar that examines the prevalence of domestic violence against women and its implications on their mental health. Findings from an Arabic study confirm that domestic abuse occurs in a variety of forms like in many other western cultures, according to Usta et al. (2007). The study examines the prevalence of domestic violence among women in Lebanon by analysing data and conducting interviews at four different primary healthcare facilities. Women reported 35% experiencing domestic violence; verbal abuse accounted for 88% of abuse and physical abuse accounted for 66%. In most cases, their spouse was the perpetrator. According to the WHO (2012a), IPV is any kind of abuse that results in physical, sexual, or psychological harm to intimately involved individuals. Approximately one in four women will experience IPV during their lifetime, according to Renzetti et al. (2017).

Ten to fifty percent of women have been physically abused or subjected to various types of violence by a partner in their lives, according to a population-based poll (Watts & Zimmerman, 2002). This is a commonly known reality, and it is for this reason that many instances of violence go unreported due to the sensitivity of the issue. IPV or types of spousal abuse seldom occur alone, since they may escalate while the victim remains in the abusive relationship. Psychological, physical, sexual, and economic abuse are the most common non-fatal kinds of abuse that occur in intimate relationships. IPV or types of spousal abuse are seldom lone occurrences, since they may escalate while the victim remains in an abusive relationship (Paulino, 2016).

A household study (Bhona et al., 2019) revealed that psychological aggression was the most prevalent type of abuse reported by victims (48.31%), followed by physical abuse (10.81%), and then sexual coercion (8%). Before they participated in the study, each of these victims had been subjected to IPV for 3 months. Undoubtedly, emotional abuse was the most prevalent sort of abuse recorded by victims in Saudi Arabia, followed by sexual and physical abuse, which were reported the least (Alquaiz et al., 2021).

The findings would have been much more convincing if they had included the preceding year in the victim's life to quantify how the frequency and severity of domestic violence impact the victim's performance on CTS-2, which may vary from their current reporting score. Domestic violence is one of the risk factors that contribute to premature death among African American females and is the seventh leading cause of death in the United States. While more severe forms of abuse, such as the murder of a spouse by an intimate partner, can have profoundly lethal consequences, domestic violence is one of the risk factors that contribute to premature death among African American females and is the seventh leading cause of death in the United States (Campbell et al., 2003). Previous research done by Berrios and Grady (1991) has shown that more severe kinds of physical assault on an intimate partner are associated with injuries requiring medical attention. One of the most widely cited early studies on the health consequences of domestic abuse found that IPV victims typically exhibit symptoms of depression, anxiety, and PTSD (Campbell, 2002). Exposure to IPV has both short-term and long-term detrimental impacts, including a high incidence of PTSD and depressive symptoms among victims, according to further studies (Sabri, 2021). According to the results of previous studies, the prevalence of anxiety and depression among victims is mostly a consequence of their exposure to domestic violence (Zlotnick et al., 2006).

There has been a lot of research done on sociodemographic and sociocultural factors, and one study indicated that the likelihood of having an intimate partner rises during pregnancy. As a consequence of this, pregnant women who are exposed at a higher level show an increased degree of anxiety symptoms (Fonseca-Machado et al., 2015). In a second study that was carried out in Wales and England with participants ranging in age from 16 to 59 years, the researchers looked at another predictor variable and found that approximately 24% of females have experienced IPV at some point in their lives. The researchers found that the predictors of IPV were a lack of education, a low-income family, and low social status (Khalifeh et al., 2013). Results retained from cross-cultural studies could vary in nature depending on socioeconomic and sociocultural factors. For instance, the findings of a systematic review carried out among the African culture (Shamu et al., 2011) were able to show that a low socioeconomic class, a young age, and pregnancy were significantly associated with IPV. It is not clear how witnessing or experiencing family-of-origin violence in their childhood affects adulthood victimisation or perpetration, and it's a detrimental leading fact that shapes adulthood behaviour, according to a comprehensive study that was made by Smith-Marek et al. (2015).

This study was included in their meta-analysis about the effects of family-of-origin violence on adulthood victimisation or perpetration. The social learning theory was unable to provide an appropriate explanation for their conclusion. This finding may be open to scrutiny due to the type of the data, which was in the form of a retrospective account; a more live kind of data may produce different signs. Several studies have been overlooked and found inconsistency about the effect of a childhood history of witnessing parental abuse due to the nature in complexity of other covariates that could influence adulthood victimisation that prevents establishing a significant association between history of a childhood abuse and their risk of IPV, however in their study they findings concluded that marital violence was noticeably indicated among females who have a history of childhood abuse (Riggs et al., 2000). A more recent argument was presented by Madruga et al. (2017) in their study on the effect of witnessing parental abuse on childhood history and future adulthood victimisation. The researchers came to the conclusion that the risk of IPV victimisation increases by four times among those who had witnessed parental abuse in comparison to their counterparts.

Women in polygamous marriages are more likely to report greater levels of physical, emotional, and sexual abuse than women in monogamous marriages, with the exception of Cameroon, according to the findings of a poll that used a cross-sectional approach and included 16 different nations. On the other hand, women who are in monogamous marriages had a decreased average probability of experiencing abuse at the hands of their partners (Ahinkorah, 2021). It is not feasible to generalise these findings due to the nature of the research, and the study would have generated a better result if it had addressed the influence of patriarchal ideology and family money on the stability of marriages. In a recent study that was carried out in Saudi Arabia, the overall rate of spousal abuse was found to be 43%. The predictor variables revealed a significant association between young age and the level of reported IPV, specifically between the ages of 30–40 and 41–50, and polygamous marriage was also found to be associated with higher levels of reported violence (Alquaiz et al., 2021). According to the findings of a study that was conducted not too long ago, there is a significant correlation between injuries and low levels of education, such as the absence of a high school certificate among abusers, as well as recent joblessness (Kyriacou et al., 2018). Gravelin et al. (2019) suggested that male-dominant cultures that are shaped by masculine ideology are more likely to seek greater authority and control in the relationship, and those who experienced sexual coercion were found to embrace conventional gender roles. These findings support the hypothesis that male dominant cultures are more likely to seek greater authority and controls in the relationship.

Another recent study that looked at the sociodemographic factors that predict domestic violence against women found that male-driven gender norms, a history of witnessing violence in the family of origin, a greater number of children, living in poverty, having a large household, an age disparity between intimate couples, and a history of witnessing violence in the family of origin were all associated with IPV (Clare et al., 2021). However, the cultural background of domestic violence among high-income communities in the Middle East is still not well recognised. An intriguing finding from a study carried out in India indicates that women's risk of abuse doubles among those who indicated they are from an arranged marriage, triples among those who came from a mixed marriage group and is at its lowest among those who are in a love marriage. Although there is still a great deal of uncertainty regarding the relationship between socioeconomic risk factors and spousal abuse, the finding is quite intriguing (Mahapatro et al., 2012). It is already common knowledge that the form of marriage has a role in determining the likelihood of violence inside marriages; however, the impact that marriage type has on Arabic culture is unclear. This difference was not statistically significant among participants from other religions such as Muslim, according to the findings of a study that was carried out in India. The study found that the risk of marital violence was higher among couples who had married within their family than among those who had married outside their family (Rahaman et al., 2021).

One research looked at the complicated nature of remarriages as well as the societal factors that play a role in them. This was done for those who wanted to give their second marriage a better chance of success. According to the findings of this research, the family is comprised of many different life changes, emotional issues, and financial concerns that might contribute to an increased risk of spousal violence (Hetherington et al., 1992). However, this does not constitute a clear result since there is still the issue of investigating the regulations that control family life. One of the most common strategies used by abusers to regain power and control in the relationship, according to survivors of IPV, was to threaten mothers about their child custody rights, visitation rights, or inability to meet with their children. This was one of the most common ways that abusers regained power and control in the relationship. This is one of the logical reasons why victims could think twice before carrying out their original plan to end the relationship (Clements et al., 2021). However, the findings did not take into consideration all the factors that impact a mother's position during the divorce process. These factors include women's awareness of their rights as divorce mothers as well as the accessibility of financial and emotional support. According to the findings of different earlier research, remarried women reported a significantly increased risk of both physical and psychological violence (Ugwuanyi et al., 2022).

The choice that female victims of domestic violence make on whether or not to leave an abusive relationship or to stay in the relationship has been identified as one of the most crucial variables by a number of authorities. Previous studies have demonstrated that women learn to put up with the abusive behaviour of their partners because they have been led to believe that the behaviour would improve in the near future. According to the findings of other research, as more time passes, women become more hesitant to leave abusive relationships. Other studies have indicated that when women do not have enough access to emotional and material resources, they experience hopelessness (Rhodes & McKenzie, 1998). One of the few systematic studies that have analysed the decision to leave an abusive relationship found that economic variables were a major predictor of a woman's decision to remain in or leave an abusive relationship. The study looked at the decision to leave an abusive relationship from the perspective of women. According to the findings of the study, women who are in abusive relationships go through a difficult decision-making process and an exhaustive psychological and emotional analysis of the benefits and drawbacks of leaving the relationship before choosing to do so (Anderson & Saunders, 2003). In spite of the fact that a recent study discovered that one of the most common strategies used by abusers to regain power and control in the relationship was to threaten mothers about their child custody rights, visitation rights, or inability to meet with children and that this was one of the rational reasons why victims would reconsider their decision to leave the relationship (Clements et al., 2021), the findings failed to take into account some contextual factors that contribute to victims reconsidering their decision to leave the relationship. For example, the investigation did not include of.

The most recent study on the topic, which was carried out in Qatar by Lari (2022), revealed that the choice of a life partner is still heavily influenced by the traditions and conventions of the family, which are primarily influenced by the patriarchal framework of the society. This was one of the findings of the study. Other kinds of marriages, such as those founded on love, are less likely to be respected by society than other kinds of marriages. Women's reasons for violent behaviour, conventional gender roles, and the expectations of Arab family obligations all seem to have a major effect on the degree of domestic violence to which women may be subjected, according to the findings of yet another research (Abu-Ras, 2007). Arab families have the propensity to preserve their cultural identity and gender roles by empowering patriarchal beliefs and prioritising the reputation of the family over the personal interests of the victims, particularly those who want to end their marriage as a result of Intimate Partner Violence, because it is considered the women's duty to ensure that the family unit continues to exist. This is because it is considered the women's duty to ensure that the family unit continues to exist, after all, it is considered the women's duty to ensure that the family unit continues as per the views of research conducted in 2019 by Aboulhassan and Brumley. There is cultural sensitivity around the matter itself, in addition to the difficulty of proving guilt within the legality of marital duties and responsibilities, often known as wifely duty (Kwiatkowski, 2019).

2.2 Key Terminologies

To establish essential understanding about the components of domestic abuse the following section will outline the key terminology employed in the current study. These terminologies will serve as a foundation for the subsequent analysis and decision.

The Institute for the Control and Prevention of infectious diseases defines IPV as any act of violence that happens inside an intimate relationship. This may involve physical, sexual, psychological, and stalking hostility towards current or previous spouses or romantic partners (CDC, 2020). According to the conclusions of this study, "violence against married or engaged women" best captures the meaning of "intimate partner violence". In this study, the terms spouse abuse, intimate partner violence, domestic violence against women, and IPV will be used interchangeably to refer to the same concept: IPV (CDC, 2020, pp. 11–12).

According to several publications, there are several definitions of what constitutes physical, sexual, and psychological violence towards a life partner (WHO, 2012a, p. 1). Bodily abuse refers to any act of slapping, striking, beating, or other external violence committed by the spouse that causes physical harm to the victim. Sexual violence is a pattern of behaviour that involves any sort of sexual coercion that happens without the agreement of the partner. Psychological abuse refers to any actions that degrade or frighten the partner in a relationship. For the inquiry, "any physical force that hurts a married or engaged woman" is synonymous with "physical abuse", "physical assault", and "physical aggression". While the terms psychological abuse, emotional violence, and aggression will be used interchangeably to mean the same thing, they are not synonymous "The term "negotiation abuse" will be used to refer to "any forms of verbal or non-verbal communication that are intended to intimidate married or encaged women". This expression is interchangeable with "sexual abuse", "sexual coercion", "sexual assault", and "sexual violence". The term "injuries" will be used throughout this study to refer to "any act of violence against a married or encaged woman that resulted in physical damage."

This study will use the terms economic control, economic exploitation, and economic sabotage to refer to three subcategories of economic abuse: economic control, economic exploitation, and economic sabotage. Economic abuse is defined as a pattern of behaviour that is primarily experienced by victims of domestic abuse for the perpetrator to maintain power and gain control over the relationship (p. 546). The phrase economic abuse is given by Adams et al. (2008). According to de Serpa Pimentel et al. (2021), the term "economic exploitation" can be defined as "Manipulating a life partner resource for own gain", whereas the terms "employment sabotage" and "economic controls" can be defined as "coercive actions by the abuser that result in the creation of barriers that prevent women from obtaining or maintaining employment" (p. 2). "Limiting or preventing women from acquiring information about the household financial status and reducing their capacity to do so. In the purpose of this study, the phrases "economic abuse", "economic violence", and "economic aggression" will be used interchangeably to refer to "any act of control over household funds from victims that hindered her ability to achieve financial stability and independence".

According to Hunnicutt (2009), a patriarchal society may be described as a systemic situation, as opposed to the individual behaviour patterns that lead to domestic violence against women (p. 557). In patriarchal societies, men have the right to command and control the power structure, whereas women are viewed as submissive to men. Patriarchal society is the cause of domestic violence against women. In the context of this study, "traditional gender role enforced by the social structure of the society that dictated and defined women and men roles and responsibilities in the Arabic culture" is synonymous with a male-dominated society, patriarchal society, men's ideology, and attitude towards women's rights. These names are interchangeable when referring to the same notion.

As recommended by the WHO, the words femicide, homicide, and women murder shall be used interchangeably in this research to refer to "prospective husband's risk of murdering his future wife". Femicide, as defined by the WHO (2012b, p. 7), refers to the purposeful death of a woman by her current or past abusive male partner.

Koepsell et al. (2007) refer to the term 'leave the abusive relationship' in their study as any notions of inactivity and temporary departure which encompass a difficult decision process to leave an abusive relationship (p. 132). Throughout this study, the terms "women remain passive", "women remain inactive", and "women remain silent" will be used interchangeably to refer to the "wife's refusal to leave her violent relationship".

According to Singh and Wassenaar (2016), the term "gatekeeper" refers to any individual or organisation that regulates or enables access to certain data (p. 43). These researchers contributed to this definition. The term "gatekeepers" will be used in the context of this study to refer to "any governmental body or institution that authorises the study to interview with potential participants, provides a venue to conduct an interview, or shares the study's link" (Singh & Wassenaar, 2016).

According to Brownridge (2006), "post-separation violence" refers to any kind of abuse a victim has endured at the hands of her ex-husband, boyfriend, or cohabiting partner following the termination of their partnership (p. 516). For this investigation, "post separation abuse", "post-separation violence", and "divorce" will be used interchangeably to refer to "any manipulative and abusive actions that tend to continue after the separation or divorce from the husband to regain control or retaliate against the victims".

According to Shahid (2013), women in the culture of the Khula have the legal right to divorce their spouses, regardless of whether the guy consents to the divorce (p. 206). According to what he indicated, after the divorce is finalised, the former husband would give payment to the former wife known as Muta'ah Al-Talaq (Iddat period) (p. 212). During this inquiry, the expression "he divorces me" will be used to refer to "a lady whose marriage has come to an end as a result of her husband's choice to divorce her". According to the findings of this study, the term "khula" refers to a kind of divorce in which the woman files for the dissolution of the marriage while simultaneously returning the dowry or wedding present to the husband. "talaq" will be used to describe "divorce" among Muslims, and "Mut'ah Al-talaq" will be used to describe "a term in marriages among Muslims that awards a gift or recompense paid by a former husband to his divorced wife in the form of money depending on court order". Both terms refer to "a term in marriages among Muslims that awards a gift or recompense paid by a former husband to his divorced wife in the form of the phrase "fault-based divorce" gives the impression that the former husband, rather than the woman, is to blame for the start of the divorce proceedings. This is not the case. Adultery is only one of the many things that may get in the way of a man fulfilling his mental and physical responsibilities as a spouse, and there are plenty of other things too. In addition, the woman does not bear any blame or responsibility for the breakup of the marriage in this scenario (Singer, 1989). Despite the designation "For this investigation, the terms "fault-based divorce" and "no-fault divorce" will mean the same thing: "a form of divorce in which one spouse proves that the other caused the dissolution of the marriage or the inability to maintain it", and "no-fault divorce" will mean the opposite of "fault-based divorce".

According to Tahirih's (2016) review of forced marriages definition can be referred to as "a marriage without consent" (p. 7), but an arranged marriage is defined as "the lack of current free choice of a life mate that is primarily planned by a guardianship and typically launched under parental supervision". According to Rashad et al. (2005), Osman, and Roudi-Fahimi's definition of consanguinity weddings, "cousins' marriages in particular are a popular sort of consanguine marriages that occur between close relatives" (p. 4), cousins marriages are the most prevalent kind of consanguine marriage (Rashad et al., 2005). According to the findings of this study, the term "arranged marriage" refers to "cultural common norms in forming the marriage, in which the life partner selection is generally prepared and offered by the men's parents". "Weddings between closely related cousins" (p. 4), on the other hand, shall be referred to as "consanguine weddings" throughout this investigation. In this investigation, you may come across terms that may give the impression that "one of the spouses was forced against their will to marry a family-recommended partner". However, it is essential to emphasise that this is not the case. Throughout the whole of this study, this definition of "forced marriage" will be used.

Abraham (2005) defines a "love marriage" as "a kind of marriage in which the choice of spouses is made without consideration to other family members" (p. 437). This type of marriage is considered problematic when the conventional system of marriage is used to build families. The term "love marriage", on the other hand, is often used to refer to "a sort of marriage that is copied by one of the emotionally linked couples, which is mainly against their engagement in official marriage".

There have been many different interpretations proposed for the difference between monogamous and polygamous marriages. According to Daoud et al. (2019), the definition of a polygamous marriage is "a legal marriage across some societies and religions in which a man marries numerous women is commonly practised" (p. 44). While the definition of a monogamous marriage is "a husband who has only one wife or no other life partner" (p. 127).

Both types of marriages are considered to be valid. There have been several reports of couples being married in either a monogamous or polygamous fashion. The terms "women who are married to a guy with numerous wives" and "polygamous spouse" will be used interchangeably throughout the course of this research. During the course of this investigation, the terms "monogamous marriages" and "a spouse who is married to only one woman" will be used interchangeably.

According to Bramlett and Mosher (2002), the term "remarry" refers to "a woman who has been in a relationship, such as marriage or cohabitation, and has since been divorced or separated, and then marries again" (p. 7). In other words, "a woman who has remarried" is a woman who has previously been married or cohabitated and who subsequently married again. The words "second marriage", "remarried wife", and "remarried lady" may all be used interchangeably for this investigation. "It is more probable for a woman to become a mother if she has been through a divorce and then remarried.

According to Dierickx et al. (2019) research, "In polygamous marriages, the first wife is often referred to as the senior lady, while another new wife is commonly referred to as the co-wife" (p. 5). In other words, the senior woman is the one who has the most senior status. The terms "first wife" and "co-wife" are discussed in the context of polygamous partnerships over the course of this research. According to the findings of this research, the first wife of a husband is also referred to as the senior wife of that husband. In a similar vein, the new wife of the husband will be referred to as both the co-wife and the second wife. This is due to the fact that following her marriage to the husband, she will need her own set of marital arrangements.

2.3 Theoretical Insights

The following section will provide the theoretical framework adopted to establish a solid foundation to examine research questions. This will help the researcher to understand the influence of the risk factors involved in intimate partner violence. A wide range of theories has been proposed as explanations for the nature of domestic abuse against women. Because of the complexity of this abuse, a more holistic approach is required in order to identify factors that may increase the likelihood of victimization (Gage & Lease, 2021; Hong & Espelage, 2012). According to Lawson (2012) ecological theory, social learning theory, and other theories of family violence point out the importance of understanding the social structures that underlie the use of violence against women, while feminist scholars commonly refer to gender-based violence as a consequence of power imbalances and gender inequality. Feminist theories considerably emphasize that patriarchal social structures are the root cause of violence against women.

The ecological theory explains domestic abuse through a structural approach. The ecological factors that result in an imbalance of power include "marital violence, underemployment, financial pressures, anxiety, and alcohol abuse" (Burgess & Draper, 1989, p. 59). The more ecological disturbance there is, the higher the rate of domestic abuse (p. 59). Another factor also includes the "reinforcement of abusive behaviour" through structural forces (Kurst-Swanger & Petcosky, 2003, p. vii).

Following the social control theory paradigm, Gordon studies child abuse in the United States in her study (Gordon, 1988, p. 523). She focuses on the structural response from the government regarding this issue and explains that child abuse exists due to the patriarchal superstructure where the father has control over all the family members due to his "monopolization of economic resources" (p. 524). She argues, however, that once children and family members become financially independent, they can escape domestic abuse (p. 524). Fagan (1988) also argues that domestic abuse and violence were viewed as personal conflicts that the authorities were not supposed to get involved in (p. 160). This stems from the patriarchal social structure where the man is responsible for his household. The gendered resource theory suggests that uneven power distributions between husband and wife influence the risk of domestic abuse (Anderson, 2010; Lawson, 2012). If men feel threatened, they use their power to regain control of women's financial resources, which in this case offers another explanation for how economic abuse occurred. A woman's lack of financial autonomy and dependency on her partner increases abuse risk (Capaldi et al., 2012).

Moder's study relies on feminist theory to explain domestic abuse; she points to patriarchy as the root cause. She argues that since God is portrayed as a "dominant male figure", it indoctrinates women to accept themselves as subordinates of men (Moder, 2019, p. 85). Another theorist, Sharma, explains domestic abuse using feminist theory's explanation of "systemic oppression and hegemony" (Sharma, 2001, p. 1405). She studies immigrant and "racially visible women" and explains what domestic abuse means; domestic abuse includes violence, controlling or restraining women's activities, physical assault, verbal harassment, emotional neglect, emotional threats, sexual coercion, and intimidation (p. 1407). She explains that patriarchal norms and practices are responsible for domestic abuse because they lay the groundwork for violence to occur at home (p. 1408). These patriarchal norms make women internalize their subordination affecting their self-worth and creating a tolerance for abuse (p. 1408).

There is ample literature that explains domestic abuse in Arab societies. Haj-Yahia (2000) explains that domestic abuse is present in all cultures and all divisions of society (p. 237). He argues that this issue is explained without keeping in mind the socio-cultural context of Arab societies (p. 238). He explains that Arab societies are deeply patriarchal and place the man as the head of the household; hence, the interference of the law to remove abusive men is perceived as bringing the family structure down (p. 238). He uses feminist theory as well as social control theory to recommend more cultural sensitivity by scholars (p. 238). Another study concludes that Arab women are subjected to domestic abuse much more than Jewish women in Israel (Ben-Porat et al., 2021, p. 26). It takes the feminist and ecological theory approach to explain why this is analysing factors such as access to gun violence, level of education, age, and employment level (pp. 26–27). There is less scholarship published on Gulf societies and domestic abuse. Albrithen (2006) studied this issue in Saudi Arabia in relation to the issue of alcohol, and his study shows that alcoholism leads to high rates of domestic abuse, especially against women (p. ii). This shows that he takes an ecological and social control theory approach. Al-Ghanim (2009) also writes about women's experience of violence in Qatari households. Her findings show that "a substantial women" have experienced violence that mostly occurs within the family from male members such as brothers, husbands, and fathers (p. 80). She argues that this is due to a "lack of legislation" and "official organisations" that protect women from violence (p. 80). Hence, she takes a feminist as well as ecological and social control theory approach.

A thorough analysis of the detrimental impacts of domestic violence against women reveals that victims who have been subjected to various kinds of domestic violence are more likely to acquire anxiety, depression, and PTSD (Lagdon et al., 2014). This is the conclusion reached from the review's findings. Although violence can occur at a variety of developmental life stages, numerous studies have measured the impact of exposure to IPV within the previous 12 months in their samples and found that depression is a commonly reported mental health disorder among victims of IPV (Chatterji & Heise, 2021). It has been suggested that both the short- and long-term effects of domestic violence increase the likelihood of developing mental health issues such as depression, anxiety, and PTSD (Braaf & Meyering, 2013). The major goal of this study is to test the hypothesis that domestic violence victims have a considerably greater risk of developing and exhibiting a larger range of symptoms associated with mood and anxiety disorders, as well as PTSD (Krause et al., 2006).

To comprehend the mental health effects of domestic abuse pathways, it is vital to study the multilayer risk factors for IPV victimisation. The choice to leave an abusive relationship puts IPV victims at a higher risk of murder, a form of crime that has been highlighted by many researchers as a particularly lethal type. The human rights approach recognises female homicide as a serious form of violence that extends beyond reported non-lethal forms of domestic abuse, whereas the feminist approach tends to emphasise that male-dominated society and gender inequalities are the primary contributors to women's victimisation or homicide (Corradi et al., 2016). Several hypotheses provide diverse explanations for a life partner's murder. Among these philosophies are the human rights and feminist approaches. Therefore, additional theoretical perspectives to understand female homicide have been overlooked by western scholars while they have been attempting to highlight the risk factors that put women's lives in danger (Graham et al., 2022). This is a secondary objective of this study, which seeks to understand when females are at a greater risk of being murdered.

Within the ecological theoretical framework, one of the well-known ideas for understanding how personal and environmental variables influence women's choice to leave an abusive spouse is investigated (Alaggia et al., 2012). A victim of IPV may fall prey to a variety of different conditions. The secondary purpose of this study is partially based on the ecological theoretical framework, which tries to determine which characteristics are most likely to be connected with IPV victimisation and why victims continue in violent relationships. This aim was selected because it relates to the study's primary purpose, which is to identify why victims remain in abusive relationships. No one strategy may provide clear information as to whether women are in danger of abuse; rather, domestic violence against women is the result of a multiplicity of connected conditions. Within the context of analysing domestic violence against women, the ecological framework theory recognises the interaction between people, relationships, communities, and societal levels (Tekkas Kerman & Betrus, 2020). Investigating cultural views on domestic violence is another method for comprehending how cultural identity might be a risk factor in cases of IPV. For instance, Zhang and Breunig (2021) found that breaching gender norms and disputing the breadwinner position seems to increase the chance of IPV victimisation. This inquiry included cultural views on domestic violence. According to Mshweshwe (2020), the fact that patriarchy is still an active influence in the majority of societies, with an inflexible gender hierarchy in which men have more privilege and entitlement than women, and an uneven distribution of power influenced by social norms that primarily derive from the distinction between men and women, can increase the risk of domestic violence against women. While patriarchy still has an active effect in the majority of nations, with an inflexible gender hierarchy in which males have more power and entitlement than women, it is becoming less prevalent.

The idea of resource theory is discussed in this article as a means of developing the theoretical considerations around domestic violence. This idea accepts that a husband who has little financial means can be able to achieve control in the home by establishing a more aggressive attitude towards his spouse to sustain the breadwinner mentality. This specific traditional belief system tends to tolerate abusive behaviour in exchange for compliance, while also enforcing the idea that men should behave in a certain way (Atkinson et al., 2005).

According to Dare et al. (2013), one principle that could keep women trapped in abusive relationships is that they have fewer alternative options to end the relationship because they have fewer financial resources and lower educational attainment. Other perspectives on understanding why abused women would remain passive in the relationship include interpersonal factors such as seeking an excuse for a husband or women who have lower educational attainment and fewer financial resources. Another explanation that has been the subject of extensive discussion among feminist theory scholars is the notion that culturally robust definitions and classifications of cultural identity emphasize the shaping of appropriate male and female roles. This is a form of social control that justifies unequal power distribution and suppers women's roles in society (De Coster & Heimer, 2021). The importance of referring to the patriarchy concept in order to understand the context of domestic violence against women is emphasised by feminist perspectives, and the prioritisation of this principle over other factors, which could be undermined by the scholars who take this approach, is also emphasised by feminist perspectives (DeKeseredy, 2021).

Having access to a wider range of viewpoints has the potential to provide a more complete picture, so enhancing one's understanding of the dynamics of domestic violence against women. Other researchers, such as DeKeseredy and Dragiewicz (2007), advocated for more integrative and holistic methods to explain the nature of domestic violence that occurs in intimate relationships, as opposed to attributing the primary source of the problem only to the patriarchal societal structure. Intimate Partner Violence (IPV) has been explained by a number of theories, including social learning theory, ecological system theory, and feminist theory, which have been examined in previous studies (Bell & Naugle, 2008). Domestic abuse is a complex issue intertwined with a variety of factors that are understood from various perspectives. The power imbalance, gender inequality, social tolerance of violence, and the cultural and societal context of domestic abuse are all aspects of domestic abuse that increase the risk of IPV.

The current variables that have been studied have been conceptualised based on an ecological theoretical framework that was proposed by Heise (1998). This framework emphasises the importance of interrelated variables that are influenced by personal and socio-cultural variables to understand when abuse may exist.

References

Abraham, M. (2005). Domestic violence and the Indian diaspora in the United States. *Indian Journal of Gender Studies, 12*(3), 427–451. https://doi.org/10.1177/097152150501200212

Abu-Ras, W. (2007). Cultural beliefs and service utilization by battered Arab immigrant women. *Violence Against Women, 13*(10), 1002–1028. https://doi.org/10.1177/1077801207306019

Adams, A. E., Sullivan, C. M., Bybee, D., & Greeson, M. R. (2008). Development of the scale of economic abuse. *Violence Against Women, 14*(5), 563–588. https://doi.org/10.1177/1077801208315529

Ahinkorah, B. O. (2021). Polygyny and intimate partner violence in sub-Saharan Africa: Evidence from 16 cross-sectional demographic and health surveys. *SSM - Population Health, 13*(December 2020), 100729. https://doi.org/10.1016/j.ssmph.2021.100729

Alaggia, R., Regehr, C., & Jenney, A. (2012). Risky business: An ecological analysis of intimate partner violence disclosure. *Research on Social Work Practice, 22*(3), 301–312. https://doi.org/10.1177/1049731511425503

Albrithen, A. A. (2006). *Alcoholism and domestic violence in Saudi society* [Doctoral dissertation, The University of Liverpool]. https://www.cawtarclearinghouse.org/storage/AttachementGender/Alcholisme%20and%20domestic%20violence%20in%20saudi%20socity.pdf

Alejo, K. (2014). Long-term physical and mental health effects of domestic violence. *Themis: Research Journal of Justice Studies and Forensic Science, 2*(1), 5. https://doi.org/10.31979/THEMIS.2014.0205

Al-Ghanim, K. A. (2009). Violence against women in Qatari society. *Journal of Middle East Women's Studies, 5*(1), 80–93. https://doi.org/10.2979/mew.2009.5.1.80

Alquaiz, A. M., Almuneef, M., Kazi, A., & Almeneessier, A. (2021). Social determinants of domestic violence among Saudi married women in Riyadh, Kingdom of Saudi Arabia. *Journal of Interpersonal Violence, 36*(3–4), NP1561–NP1585. https://doi.org/10.1177/0886260517746128

Anderson, D. K., & Saunders, D. G. (2003). Leaving an abusive partner: An empirical review of predictors, the process of leaving, and psychological Well-being. *Trauma, Violence & Abuse, 4*(2), 163–191. https://doi.org/10.1177/1524838002250769

Anderson, K. L. (2010). Conflict, power, and violence in families. *Journal of Marriage and Family, 72*(3), 726–742. https://doi.org/10.1111/j.1741-3737.2010.00727.x

Atiyat, R. B. A. R. (2015). *No redress? Investigating wife abuse through the lens of Feminist Theory and Resource Theory in Jordan* [Doctoral dissertation, University of York]. White Rose eTheses Online. https://etheses.whiterose.ac.uk/10524/

Atkinson, M. P., Greenstein, T. N., & Lang, M. M. (2005). For women, breadwinning can be dangerous: Gendered resource theory and wife abuse. *Journal of Marriage and Family, 67*(5), 1137–1148. https://doi.org/10.1111/j.1741-3737.2005.00206.x

Bacchus, L. J., Ranganathan, M., Watts, C., & Devries, K. (2018). Recent intimate partner violence against women and health: A systematic review and meta-analysis of cohort studies. *BMJ Open, 8*(7), e019995. https://doi.org/10.1136/bmjopen-2017-019995

Bell, K. M., & Naugle, A. E. (2008). Intimate partner violence theoretical considerations: Moving towards a contextual framework. *Clinical Psychology Review, 28*(7), 1096–1107. https://doi.org/10.1016/j.cpr.2008.03.003

Bellali, N., Laboudi, F., & Ouanass, A. (2019). Domestic violence and psychopathological impact. *Austin Journal of Psychiatry and Behavioral Sciences, 6*(1), 1070. https://austinpublishinggroup.com/psychiatry-behavioral-sciences/fulltext/ajpbs-v6-id1070.php

Ben-Porat, A., Levy, D., Kattoura, O., Dekel, R., & Itzhaky, H. (2021). Domestic violence in Arab society: A comparison of Arab and Jewish women in shelters in Israel. *Journal of Interpersonal Violence, 36*(1–2), NP26–NP45. https://doi.org/10.1177/0886260517731789

Berrios, D. C., & Grady, D. (1991). Domestic violence: Risk factors and outcomes. *Western Journal of Medicine, 155*(2), 133–135. https://pubmed.ncbi.nlm.nih.gov/1926841/

Bhona, F. M. C., Gebara, C. F. P., Noto, A. R., Vieira, M. D. T., & Lourenço, L. M. (2019). Socioeconomic factors and intimate partner violence: A household survey. *Trends in Psychology, 27*(1), 205–218. https://doi.org/10.9788/TP2019.1-15

Braaf, R., & Meyering, I. B. (2013, June 4). *Domestic violence and mental health.* Australian Domestic and Family Violence Clearing House. https://www.nifvs.org.au/wp-content/uploads/2015/01/Domestic-Violence-and-Mental-Health.pdf

Bramlett, M. D., & Mosher, W. D. (2002). Cohabitation, marriage, divorce, and remarriage in the United States. *Vital and Health Statistics, 23*(22), 1–93. https://pubmed.ncbi.nlm.nih.gov/12183886/

Breiding, M. J., Basile, K. C., Smith, S. G., Black, M. C., & Mahendra, R. R. (2015). *Intimate partner violence surveillance: Uniform definitions and recommended data elements, Version 2.0.* National Center for Injury Prevention and Control, Centers for Disease Control and Prevention. https://www.cdc.gov/violenceprevention/pdf/ipv/intimatepartnerviolence.pdf

Brownridge, D. A. (2006). Violence against women post-separation. *Aggression and Violent Behavior, 11*(5), 514–530. https://doi.org/10.1016/j.avb.2006.01.009

Bureau of Justice Statistics. (2013). *Intimate partner violence: Attributes of victimization, 1993-2011.* https://bjs.ojp.gov/press-release/intimate-partner-violence-attributes-victimization-1993-2011

Burgess, R., & Draper, P. (1989). The explanation of family violence: The role of biological, behavioral, and cultural selection. In L. Ohlin & M. Tonry (Eds.), *Family violence, crime and justice: A review of research* (Vol. II, pp. 59–116). University of Chicago Press. https://www.jstor.org/stable/1147526

Campbell, J. C. (2002). Health consequences of intimate partner violence. *Lancet (London, England), 359*(9314), 1331–1336. https://doi.org/10.1016/S0140-6736(02)08336-8

Campbell, J. C., Webster, D., Koziol-McLain, J., Block, C., Campbell, D., Curry, M. A., Gary, F., Glass, N., McFarlane, J., Sachs, C., Sharps, P., Ulrich, Y., Wilt, S. A., Manganello, J., Xu, X., Schollenberger, J., Frye, V., & Laughon, K. (2003). Risk factors for femicide in abusive relationships: Results from a multisite case control study. *American Journal of Public Health, 93*(7), 1089–1097. https://doi.org/10.2105/ajph.93.7.1089

Capaldi, D. M., Knoble, N. B., Shortt, J. W., & Kim, H. K. (2012). A systematic review of risk factors for intimate partner violence. *Partner Abuse, 3*(2), 231–280. https://doi.org/10.1891/1946-6560.3.2.231

Carbone-López, K., Kruttschnitt, C., & Macmillan, R. (2006). Patterns of intimate partner violence and their associations with physical health, psychological distress, and substance use. *Public Health Reports, 121*(4), 382–392. https://doi.org/10.1177/003335490612100406

CDC. (2020, October 9). *Centers for disease control and prevention.* Intimate Partner Violence, Violence Prevention Injury Center. https://www.cdc.gov/violenceprevention/intimatepartnerviolence/index.html

Chatterji, S., & Heise, L. (2021). Examining the bi-directional relationship between intimate partner violence and depression: Findings from a longitudinal study among women and men in rural Rwanda. *SSM - Mental Health, 1*(March), 100038. https://doi.org/10.1016/j.ssmmh.2021.100038

Clare, C. A., Velasquez, G., Mujica Martorell, G. M., Fernandez, D., Dinh, J., & Montague, A. (2021). Risk factors for male perpetration of intimate partner violence: A review. *Aggression and Violent Behavior, 56*(November 2020), 101532. https://doi.org/10.1016/j.avb.2020.101532

Clements, C. M., Bennett, V. E., Hungerford, A., Clauss, K., & Wait, S. K. (2019). Psychopathology and coping in survivors of intimate partner violence: Associations with race and abuse severity. *Journal of Aggression, Maltreatment & Trauma, 28*(2), 205–221. https://doi.org/10.1080/10926771.2018.1470588

Clements, K. A. V., Sprecher, M., Modica, S., Terrones, M., Gregory, K., & Sullivan, C. M. (2021). The use of children as a tactic of intimate partner violence and its relationship to survivors' mental health. *Journal of Family Violence, 37*, 1049–1055. https://doi.org/10.1007/s10896-021-00330-0

Corradi, C., Marcuello-Servós, C., Boira, S., & Weil, S. (2016). Theories of femicide and their significance for social research. *Current Sociology, 64*(7), 975–995. https://doi.org/10.1177/0011392115622256

Daoud, N., Berger-Polsky, A., Abu-Kaf, S., & Sagy, S. (2019). Sense of coherence among Bedouin women in polygamous marriages compared to women in monogamous marriages. *Women & Health, 60*(1), 43–59. https://doi.org/10.1080/03630242.2019.1610826

Dare, B., Guadagno, R., & Muscanell, N. (2013). Commitment: The key to women staying in abusive relationships. *Journal of Interpersonal Relations, Intergroup Relations and Identity, 6*(January 2013), 58–63. https://www.researchgate.net/publication/236647230

De Coster, S., & Heimer, K. (2021). Unifying theory and research on intimate partner violence: A feminist perspective. *Feminist Criminology, 16*(3), 286–303. https://doi.org/10.1177/1557085120987615

de Serpa Pimentel, A., Mshana, G., Aloyce, D., Peter, E., Mchome, Z., Malibwa, D., Dwarumpudi, A., Kapiga, S., & Stöckl, H. (2021). Women's understanding of economic abuse in North-Western Tanzania. *Women's Health, 17*, 1–11. https://doi.org/10.1177/17455065211042180

DeKeseredy, W. S. (2021). Bringing feminist sociological analyses of patriarchy back to the forefront of the study of woman abuse. *Violence Against Women, 27*(5), 621–638. https://doi.org/10.1177/1077801220958485

DeKeseredy, W. S., & Dragiewicz, M. (2007). Understanding the complexities of feminist perspectives on woman abuse a commentary on Donald G. Dutton's rethinking domestic violence. *Violence Against Women, 13*(8), 874–884. https://doi.org/10.1177/1077801207304806

Dierickx, S., Coene, G., Jarju, B., & Longman, C. (2019). Women with infertility complying with and resisting polygyny: An explorative qualitative study in urban Gambia. *Reproductive Health, 16*(1), 1–11. https://doi.org/10.1186/s12978-019-0762-1

Dillon, G., Hussain, R., Loxton, D., & Rahman, S. (2013). Mental and physical health and intimate partner violence against women: A review of the literature. *International Journal of Family Medicine, 2013*, 313909. https://doi.org/10.1155/2013/313909

Dokkedahl, S. B., Kirubakaran, R., Bech-Hansen, D., Kristensen, T. R., & Elklit, A. (2022). The psychological subtype of intimate partner violence and its effect on mental health: A systematic review with meta-analyses. *Systematic Reviews, 11*(1), 163. https://doi.org/10.1186/s13643-022-02025-z

Dutton, M. A., James, L., Langhorne, A., & Kelley, M. (2015). Coordinated public health initiatives to address violence against women and adolescents. *Journal of Women's Health, 24*(1), 80–85. https://doi.org/10.1089/jwh.2014.4884

Fagan, J. (1988). Contributions of family violence research to criminal justice policy on wife assault: Paradigms of science and social control. *Violence and Victims, 3*(3), 159–186. https://pubmed.ncbi.nlm.nih.gov/3154178/

Flynn, A., & Graham, K. (2010). "Why did it happen?" A review and conceptual framework for research on perpetrators' and victims' explanations for intimate partner violence. *Aggression and Violent Behavior, 15*(3), 239–251. https://doi.org/10.1016/j.avb.2010.01.002

Fonseca-Machado, M. d. O., Monteiro, J. C. d. S., Haas, V. J., de Vilhena, A. C. F. A., & Gomes-Sponholz, F. (2015). Intimate partner violence and anxiety disorders in pregnancy: The importance of vocational training of the nursing staff in facing them. *Revista Latino-Americana de Enfermagem, 23*(5), 855–864. https://doi.org/10.1590/0104-1169.0495.2624

Gage, A. N., & Lease, S. H. (2021). An exploration of the link between masculinity and endorsement of IPV myths in American men. *Journal of Interpersonal Violence, 36*(13–14), 6145–6165. https://doi.org/10.1177/0886260518818430

Gordon, L. (1988). *Heroes of their own lives: The history and politics of family violence*. Viking/Penguin.

Graham, L. M., Macy, R. J., Rizo, C. F., & Martin, S. L. (2022). Explanatory theories of intimate partner homicide perpetration: A systematic review. *Trauma, Violence & Abuse, 23*(2), 408–427. https://doi.org/10.1177/1524838020953800

Gravelin, C. R., Biernat, M., & Bucher, C. E. (2019). Blaming the victim of acquaintance rape: Individual, situational, and sociocultural factors. *Frontiers in Psychology, 9*(JAN), 1–22. https://doi.org/10.3389/fpsyg.2018.02422

Haj-Yahia, M. M. (2000). Wife abuse and battering in the sociocultural context of Arab society. *Family Process, 39*(2), 237–255. https://doi.org/10.1111/j.1545-5300.2000.39207.x

Heise, L. L. (1998). Violence against women: An integrated, ecological framework. *Violence Against Women, 4*(3), 262–290. https://doi.org/10.1177/1077801298004003002

Hetherington, E. M., Bridges, M., & Insabella, G. M. (1992). What matters? What does not? *American Psychologist, 53*(2), 167–184.

Holmes, S. C., King, K. C., Gonzalez, A., Norton, M. K., Silver, K. E., Sullivan, T. P., & Johnson, D. M. (2023). Associations among intimate partner violence, posttraumatic stress disorder symptoms, and disordered eating among women intimate partner violence survivors residing in shelter. *Journal of Interpersonal Violence, 38*(1–2), NP2135–NP2158. https://doi.org/10.1177/08862605221098968

Hong, J. S., & Espelage, D. L. (2012). A review of research on bullying and peer victimization in school: An ecological system analysis. *Aggression and Violent Behavior, 17*(4), 311–322. https://doi.org/10.1016/j.avb.2012.03.003

Hunnicutt, G. (2009). Varieties of patriarchy and violence against women. *Violence Against Women, 15*(5), 553–573. https://doi.org/10.1177/1077801208331246

Karakurt, G., Whiting, K., Jones, S. E., Lowe, M. J., & Rao, S. M. (2021). Brain injury and mental health among the victims of intimate partner violence: A case-series exploratory study. *Frontiers in Psychology, 12*(October). https://doi.org/10.3389/fpsyg.2021.710602

Khalifeh, H., Hargreaves, J., Howard, L. M., & Birdthistle, I. (2013). Intimate partner violence and socioeconomic deprivation in England: Findings from a national cross-sectional survey. *American Journal of Public Health, 103*(3), 462–472. https://doi.org/10.2105/AJPH.2012.300723

Koepsell, J. K., Kernic, M. A., & Holt, V. L. (2007). Factors that influence battered women to leave their abusive relationships. *Violence and Victims, 21*(2), 131–147. https://doi.org/10.1891/088667006780644299

Krause, E. D., Kaltman, S., Goodman, L., & Dutton, M. A. (2006). Role of distinct PTSD symptoms in intimate partner reabuse: A prospective study. *Journal of Traumatic Stress, 19*(4), 507–516. https://doi.org/10.1002/jts.20136

Kurst-Swanger, K., & Petcosky, J. L. (2003). *Violence in the home: Multidisciplinary perspectives*. Oxford Academic. https://doi.org/10.1093/acprof:oso/9780195165180.001.0001

Kwiatkowski, L. (2019). A "wife's duty" and social suffering: Sexual assault in marital relationships in Vietnam. *Journal of Aggression, Maltreatment and Trauma, 28*(1), 68–84. https://doi.org/10.1080/10926771.2018.1494237

Kyriacou, D. N., Anglin, D., Taliaferro, E., Stone, S., Tubb, T., Linden, J. A., Muelleman, R., Barton, E., & Kraus, J. F. (2018). Risk factors for injury to women from domestic violence. In M. Natarajan (Ed.), *Domestic violence* (pp. 145–151). Routledge. https://doi.org/10.4324/9781315264905-10

Lagdon, S., Armour, C., & Stringer, M. (2014). Adult experience of mental health outcomes as a result of intimate partner violence victimisation: A systematic review. *European Journal of Psychotraumatology, 5*(1), 24794. https://doi.org/10.3402/ejpt.v5.24794

Lari, N. (2022). Toward marriage sustainability: Impacts of delayed marriages in Qatar. *Cogent Social Sciences, 8*(1). https://doi.org/10.1080/23311886.2022.2083480

Lawson, J. (2012). Sociological theories of intimate partner violence. *Journal of Human Behavior in the Social Environment, 22*(5), 572–590. https://doi.org/10.1080/10911359.2011.598748

Levendosky, A. A., Lannert, B., & Yalch, M. (2012). The effects of intimate partner violence on women and children survivors: An attachment perspective. *Psychodynamic Psychiatry, 40*(3), 397–434. https://doi.org/10.1521/pdps.2012.40.3.397

Madruga, C. S., Viana, M. C., Abdalla, R. R., Caetano, R., & Laranjeira, R. (2017). Pathways from witnessing parental violence during childhood to involvement in intimate partner violence in adult life: The roles of depression and substance use. *Drug and Alcohol Review, 36*(1), 107–114. https://doi.org/10.1111/dar.12514

Mahapatro, M., Gupta, R. N., & Gupta, V. (2012). The risk factor of domestic violence in India. *Indian Journal of Community Medicine, 37*(3), 153–157. https://doi.org/10.4103/0970-0218.99912

Moder, A. (2019). Women, personhood, and the male God: A feminist critique of patriarchal concepts of God in view of domestic abuse. *Feminist Theology, 28*(1), 85–103. https://doi.org/10.1177/0966735019859471

Mshweshwe, L. (2020). Understanding domestic violence: Masculinity, culture, traditions. *Heliyon, 6*(10), e05334. https://doi.org/10.1016/j.heliyon.2020.e05334

Ogden, S. N., Dichter, M. E., & Bazzi, A. R. (2022). Intimate partner violence as a predictor of substance use outcomes among women: A systematic review. *Addictive Behaviors, 127*, 107214. https://doi.org/10.1016/j.addbeh.2021.107214

Paulino, M. (2016). The different forms of spousal violence. In *Forensic psychology of spousal violence* (pp. 33–43). Elsevier. https://doi.org/10.1016/b978-0-12-803533-7.00003-x

Pinto, I. V., Bernal, R. T. I., Souza, M. d. F. M. d., & Malta, D. C. (2021). Fatores associados ao óbito de mulheres com notificação de violência por parceiro íntimo no Brasil. *Ciência & Saúde Coletiva, 26*(3), 975–985. https://doi.org/10.1590/1413-81232021263.00132021

Priestley, S., & Lee, K. A. (2021). Understanding IPV perpetration among young Jamaican men: The role of socialization and attitudinal factors. *Journal of Interpersonal Violence, 36*(17–18), NP9053–NP9077. https://doi.org/10.1177/0886260519854553

Rahaman, M., Sen, S., Rana, M. J., & Ghosh, S. (2021). Is consanguineous marriage related to spousal violence in India? Evidence from the National Family Health Survey, 2015–16. *Journal of Biosocial Science, 1–16*, 959–974. https://doi.org/10.1017/S0021932021000626

Rashad, H., Osman, M., & Roudi-Fahimi, F. (2005). Marriage in the Arab World. *Population Reference Bureau*, 2–8. https://citeseerx.ist.psu.edu/viewdoc/download?doi=10.1.1.738.1360&rep=rep1&type=pdf

Renzetti, C. M., Follingstad, D. R., & Coker, A. L. (Eds.). (2017). *Preventing intimate partner violence: Interdisciplinary perspectives* (1st ed.). Bristol University Press. https://doi.org/10.2307/j.ctt1t89gf6

Rhodes, N. R., & McKenzie, E. B. (1998). Why do battered women stay?: Three decades of research. *Aggression and Violent Behavior, 3*(4), 391–406. https://doi.org/10.1016/S1359-1789(97)00025-6

Riggs, D. S., Caulfield, M. B., & Street, A. E. (2000). Risk for domestic violence: Factors associated with perpetration and victimization. *Journal of Clinical Psychology, 56*(10), 1289–1316. https://doi.org/10.1002/1097-4679(200010)56:10<1289::AID-JCLP4>3.0.CO;2-Z

Rioli, G., Sgarbi, C., Moretti, V., & Sinisi, A. (2017). An update on intimate partner violence and mental health. *Minerva Psichiatrica, 58*(4), 216–233. https://doi.org/10.23736/S0391-1772.17.01943-4

Rizo, C. F., Givens, A., & Lombardi, B. (2017). A systematic review of coping among heterosexual female IPV survivors in the United States with a focus on the conceptualization and measurement of coping. *Aggression and Violent Behavior, 34*, 35–50. https://doi.org/10.1016/j.avb.2017.03.006

Sabri, Y. (2021). Depression and post-traumatic stress disorder in females exposed to intimate partner violence. *Middle East Current Psychiatry, 28*(1). https://doi.org/10.1186/s43045-021-00157-x

Sezgin, A. U., & Punamäki, R. L. (2021). Type of traumatic events, mental health problems, and posttraumatic cognitions among eastern Anatolian women. *Journal of Interpersonal Violence, 36*(17–18), NP9501–NP9525. https://doi.org/10.1177/0886260519858385

Shahid, A. (2013). Post-divorce maintenance for Muslim women in Pakistan and Bangladesh: A comparative perspective. *International Journal of Law, Policy and the Family, 27*(2), 197–215. https://doi.org/10.1093/lawfam/ebt004

Shamu, S., Abrahams, N., Temmerman, M., Musekiwa, A., & Zarowsky, C. (2011). A systematic review of African studies on intimate partner violence against pregnant women: Prevalence and risk factors. *PLoS One, 6*(3), 1–9. https://doi.org/10.1371/journal.pone.0017591

Sharma, A. (2001). Healing the wounds of domestic abuse: Improving the effectiveness of feminist therapeutic interventions with immigrant and racially visible women who have been abused. *Violence Against Women, 7*(12), 1405–1428. https://doi.org/10.1177/10778010122183928

Singer, J. B. (1989). Divorce reform and gender justice. *North Carolina Law Review, 67*(5), 1103–1121. https://scholarship.law.unc.edu/nclr/vol67/iss5/8

Singh, S., & Wassenaar, D. (2016). Contextualising the role of the gatekeeper in social science research. *South African Journal of Bioethics and Law, 9*(1), 42. https://doi.org/10.7196/sajbl.2016.v9i1.465

Smith-Marek, E. N., Cafferky, B., Dharnidharka, P., Mallory, A. B., Dominguez, M., High, J., Stith, S. M., & Mendez, M. (2015). Effects of childhood experiences of family violence on adult partner violence: A meta-analytic review. *Journal of Family Theory & Review, 7*(4), 498–519. https://doi.org/10.1111/jftr.12113

Stöckl, H., Devries, K., Rotstein, A., Abrahams, N., Campbell, J., Watts, C., & Moreno, C. G. (2013). The global prevalence of intimate partner homicide: A systematic review. *The Lancet, 382*(9895), 859–865. https://doi.org/10.1016/S0140-6736(13)61030-2

Stuart, G. L., Moore, T. M., Gordon, K. C., Ramsey, S. E., & Kahler, C. W. (2006). Psychopathology in women arrested for domestic violence. *Journal of Interpersonal Violence, 21*(3), 376–389. https://doi.org/10.1177/0886260505282888

Tahirih. (2016, October 20). *Arranged marriage*. Tahirih Justice Center. Forced Marriage Initiative. https://preventforcedmarriage.org/understanding-arranged-and-forced-marriage/.

Tekkas Kerman, K., & Betrus, P. (2020). Violence against women in Turkey: A social ecological framework of determinants and prevention strategies. *Trauma, Violence & Abuse, 21*(3), 510–526. https://doi.org/10.1177/1524838018781104

Ugwuanyi, B. C., Formella, Z., & Szadejko, K. (2022). *Reporting domestic violence on women. An exploratory research in Igboland of Nigeria* (No.:16). Transdisciplinary Studies on Culture and Education. Scientific Yearbook of the Kuyavian-Pomeranian University in Bydgoszcz. https://www.researchgate.net/publication/358187209_REPORTING_DOMESTIC_VIOLENCE_ON_WOMEN_AN_EXPLORATORY_RESEARCH_IN_IGBOLAND_OF_NIGERIA

Ulloa, E. C., & Hammett, J. F. (2016). The effect of gender and perpetrator–victim role on mental health outcomes and risk behaviors associated with intimate partner violence. *Journal of Interpersonal Violence, 31*(7), 1184–1207. https://doi.org/10.1177/0886260514564163

Umubyeyi, A., Mogren, I., Ntaganira, J., & Krantz, G. (2014). Intimate partner violence and its contribution to mental disorders in men and women in the post genocide Rwanda: Findings from a population based study. *BMC Psychiatry, 14*, Article 315. https://doi.org/10.1186/s12888-014-0315-7

Usta, J., Farver, J. A., & Pashayan, N. (2007). Domestic violence: The Lebanese experience. *Public Health, 121*(3), 208–219. https://doi.org/10.1016/j.puhe.2006.09.014

Watts, C., & Zimmerman, C. (2002). Violence against women: Global scope and magnitude. *Lancet, 359*(9313), 1232–1237. https://doi.org/10.1016/S0140-6736(02)08221-1

World Health Organization (WHO). (2012a, November 23). *Understanding and addressing violence against women: Intimate partner violence*. 1–12. https://apps.who.int/iris/bitstream/handle/10665/77432/WHO_RHR_12.36_eng.pdf

World Health Organization (WHO). (2012b, November 23). *Understanding and addressing violence against women: Femicide*. 1–8. https://apps.who.int/iris/bitstream/handle/10665/77421/WHO_RHR_12.38_eng.pdf

Yadav, A., Kumar, P., & Kumar, J. (2022). Domestic violence: Consequences, causes and preventive measures. *Indian Journal of Psychology and Education, 12*(2), 40–43. https://www.researchgate.net/publication/362760828_Domestic_Violence_Consequences_Causes_and_Preventive_Measures

Zhang, Y., & Breunig, R. V. (2021). Gender norms and domestic abuse: Evidence from Australia (March 31, 2021). Tax and transfer policy institute - working paper 5/2021. *SSRN Electronic Journal*. https://doi.org/10.2139/ssrn.3824466

Zlotnick, C., Johnson, D. M., & Kohn, R. (2006). Intimate partner violence and long-term psychosocial functioning in a national sample of American women. *Journal of Interpersonal Violence, 21*(2), 262–275. https://doi.org/10.1177/0886260505282564

Chapter 3
Research Setting and Design

This chapter presents and discusses methods for conducting an explanatory sequential mixed methods study. Figure 3.1 presents visual representation of explanatory sequential mixed methods protocol. The first section will provide the rational and theoretical position of utilizing an explanatory sequential mixed method approach. The second section will describe the research design and the third section will present the rationale for data analysis implementation. This study adopted an explanatory sequential mixed methods study conducted in Doha, the capital city of Qatar which served as the location for the data gathering procedure, which took place during the months of December 2020 and March 2021. This is a subject that has not received enough research, and this approach adds greater understanding by merging both data and contextualized research questions. This will provide a rich understanding of the phenomena by explaining the findings from the quantitative approach (Bowen et al., 2017) and as a result, in the Quantitative phase, the primary and secondary aims of this study presented to evaluate the impact of various forms of domestic abuse actions on mental health issues in Qatari women by analysing the levels of anxiety, depression, and PTSD that these women experience.

As a secondary aim investigates factors associated with domestic abuse victims most likely to occur. Individuals who were interested in the study were directed to a website where they could find out every piece of information through the announcements that were made at each institution as well as the promotional posters that were shown for the research. Participants were asked to sign an electronic consent form to participate in the survey, which they did after finishing the questionnaire. Recruitment was based on snowball sampling and the analysis of the study was based on the primary data that was collected and recreated through the composition of the general population and victims of domestic abuse to have a representative sample that could help in reaching hidden population were people might be harder to be recruited (Etikan, 2016). The gatekeepers such as AMAN (Protection and Rehabilitation), WIFAQ (Family Consulting Centre), Community college, and the public

K. Al-Naama, *Domestic Abuse and Mental Health in Qatar*, Gulf Studies 23,
https://doi.org/10.1007/978-981-96-7392-6_3

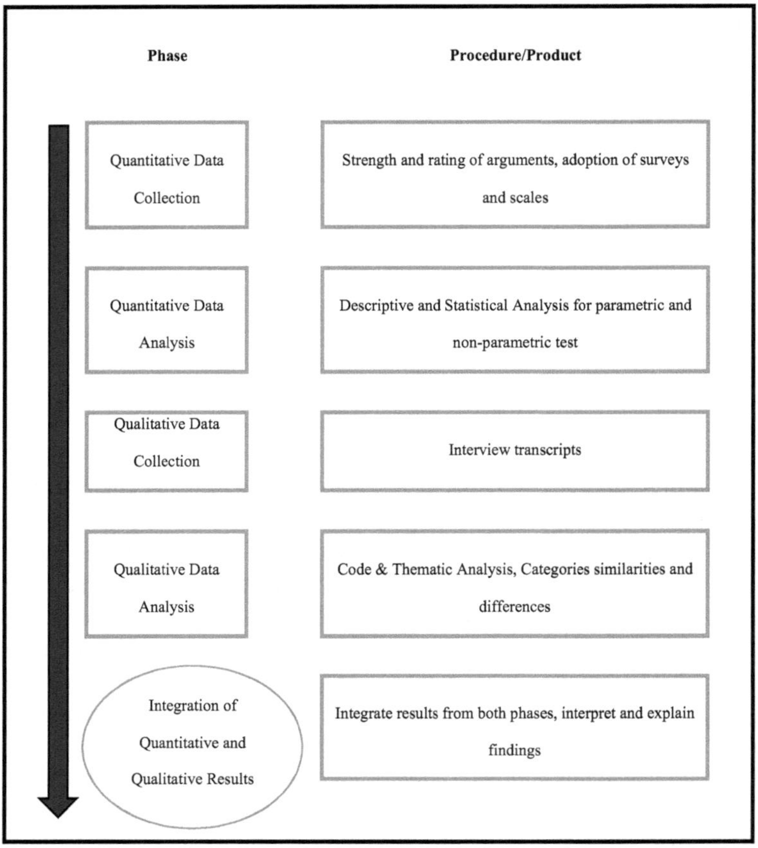

Fig. 3.1 Visual Representation of Explanatory Sequential Mixed Methods Protocol

domain invited participants by sharing the link of the questionnaire in the Quantitative phase, and those who were willing to participate in face-to-face interviews were requested to share their personal emails or phone numbers in order to arrange for the interview.

The interviews with the victims were done at WAYAK (Mental Health Friends Association), in a small room designated for consultation but used for the interview to ensure the safety and privacy of the participants. The interviews were conducted without the spouses of the victims present. Before commencing the interviewing procedure, the researcher had attended many CITI training sessions and negotiated a non-disclosure agreement with the gatekeepers.

In the Qualitative phase, the subcategory objectives of this research were to investigate the reasons why people who have been abused in their homes continue to be in violent relationships and, and to evaluate the risk of homicide among victims of domestic abuse. In addition, the rights and roles of women in society were examined from the perspective of victims. After considering my request, both the Hamad

Psychiatric Hospital and the Mental Health Advisory Group denied my request for authorization to collect data. Because of the delicate nature of the research that was being carried out, this was necessary.

3.1 Research Design

Within the context of a phenomenological and correlational case study, the research in question makes use of explanatory sequential mixed methodology which compose of two phases that began with quantitative followed-up by a second phase of collecting and analysing qualitative data to develop the quantitative findings that offset the limitations of each approach and provide a profound understanding of a research problem than a mono-method approach (Ivankova et al., 2006). A triangulation approach was adopted during the integration process, collected and analysed simultaneously to provide a more comprehensive understanding of the proposed study questions (Creswell & Plano Clark, 2018). The use of both quantitative and qualitative methodologies provides the greatest opportunity to answer research questions (Malina et al., 2011).

The theoretical position of the mixed method approach argues that it could help researchers to elaborate more on the quantitative results from the first phase and gain a better understanding of participants' views in depth by reflecting on the statistical results (Creswell & Plano Clark, 2011, as cited in Guest & Fleming, 2015). In addition, Creswell and Plano Clark (2011) mention the research issues that are alleviated by integrating methods. A mono method approach may not be enough to answer a question, explain initial findings, broaden exploratory results, advance research with more methods, issue a theoretical stance, or comprehend the objective of research using many research phases (Creswell & Plano Clark, 2011, as cited in Guest & Fleming, 2015). According to Creswell (2014), a sequential mixed method approach is based on the belief that researchers can gain a deeper understanding of a phenomenon or a research question by combining various methodologies. It is also recognized in this method that different kinds of data may offer unique insights and perspectives. According to Tashakkori et al. (2020), sequential mixed methods provide an in-depth understanding and answers to the research questions or phenomena studied. Moreover, an explanation-sequential mixed methods research design emphasizes the importance of practical problem solving within a flexible context-based framework (Johnson & Onwuegbuzie, 2004). The variables considered in the study were not explored in Qatar. Therefore, it is a useful approach to conduct an explanatory sequential design when the variables have not been examined quantitatively. Therefore, priority is given to analysing quantitative data, followed by qualitative data (Creswell et al., 2004; Hanson et al., 2005)

3.2 Quantitative Phase

The purpose of this phase was to determine the relationship between the proposed variables, which is something that has been investigated in previous research and has been tested in several western and cross-cultural studies, as well as in Arab studies (Ivankova et al., 2006; Straus et al., 1996, 2009).To conduct this evaluation, a slightly adjusted version of the Conflict Tactic Scale (CTS-2) for victimisation was used as the measuring tool. To make predictions about the many forms of domestic violence that were seen within the cultural setting of the research, the independent factors had to be defined (Afifi et al., 2011; Almubaddel, 2022). In western civilizations, these independent factors have been discovered, and their theoretical interpretations have been developed.

The process of data collection was broken down into two primary steps for the most part. The next step in the quantitative phase was to define the demographic profile of the participants by evaluating the impact of domestic violence using a set of measures. This was done by first identifying the various types of abuse (sexual, physical, psychological, and financial), and then moving on to the next step in the process. Following a predetermined set of guidelines allowed us to complete this task.

The demographic profile questionnaire included the following categories: marital status, marriage classification, the husband's and wife's respective ages when they were married, their current ages, the number of children, the educational level of both partners, household income, and the employment status of both partners. They were questioned about how long they had been in a relationship with the person who had abused them, whether or not they were pregnant at the time of the assault, and whether or not they had miscarried an unborn child as a result of the violence. In addition, they were questioned on whether or not the offender had seen his father physically abusing his mother when he was a little child. The question of whether or not this was the couple's first marriage was posed to them. They were questioned about whether or not they had seen their father verbally or physically assaulting their mother, and they were also questioned about whether or not their father had been married to more than one woman. The very last question that was asked was whether or not the person's spouse was a monogamist or a polygamist.

3.2.1 Revised Conflict Tactics Scale (CTS-2)

The CTS-2 is a self-report measure that is often given to victims of domestic violence as well as their partners in the course of its administration. It examines hostile behaviours and behaviours that occurred during the previous year from the date of the test or evaluates whether it has occurred at any point in the victims' lives. The participants were requested to identify how often they had been subjected to abusive behaviour during the course of the previous year. A CTS-2 scale is a thorough instrument that takes into account five distinct types of abuse.

The first subscale is called the Negotiation items, and it consists of six questions. These questions represent cognitive problem-solving behaviours, such as explanation, compromise, and openness to suggestions. Additionally, these questions all involve the expression of emotional support and care, optimism, and respect. The second subscale is called the Psychological Aggression subscale, and it consists of eight questions, four of which are rated as mild and four of which are rated as severe. This subscale analyses symbolic behaviours that are meant to induce partners to dread and live in psychological agony. The Psychological Aggression subscale is comprised of eight different methods that are utilised by predators. These tactics include loud, aggressive displays and threats, as well as varied assaults, insults, and other forms of verbal aggression. The third subscale is made up of 12 different questions that pertain to physical assault, and these items are divided into two categories to evaluate the severity of the attack (whether it was mild or severe), as well as define the amount of risk that the victims are now facing. The degree of injuries sustained during violent disputes is rated on the fourth subscale, with two mild and four severe items. The sexual coercion subscale is the sixth one, and it brings attention to sexual actions that do not have the participant's consent, such as oral, anal, or unprotected intercourse. Depending on the behaviours that were demonstrated, the coercion items divided sexual assault into either a severe category (four items) or a minor category (three items).

The respondents indicated the frequency of abusive behaviours based on a 7-point rating scale ranging from occurred once, twice, 3–5 times, 6–10 times, 11–20 times, more than 20 times, and never. The range for this scale is: once, twice, 3–5 times, 6–10 times, 11–20 times, and more than 20 times. The sum of the total values for each answer was added together, and that was how the overall scores for each category were determined.

The current study employed the CTS-2 victimisation tool, which consisted of 39 self-rated questionnaires given solely to female victims (items directed at perpetrators were not included). Another study of western culture used the victimisation scale, and an Italian translation was also completed. The research sample size was composed of 209 female victims of domestic violence. In this period, the questionnaire's grading indicated strong reliability of the subscales, which ranged from 0.78 to 0.96. It is evident from the study that the scale is adaptable to clinical settings and can be used for research to identify domestic violence cases (Signorelli et al., 2014).

This measure, based on Arabic culture, was administered to 622 Palestinian women who had experienced domestic violence. The scale score during this period had an alpha value of 0.88 for the injury subscale and 0.89 for the sexual coercion subscale. Psychological aggression showed a coefficient of 0.88, while physical violence showed a coefficient of 0.92 (Thabet et al., 2015).

In 2012, the Conflict Tactics Scale was updated for use in a male-dominated culture to measure the frequency of domestic abuse among college students. The sample consisted of college students from 32 nations and 14 published studies. These countries varied from those with an egalitarian social structure, such as Sweden, to those with a patriarchal social structure, such as Iran (Straus, 2008). The findings of the study suggested that male-dominant nations had a higher frequency of physical abuse by male partners. This finding revealed that the scale had a high degree of sensitivity and internal consistency in both male-dominated civilizations and cross-cultural contexts. According to the 14 published research, the median range for the proportion of physically abused women was between 0.4% and 45.0%. According to the injury score data, the alpha coefficient of dependability for female patients was determined to be 0.59. In addition, it has been shown that female victims of male-dominated societies are more prone to PTSD and depression than female victims of more egalitarian countries.

3.2.2 *Scale of Economic Abuse (SEA-12)*

For the present study's purpose, tactics and control actions of economic abuse were assessed by administering the Scale of Economic Abuse-12 (SEA-12), which measures a wide range of controls and strategies used against victims to impose certain control on the victims' lives based on three major criteria. The scale comprises 12 items rated on a 5-point Likert scale ranging from 1 (Never) to 5 (Quite Often), which is used to assess the frequency of those actions in the last 12 months. The average and mean scores were calculated based on the frequency indicated by the victims. In 2008, a study was conducted (Adams et al., 2008) to develop a tool to measure different forms of economic abuse. The study's findings resulted in the development of the Scale of Economic Abuse. The sample size of the study participants was 103 female victims of domestic abuse. This scale has good face validity, and the total SEA demonstrates a reliability coefficient of 0.93. Their study findings outlined a positive correlation with an elevated level of psychological and physical abuse based on the modified CTS indicator.

Another study adapted SEA-12 to assess depression among victims of IPV who have been exposed to economic abuse. The scale was administered among 457 IPV victims from seven states in the USA (Stylianou, 2018). Their scoring showed strong reliability among the study sample with an alpha coefficient of 0.89.

Similar results were reached by different research conducted in the United States, which are supported by the present findings. In that research, 120 domestic violence survivors were administered the Economic Abuse scale to verify its psychometric assessment as a separate kind of domestic abuse. Similar significant conclusions were reached from the outcomes of the present investigation and the prior study. A longitudinal and exploratory study test of a programme designed to reduce domestic violence in the United States This was a section of the research (Postmus et al., 2016). The average age of the female participants was 39 (standard deviation = 11.5 years), 65% of them were employed, and 60% of the women had sought psychiatric or counselling support as a consequence of being a victim. The findings indicate that the mean score for economic control was 3.40 (SD = 1.26), the mean score for employment sabotage was 2.36 (SD = 1.21) and the mean score for economic exploitation was 2.95 (SD = 1.49) This correlation was statistically significant (r = 0.775; p,01) and demonstrated that a higher level of both physical and psychological violence was substantially connected with economic abuse. Cronbach's alpha for the SAE-12 was determined to be 0.89. The study indicates that the economic abuse scale-12, in its abbreviated form, is a reliable and valid instrument for measuring the severity of economic abuse.

In a study including 504 Chinese women, with a mean age of 49 and a standard deviation of 8.02 years, researchers investigated the effects of economic abuse as well as the characteristics that put people at risk for it. The Chinese version of the scale of economic abuse (C-SEA-12) was used to conduct the investigation and analysis of economic abuse (Yau et al., 2020). The data indicated that a greater proportion of women with higher levels of educational attainment were victims of financial abuse compared to those with educational levels of a high school diploma or less (95% confidence interval = 1.13 – 5.78, p = 0.02). When compared to females who were not victims of economic abuse, those who were victims of economic abuse had a 95% confidence interval that ranged from 1.02 to 1.17, and this difference was significant (p = 0.02). Depression was more prevalent among individuals who had been subjected to economic abuse as compared to their counterparts who had not been subjected to economic abuse (95% confidence interval = 1.48 – 4.08, p. 001).

Several studies used the economic abuse scale to assess economic abuse influence on victims' psychopathology. For example, exploratory research was conducted in Puerto Rico and 10 other states in 2018. In a domestic violence program, 457 domestic abuse victims were assessed for the relationship between economic violence and depression. SAE-12 was useful for analysing financial abuse among participants during a year-long period using data collected over the previous year (Stylianou, 2018). Participants reported psychological aggression as the most prevalent kind of violence (96.3%). Financial abuse accounts for 93% of all cases, and depression is associated with economic violence. A similar conclusion was made by a study conducted on 103 survivors of domestic violence who had responded to several screening measures of domestic violence, including the modified Conflict Tactics Scale (23 items). The study focused on a field that had not received a lot of attention in the past (Adams et al., 2008). Participants came from organisations in states located in the Midwest that assists those who have been victims of domestic abuse. Participants varied in age from 18 to 85 years old, and their families typically consisted of two kids each. Eighty-eight percent had either completed high school or college, while 16% were employed, and 84% were unemployed. In addition, 20% of the participants had annual household incomes of between fifteen thousand dollars and three hundred thousand dollars, while more than half of the participants earned less than or equal to fifteen thousand dollars, and 23% earned more than three hundred thousand dollars. The Cronbach's alpha for the SAE scale came in at 0.93. The findings showed that there was a significant association between the modified version of the CTS and the economic abuse scale (r = 0.61, p = 0.01). According to the CTS scores, psychological aggression was positively related with physical violence (r = 0.56, p = 0.01) and economic abuse was positively connected with physical violence (r = 0.52, p = 0.01). In other words, if both psychological and physical violence are present in the victim's case, her assets will likely be under her spouse's control, and she will not have access to financial resources.

3.2.3 Danger Assessment Scale

The Danger Assessment Scale (DA) is a self-administered assessment that may be used to assess the amount of danger presented to female victims living with an abusive partner, especially the likelihood of being killed (Campbell et al., 2008). The goal of the scale is to equip victims with a better knowledge of the likelihood that they may be severely injured or murdered by an intimate partner. This study did not include the calendar component of the scale; nonetheless, it is vital to include it since it supports victims in remembering the frequency of partner violence and because victims tend to underestimate the severity of their spouse's violent behaviour. Respondents were given a list of 20 questions, each with a Yes or No box next to it and were asked to report any instances of abuse. The previously calculated cutoff scores were changed to classify the responses into four unique categories: a score of 7 indicates a variable degree of risk, 8–13 shows a growing level of risk, 14–17 indicates a severe level of risk, and >18 indicates an exceedingly hazardous level of risk. Using this scale, the user may indicate the approximate date of the abuse that happened during the last year.

This scale has been employed within the setting of western civilization. In 2008, a study was conducted to determine the effect of IPV on the likelihood of miscarriage among women who had been the victims of physical and psychological domestic abuse (Morland et al., 2008). The sample included 118 women from diverse ethnic and cultural backgrounds. Although there was no published cutoff score and a higher score indicated a significant probability of murder, abused women scored 9.30 while non-abused women scored 0.75. This suggests that mistreated women are at a much higher risk of being killed.

Campbell et al. (1999) used a 15-item version of the Danger Assessment Scale in her 1999 analysis to estimate the likelihood that victims of intimate relationship abuse would be sexually attacked. The purpose of Campbell's (1999) research was to determine the odds of such an occurrence. The sample comprised 159 American women who were pressured into establishing an intimate connection by a current or past lover. Among the sample of participants, the results of the scoring indicated an internal consistency coefficient of 0.68 (Campbell et al., 1999).

3.2.4 PHQ-9

The Patient Health Questionnaire-9 is (Appendix 7) a self-screening tool that may assess, evaluate, and diagnose the degree and presence of depression within two weeks. Respondents are asked to choose various depression symptoms from four categories ranging from "not at all" to "nearly every day". The responders are provided with the ranges on a sliding scale. By asking participants whether they have "Thoughts that they would be better off dead or injuring themselves in some way", the last question seeks to assess if suicidal ideation is present and for how long it has been prevalent. The total score for each item may range from 0 to 27, with a score of 5 indicating mild depression, 10 indicating moderate depression, 15 indicating moderately severe depression, and 16 or above indicating severe depression.

This scale has been employed within the setting of western civilization. In Greece, for example, a sample of 140 persons of both sexes was employed to explore the consequences of intimate relationship violence on mental health (Dami et al., 2017). According to the findings of their study, the range of internal consistency and dependability was between 86% and 100%, with a standard deviation of 5.01. In 2019, a second study was conducted in Syria to identify the prevalence of depressive symptoms among Syrian women who had been exposed to several risk factors, including IPV (Falb et al., 2019). There were 214 total married women in the sample. The depressive symptomology was given a score of 10.5, with a standard deviation of 4.9 and a range of 2–27. Cronbach's alpha indicated that the reliability of the data was adequate at 0.72.

These results build on existing evidence that PHQ-9 is a useful tool in a culture setting comparable to that of Qatar, research was undertaken in Oman to examine the validity and reliability of the PHQ-9 in diagnosing depression in a cross-cultural population (Al-Ghafri et al., 2014). Participants were medical students from the College of Medicine and Health Sciences at Sultan Qaboos University and medical residents from the OMAN training programme. Comparisons were made between depressed and non-depressed students. Cronbach's alpha was 0.88, the PHQ-9 had a sensitivity rate of 80.6% and a specificity rate of 94.0%, and the rate of depression among the individuals was 11.4%. The research concluded that the PHQ-9 was a valid instrument for assessing depression in a cross-cultural population of Oman. Another research gave the PHQ-9 to Iranian outpatients to determine its reliability and validity (Dadfar et al., 2018). The mean age of the participants was 31.40 (standard deviation = 8.20) and the total number of participants was 130 Iranians; 96% of the participants were female and the other 4% were male patients. The bulk of participants (48%) were single, followed by those who were married (36%) and widowed and divorced (18%). The mean score on the PHQ-9 was 12.83 (standard deviation = 6.25), and Cronbach's alpha for the PHQ-9 was 0.91, indicating a high degree of internal consistency.

3.2.5 PCL-C

Post-Traumatic Stress Disorder (PTSD) was evaluated by adapting a self-administered tool: the PTSD checklist civilian version (PCL-C), which comprises 17 items that assess three symptomology clusters, i.e., intrusion re-experiencing, hyper-arousal, and avoidance of traumatized individuals, or it is used for people who have been through a stressful life experience that has troubled them in the previous month.

Each item is rated on a 5-point Likert scale ranging from 1 (not at all) to 5 (Extremely). The total sum of the scores is equal to 85 while sum scores report the following interpretations: 28–29 represent some PTSD symptoms, 30–44 demonstrate moderate to moderately high severity of PTSD symptoms, whereas 45–85 represent victims with high severity of PTSD symptoms and the cutoff point of 17–27 sores shows little to no severity.

PCL-C has been validated in Arabic studies, where it shows high internal consistency of alpha = 0.85 (Ibrahim et al., 2018). This scale has also been administered in eastern cultural studies. For example, it was applied in a mixed-method study by adapting the Chinese version of the PCL-C scale to assess the different effects of terrorism on mental health outcomes among female Chinese victims of domestic abuse. The sample size of this study was 613 abused women. The scoring showed that 65.6% of the participants had experienced PTSD symptoms based on the PCL-C score shown beta = 22.4, $p < 0.001$ (Tiwari et al., 2015).

In another study, the validity and reliability of the scale was applied to non-clinical sample groups (Conybeare et al., 2012). The average age of all 471 participants was 19.33 years old (standard deviation equal to 2.54 years), and there were both male and female participants. Females comprised 67% of the total participants, making up the overwhelming majority of those who took part in the study. The PCL-C revealed that the average PTSD score among the subjects was 29.12, with a standard deviation of 12.31 points. According to the results of the research, the PCL-C scale had a correlation with traumatic experiences that was much stronger than those of other types of mental illnesses, such as general anxiety disorder and social anxiety.

3.2.6 *Taylor Manifest Anxiety Scale*

Taylor's Manifest Anxiety Scale (TMAS) has fifty questions in all. To determine each individual's degree of anxiety, a true-false response scale (with yes equalling one and no equalling zero) was utilised. It was agreed to use the existing cutoff values, which specify that a total score between 0 and 16 indicates "No Anxiety", 17–20 corresponds to "Mild Anxiety", 21–26 to "Moderate Anxiety", 27–29 to "Severe Anxiety", and 30–50 to "Very Severe Anxiety".

This scale has been employed within the setting of western civilization. In 2014, a study was conducted in the United States to determine the individual differences associated with disclosing sexual, physical, and emotional abuse as a child, as well as the influence of witnessing domestic violence. The Taylors Manifest Anxiety assessments were administered to a total of 1679 college students who participated in the research project. This investigation's sample indicates that = 0.83, the mean score was 9.74, and the standard deviation was 3.50 (Bottoms et al., 2016).

The original English version has been translated into Arabic, and the Arabic version has been used in a study conducted in Gaza, Palestine, to assess the anxiety levels of battered women (Thabet et al., 2015). All of the 622 Palestinian women who participated in this study were questioned. Their investigation yielded a mean anxiety score of 25.11 and a standard deviation of 9.57. In addition, Cronbach's alpha score of 0.79 revealed a high degree of internal consistency and validity.

A variety of populations were assessed using the current anxiety scale, demonstrating the scale's credibility and reliability in different settings. The original version of the modified manifest anxiety scale was produced by Taylor and was based on 200 items that were generated from the Minnesota Multiphasic Personality Inventory. This version of the scale was utilised in the current investigation. In 1948, research was carried out to evaluate the accuracy of the scale by applying it to a student population that included 1971 male and female students (Taylor, 1953). The students were drawn from an introductory psychology course offered at the State University of Iowa. The distribution of the results showed a positive skew, and the mean score was 14.56. Although the difference between male and female students was not statistically significant, the gap between male and female students was somewhat larger for female students.

A group consisting of 400 adult Athenians, both male and female, had their anxiety levels measured in order to investigate the influence of age, sex, and education (Vassiliou et al., 1967). Participants had to be at least 18 years old and were living in their own homes at the time of the study. Throughout the course of the research, participants were asked to complete the Taylor Manifest Anxiety Scale. The findings showed that the female anxiety score was greater than the male anxiety score and that the anxiety score was lower the higher the participants' levels of education. When the age differences of the participants were included in the calculation of the mean score, it was found that the mean score for anxiety levels among male participants was 16.23, but the mean score for anxiety levels among female participants was 21.50.

Another study administered the short form of the Taylor Manifest Anxiety scale to understand the negative effects of a different form of childhood abuse in participants' adult lives (Bottoms et al., 2016). 1679 adult women aged between 17 and 60 years old were anonymously surveyed. The anxiety mean score among the participants was 8.87 and SD = 4.68.

3.2.7 Attitude Towards Women Scale (AWS-25)

The Attitudes Towards Women's Rights and Responsibilities in Society (AWS-25) is a scale consisting of 25 items that compare the attitudes of female and male respondents towards women's rights and roles in society. On a four-point Likert scale ranging from (A) Strongly Agree to (D) Disagree Strongly, respondents were asked to indicate their stance towards the questioned statement. It evaluates a wide range of factors, such as intellectual responsibility, freedom, courtship, cursing, filthy jokes, sexual behaviour, marital relations and responsibilities, educational attainment, and professional position. As stipulated by the AWS Scale's coding requirements, in order to arrive at the final score, the positive items were subjected to reverse coding, and this score was then added to the negative score. The highest possible score on the

AWS questionnaire is 75, while the minimum score at which candidates are rejected is 37.5.

This scale has been employed within the setting of western civilization. In 2018, for instance, a study was conducted to determine the prevalence of sexual assault among 229 persons from the United Kingdom and India (Hill & Marshall, 2018). In the course of their inquiry, they used the Attitude Towards Women Scale to compare the rights and roles provided to women among two separate ethnic groups. During that period, Cronbach's alpha was determined to be 0.87 for Indian participants, but 0.82 for British participants using the same scale. This scale has also been used in Arabic-speaking nations. For instance, it was used in a study done in Lebanon, which included 206 university students whose viewpoints on the topic of wife abuse were analysed (Obeid et al., 2010). According to their study, the dependability of the scale was 0.74 on Cronbach's alpha scale.

In a comparable manner, the scale was employed within the Thai community to analyse gender roles, encompassing an assessment of diverse elements such as marital status, degree of dedication, and the caliber of available choices. The gender roles score is towards a more traditional mindset and lower quality alternatives, raising concerns about the concept of happy marriage (Suntornkanit & Varma, 2018). Another study found that those of younger age, women, and those with higher social status have a more liberal sex role attitude than those of the opposite gender (Nelson, 1988).

3.3 Qualitative Phase

Twenty Qatari women were interviewed based on semi-structured interviews protocol and guided by the study's aim and objectives, including the following topics: their experience with domestic violence, family and community, and their effects on their mental and physical health, comments on the results from the quantitative phase which has been examined and tested in peer-reviewed articles and literature. To understand participants' experiences with IPV, a qualitative thematic analysis method was used. It was designed to collect data using open-ended and semi-structured interviews to gain a deeper understanding of the quantitative findings and to expand upon them (McIntosh & Morse, 2015). Each interview lasted approximately 45 min in line with previous standards of interviewing (Creswell & Creswell, 2018).

3.3.1 Interview Technique

A follow-up interview was conducted with participants who agreed to attend a face-to-face interview, as indicated by their responses in the quantitative phase. Each was given a fictitious name in order to conceal their identities, and they were also given the option of having someone they know, and trust accompany them during the interview (Jacob & Furgerson, 2012). Following the interview, debriefing sessions were conducted, and participants were offered free psychological help from WAYAK if they want to continue their counselling sessions. Participants were given one week to withdraw from the research after reading the transcript to check the correctness of the information.

Following a lecture to the participants regarding their rights and a thank you for their participation, the interview procedure moved on to the next step, which was to ask open-ended questions. It was requested that victims provide their perspectives on what they believed domestic violence to be and about their personal experience with it. The qualitative phase focused mainly on understanding the connection between forms of domestic abuse and physical and mental health, and why abused women remain passive. In the quantitative phase, several factors were examined and interpreted by the participants. This allowed to comment on several factors studied and gain better understanding.

The Serious consequences of domestic abuse which could result in homicide were explored with participants as well as the role of women's mindset in influencing their risk of abuse and why, which was crucial to understanding the quantitative findings on women's attitudes and rights in society. As a result of the questionnaire design, it was possible to elaborate on the manifestation of economic abuse among the current participants, as it was prevalent according to the quantitative phase, among other factors. After they gave their answer, the researcher questioned them further and asked them to illustrate what they meant by their response. During the concluding comments, they have been briefed on the last step that was required before their screenplay could be approved. They were told that the researcher would be evaluating the information that they had contributed, and if they were interested, they were allowed to have a copy of the analysis sent to them.

3.3.2 Analysis

Each interview transcribed was given to participants for final review to improve the accuracy of the transcripts and serve as a reliability tool in qualitative studies (Creswell, 2003). An inductive thematic analysis was employed, and each transcript was reviewed several times to develop a better understanding of the participant's narratives. All the interview inputs were transcribed with the help of Intelligent Verbatim Transcription, which helps to reduce verbal filers and word repetition to give more reliable and accurate data (McMullin, 2023).

The researcher generated initial codes from transcripts and recorded them as individual notes. To identify potential patterns in these coded data, similarities and overlaps in the codes were examined and their relevance to the entire set of data was examined (Alhojailan, 2012). After analysing the data for a while, temporary themes emerged and were enhanced throughout the data analysis. To improve the link between themes and subthemes, a theme map was developed with the intention of identifying patterns and combining them to form meaningful units or what are called themes. Similar approaches were employed in previous literature that investigate the topic of domestic abuse (Christian et al., 2011; Collins & Dressler, 2008).

During the interview, individual notes were taken and none of the participants consented to videotaping or recording the conversation. Thematic analysis was the aiming procedure to point out patterns or concepts within qualitative information (Maguire & Delahunt, 2017). it is flexible as it is not bounded to a theoretical approach because it is a mechanism rather than a methodology (Braun & Clarke 2006; Clarke & Braun, 2013). That is, the purpose of thematic analysis is to recognize significant patterns in the information to provide information about a certain subject or problem. This is done by analysing and explaining rather than summarizing data (Clarke & Braun, 2013). Thematic analysis is conducted based on six phases beginning with becoming familiar with the data, generating initial codes, searching for themes, reviewing themes, defining themes and writing up phase (Braun & Clarke 2006).

3.3.3 *Integration Phase*

The quantitative and qualitative data were analysed and presented separately in each chapter. As a means of understanding research problems through the adoption of a triangulation approach, findings from both phases were integrated into a discussion chapter (Bekhet & Zauszniewski, 2012) that helped to comprehend and confirm the findings from both method by discussing Similarities and differences. It is possible to integrate into three different ways, connecting, merging, and embedding, depending on the objective of the research, to support and expand on other data findings from the quantitative phase, embedding was used in the study as a means of integrating data. In this regard, the explanatory mixed methods approach played a significant role in rationalizing the type of integration used (Creswell & Creswell, 2018). Therefore, as a means of ensuring the overall coherence, validity, and reliability of data, a triangulation approach that involved data integration was utilized (Golafshani, 2003). During the integration phase, the results from the two phases are connected and constructed into meaningful conclusions. Using a mixed method approach, which integrates quantitative and qualitative approaches, according to Bulsara's (2015) research, leads to greater data validity since it addresses the question from different perspectives, reducing potential bias in the researcher and ensuring there are no gaps in data collection (p. 4).

The interpretation and explanation are discussed in this phase followed by research implications and recommendations for future research. To conclude this section, an explanatory mixed methods study was adopted and involves the collection and analysis of both quantitative and qualitative data. The study is therefore able to gain a deeper understanding of the subject matter through this approach. As a result of this procedure, findings can also be incorporated, which contributes to a more comprehensive and accurate analysis.

3.4 Population, Pilot Study, and Ethical Issues

Three hundred fifty people gave their time to help with the study voluntarily. Thirty five women were asked to take part in the study, but they chose not to do so. The remaining 45 individuals were unable to do so because they had a history of neurological disease, cognitive impairment, psychosis, or a head injury that resulted in unconsciousness that lasted for more than ten minutes. It is unlikely that these persons will be able to finish the survey since they have trouble concentrating or recalling specific instances of abuse. It is also unlikely that they will be able to answer all of the questions. This is because not all of the respondents finished the survey and provided their feedback. As a consequence of this, the study included 165 Qatari adult females who were recruited, included because they satisfied all of the inclusion criteria, and obtained data because they completed all of the scales. They were above the age of 18 and either had been a victim of domestic violence themselves or had seen it in a member of their own family or a life partner. Twenty women from Qatar gave their permission for a follow-up interview in which they were asked about their experiences with domestic abuse.

Often, pilot studies are used to refine the research question and to test the feasibility of methodology approaches. In this way, problems that may arise during the main study can be minimized. Van Teijlingen and Hundley (2002) point out the importance of pilot studies in their article, saying that pilot studies are essential to any research. Participants were asked to take part in the survey over the phone and asked to complete self-reporting questionnaires prior conducting the study. Fifteen female volunteers between the ages of 23 and 45 were recruited for the pilot study, which aided in establishing or revising the research goals and choosing which instrument should be considered. Consequently, each scale was subjected to preliminary testing before the survey was undertaken. This enabled any slight misunderstandings in the surveys to be explained and the language to be streamlined, making the survey much easier to comprehend and it helped to uncover any sensitive issues that might affect negatively the data collection process (Kim, 2011).

To use the received questionnaire and, if necessary, translate it, the author's permission was required; however, certain surveys were in the public domain and did not need author permission. Both the translation and the back-translation were performed separately in Qatar by two unique translation agencies, however, both translations were performed in Qatar. Sheen Service WLL and Nellai Services both contributed to the Arabic translation's completion. The back translation was accomplished by Nellai Services.

When reviewing the replies submitted by participants throughout the survey completion process, additional discoveries were clear. General anxiety disorder obtained the lowest score on the GAD-7 scale, which prompted questions about continuing to evaluate GAD among the victims or the potential of replacing it with other dependent variables, such as anxiety disorder. Since generalised anxiety disorder obtained the lowest GAD-7 score. As a normal reaction to domestic abuse,

GAD has gotten relatively little attention from academics. The scale was thus abandoned in favour of Taylor's evident anxiety scale. A second common participant critique was that some components of the Harassment in Abusive Relationships report were insufficiently addressed. The Self Report Scale (HARASS) findings were inapplicable to the cultural attitudes of Arabs. We opted to omit it from the questionnaire collection since it is too wordy.

Participants were given the chance to submit immediate feedback after completing the survey, and their replies, along with any further comments, were considered. They examined the particulars of their experience, which led to a discussion about the perspectives of different cultures on the rights of women in society. Therefore, the Attitude Towards Women Scale (ATW) was created to explore and assess the situation of women in modern society. Due to the delicate and personal nature of the questionnaire, participation in the survey was entirely optional. This was done to encourage women to continue completing the survey, which was an additional contribution made by the pilot study.

This research follows research ethical issues and carries out research as per university IRB and research ethics requirements. All necessary ethical approvals have been obtained from the Human and Health Science School of Research Ethics Committee - the institutional review board at the University of Huddersfield, in May 2020. Additional permission to collect data was successfully obtained from WAYAK (Mental Health Friends Association), WIFAQ (Family Consulting Centre), and AMAN – (Protection & Rehabilitation), along with the CCQ. I have signed a mandatory non-disclosure agreement with all gatekeepers before commencing the data collection process.

References

Adams, A. E., Sullivan, C. M., Bybee, D., & Greeson, M. R. (2008). Development of the scale of economic abuse. *Violence Against Women, 14*(5), 563–588. https://doi.org/10.1177/1077801208315529

Afifi, Z. E., Al-Muhaideb, N. S., Hadish, N. F., Ismail, F. I., & Al-Qeamy, F. M. (2011). Domestic violence and its impact on married women's health in Eastern Saudi Arabia. *Saudi Medical Journal, 32*(6), 612–620. http://www.emro.who.int/imemrf/Saudi_Med_J/Saudi_Med_J_2011_32_6_612_620.pdf

Al-Ghafri, G., Al-Sinawi, H., Al-Muniri, A., Dorvlo, A. S. S., Al-Farsi, Y. M., Armstrong, K., & Al-Adawi, S. (2014). Prevalence of depressive symptoms as elicited by patient health questionnaire (PHQ-9) among medical trainees in Oman. *Asian Journal of Psychiatry, 8*(1), 59–62. https://doi.org/10.1016/j.ajp.2013.10.014

Alhojailan, M. I. (2012). Thematic analysis: A critical review of its process and evaluation. *West East Journal of Social Sciences, 1*(1), 39–47. https://faculty.ksu.edu.sa/sites/default/files/ta_thematic_analysis_dr_mohammed_alhojailan.pdf

Almubaddel, A. (2022). Psychometric properties of a Saudi Arabian version of the Positive Mental Health (PMH) scale. *Psicologia: Reflexao e Critica, 35*(1), 29. https://doi.org/10.1186/s41155-022-00232-0

Bekhet, A. K., & Zauszniewski, J. A. (2012). Methodological triangulation: An approach to understanding data. *Nurse Researcher, 20*(2), 40–43. https://doi.org/10.7748/nr2012.11.20.2.40.c9442

Bottoms, B. L., Peter-Hagene, L. C., Epstein, M. A., Wiley, T. R. A., Reynolds, C. E., & Rudnicki, A. G. (2016). Abuse characteristics and individual differences related to disclosing childhood sexual, physical, and emotional abuse and witnessed domestic violence. *Journal of Interpersonal Violence, 31*(7), 1308–1339. https://doi.org/10.1177/0886260514564155

Bowen, P. W., Rose, R., & Pilkington, A. (2017). Mixed methods - Theory and practice. Sequential, explanatory approach. *International Journal of Quantitative and Qualitative Research Methods, 5*(2), 10–27. http://www.eajournals.org/wp-content/uploads/Mixed-Methods-Theory-and-Practice.-Sequential-Explanatory-Approach.pdf

Braun, V., & Clarke, V. (2006). Using thematic analysis in psychology. *Qualitative Research in Psychology, 3*(2), 77–101. https://doi.org/10.1191/1478088706qp063oa

Bulsara, C. (2015). *Using a mixed methods approach to enhance and validate your research. Brightwater Group Research Centre,* Notre Dame University, 1–82. https://www.academia.edu/23767180/USING_A_MIXED_METHODS_APPROACH_TO_ENHANCE_AND_VALIDATE_YOUR_RESEARCH

Campbell, J. C., Webster, D. W., & Glass, N. (2008). The danger assessment. *Journal of Interpersonal Violence, 24*(4), 653–674. https://doi.org/10.1177/0886260508317180

Campbell, J., Torres, S., Ryan, J., King, C., Campbell, D. W., Stallings, R. Y., & Fuchs, S. C. (1999). Physical and nonphysical partner abuse and other risk factors for low birth weight among full term and preterm babies: A multiethnic case-control study. *American Journal of Epidemiology, 150*(7), 714–726. https://doi.org/10.1093/oxfordjournals.aje.a010074

Christian, M., Safari, O., Ramazani, P., Burnham, G., & Glass, N. (2011). Sexual and gender based violence against men in the Democratic Republic of Congo: Effects on survivors, their families and the community. *Medicine, Conflict and Survival, 27*(4), 227–246. https://doi.org/10.1080/13623699.2011.645144

Clarke, V., & Braun, V. (2013). Teaching thematic analysis: Overcoming challenges and developing strategies for effective learning. *The Psychologist, 26*(2), 120–123. https://uwe-repository.worktribe.com/output/937596

Collins, C. C., & Dressler, W. W. (2008). Cultural consensus and cultural diversity. *Journal of Mixed Methods Research, 2*(4), 362–387. https://doi.org/10.1177/1558689808322766

Conybeare, D., Behar, E., Solomon, A., Newman, M. G., & Borkovec, T. D. (2012). The PTSD Checklist-Civilian Version: Reliability, validity, and factor structure in a nonclinical sample. *Journal of Clinical Psychology, 68*(6), 699–713. https://doi.org/10.1002/jclp.21845

Creswell, J. W. (2003). Research design: Qualitative, quantitative and mixed methods approach. *Sage Publications.*

Creswell, J. W. (2014). *Research design. Qualitative, quantitative and mixed method approaches* (4th ed.). SAGE.

Creswell, J. W., & Creswell, J. D. (2018). Research design: Qualitative, quantitative, and mixed methods approaches. *Sage Publications.*

Creswell, J. W., & Plano Clark, V. L. (2018). *Designing and conducting mixed methods research* (3rd ed.). SAGE.

Creswell, J. W., Fetters, M. D., & Ivankova, N. V. (2004). Designing a mixed methods study in primary care. *Annals of Family Medicine, 2*(1), 7–12. https://doi.org/10.1370/afm.104

Dadfar, M., Kalibatseva, Z., & Lester, D. (2018). Reliability and validity of the Farsi version of the patient health questionnaire-9 (PHQ-9) with Iranian psychiatric outpatients. *Trends in Psychiatry and Psychotherapy, 40*(2), 144–151. https://doi.org/10.1590/2237-6089-2017-0116

Dami, C., Karathanos, V., Dimitakopoulou, V. I., Damigos, D., & Gouva, M. (2017). Intimate Partner violence in primary settings and consequences in mental health. *International Journal of Caring Sciences, 10*(1), 17–29. http://www.internationaljournalofcaringsciences.org/docs/3_gouva_original_10_1.pdf

Etikan, I. (2016). Comparison of snowball sampling and sequential sampling technique. *Biometrics & Biostatistics International Journal, 3*(1), 1–2. https://doi.org/10.15406/bbij.2016.03.00055

Falb, K. L., Blackwell, A., Stennes, J., Hussein, M., & Annan, J. (2019). Depressive symptoms among women in Raqqa Governorate, Syria: associations with intimate partner violence, food insecurity, and perceived needs. *Global Mental Health (Cambridge, England), 6*, e22. https://doi.org/10.1017/gmh.2019.20

Golafshani, N. (2003). Understanding reliability and validity in qualitative research. *The Qualitative Report, 8*(4), 597–607. https://doi.org/10.46743/2160-3715/2003.1870

Guest, G., & Fleming, P. J. (2015). Mixed methods research. In G. Guest & E. Namey (Eds.), *Public health research methods* (pp. 581–610). Sage. https://doi.org/10.4135/9781483398839.n19

Hanson, W. E., Plano Clark, V. L., Petska, K. S., Creswell, J. W., & Creswell, J. D. (2005). Mixed methods research designs in counseling psychology. *Journal of Counseling Psychology, 52*(2), 224–235. https://doi.org/10.1037/0022-0167.52.2.224

Hill, S., & Marshall, T. C. (2018). Beliefs about sexual assault in India and Britain are explained by attitudes toward women and hostile sexism. *Sex Roles, 79*(7–8), 421–430. https://doi.org/10.1007/s11199-017-0880-6

Ibrahim, H., Ertl, V., Catani, C., Ismail, A. A., & Neuner, F. (2018). The validity of Posttraumatic Stress Disorder Checklist for DSM-5 (PCL-5) as screening instrument with Kurdish and Arab displaced populations living in the Kurdistan region of Iraq. *BMC Psychiatry, 18*(1), 1–8. https://doi.org/10.1186/s12888-018-1839-z

Ivankova, N. V., Creswell, J. W., & Stick, S. L. (2006). Using mixed-methods sequential explanatory design: From theory to practice. *Field Methods, 18*(1), 3–20. https://doi.org/10.1177/1525822X05282260

Jacob, S. A., & Furgerson, S. P. (2012). Writing interview protocols and conducting interviews: Tips for students new to the field of qualitative research. *Qualitative Report. ERIC*, 1–10. https://doi.org/10.1016/0168-1702(91)90033-R

Johnson, R. B., & Onwuegbuzie, A. J. (2004). Mixed methods research: A research paradigm whose time has come. *Educational Researcher, 33*(7), 14–26. https://doi.org/10.3102/0013189X033007014

Kim, Y. (2011). The pilot study in qualitative inquiry: Identifying issues and learning lessons for culturally competent research. *Qualitative Social Work, 10*(2), 190–206. https://doi.org/10.1177/1473325010362001

Maguire, M., & Delahunt, B. (2017). Doing a thematic analysis: A practical, step-by-step guide for learning and teaching scholars. *AISHE-J, 9*, 3351. https://ojs.aishe.org/index.php/aishe-j/article/view/335

McIntosh, M. J., & Morse, J. M. (2015). Situating and constructing diversity in semi-structured interviews. *Global Qualitative Nursing Research, 2*. https://doi.org/10.1177/2333393615597674

McMullin, C. (2023). Transcription and qualitative methods: Implications for third sector research. *Voluntas, 34*(1), 140–153. https://doi.org/10.1007/s11266-021-00400-3

Morland, L. A., Leskin, G. A., Rebecca Block, C., Campbell, J. C., & Friedman, M. J. (2008). Intimate partner violence and miscarriage: Examination of the role of physical and psychological abuse and posttraumatic stress disorder. *Journal of Interpersonal Violence, 23*(5), 652–669. https://doi.org/10.1177/0886260507313533

Nelson, M. C. (1988). Reliability, validity, and cross-cultural comparisons for the simplified attitudes toward women scale. *Sex Roles, 18*(5), 289–296. https://doi.org/10.1007/BF00288291

Obeid, N., Chang, D. F., & Ginges, J. (2010). Beliefs about wife beating: An exploratory study with Lebanese students. *Violence Against Women, 16*(6), 691–712. https://doi.org/10.1177/1077801210370465

Postmus, J. L., Plummer, S. B., & Stylianou, A. M. (2016). Measuring economic abuse in the lives of survivors: Revising the scale of economic Abuse. *Violence Against Women, 22*(6), 692–703. https://doi.org/10.1177/1077801215610012

Signorelli, M. S., Arcidiacono, E., Musumeci, G., Di Nuovo, S., & Aguglia, E. (2014). Detecting domestic violence: Italian validation of Revised Conflict Tactics Scale (CTS-2). *Journal of Family Violence, 29*(4), 361–369. https://doi.org/10.1007/s10896-014-9594-5

Straus, H., Cerulli, C., McNutt, L. A., Rhodes, K. V., Conner, K. R., Kemball, R. S., Kaslow, N. J., & Houry, D. (2009). Intimate partner violence and functional health status: Associations with severity, danger, and self-advocacy behaviors. *Journal of Women's Health, 18*(5), 625–631. https://doi.org/10.1089/jwh.2007.0521

Straus, M. A. (2008). Dominance and symmetry in partner violence by male and female university students in 32 nations. *Children and Youth Services Review, 30*(3), 252–275. https://doi.org/10.1016/j.childyouth.2007.10.004

Straus, M. A., Hamby, S. L., Boney-McCoy, S., & Sugarman, D. B. (1996). The Revised Conflict Tactics Scales (CTS2): Development and preliminary psychometric data. *Journal of Family Issues, 17*(3), 283–316. https://doi.org/10.1177/019251396017003001

Stylianou, A. M. (2018). Economic abuse experiences and depressive symptoms among victims of intimate partner violence. *Journal of Family Violence, 33*(6), 381–392. https://doi.org/10.1007/s10896-018-9973-4

Suntornkanit, N., & Varma, P. (2018). Influence of gender role attitude, quality of alternatives, investment size, and commitment on marital satisfaction between Thai women who married Thai men and Thai women who married foreign men. *Scholar: Human Sciences, 9*(2), 106–119. https://core.ac.uk/download/pdf/233619845.pdf

Tashakkori, A., Johnson, R. B., & Teddlie, C. (2020). *Foundations of mixed methods research: Integrating quantitative and qualitative approaches in the social and behavioral sciences* (2nd ed.). Sage Publications.

Taylor, J. A. (1953). A personality scale of manifest anxiety. *Journal of Abnormal and Social Psychology, 48*(2), 285–290. https://doi.org/10.1037/h0056264

Thabet, A., Tawahina, A., Victoria, T., & Vostanis, P. (2015). PTSD, depression, and anxiety among Palestinian women victims of domestic violence in the Gaza strip. *British Journal of Education, Society & Behavioural Science, 11*(2), 1–13. https://doi.org/10.9734/bjesbs/2015/18960

Tiwari, A., Chan, K. L., Cheung, D. S. T., Fong, D. Y. T., Yan, E. C. W., & Tang, D. H. M. (2015). The differential effects of intimate terrorism and situational couple violence on mental health outcomes among abused Chinese women: A mixed-method study. *BMC Public Health, 15*(1), 1–12. https://doi.org/10.1186/s12889-015-1649-x

van Teijlingen, E., & Hundley, V. (2002). The importance of pilot studies. *Nursing Standard, 16*(40), 33–36. https://doi.org/10.7748/ns2002.06.16.40.33.c3214

Vassiliou, V., Georgas, J. G., & Vassiliou, G. (1967). Variations in manifest anxiety due to sex, age, and education. *Journal of Personality and Social Psychology, 6*(2), 194–197. https://doi.org/10.1037/h0024572

Yau, J. H. Y., Fong, D. Y. T., & Wong, J. Y. H. (2020). Risk factors for and mental well-being outcomes of economic abuse in Hong Kong Chinese population. *Violence and Victims, 35*(2), 246–265. https://doi.org/10.1891/VV-D-18-00057

Chapter 4
Domestic Abuse Against Women: Correlates and Conundrums

This chapter presents the quantitative results of the study, which examined the relationship between various variables. Descriptive analysis and four statistical analyses were based on the current nature of the violet normal distribution for some scales, as well as the limitations of the small sample size. This was explained in detail previously in the methodology chapter. To analyse the data, parametric and non-parametric tests including ANOVA, Pearson correlation, Kruskal-Wallis test, and Mann-Whitney U test were necessary when the assumptions of normality were not satisfied (Chan, 2003; Song & Lu, 2015). Its purpose is to provide a detailed analysis and answer research questions and achieve greater power efficiency as stated by Siegel (2012). Therefore, this was the rationale for employing a variety of statistical measures in the quantitative chapter.

Multiple regression has been used to determine whether or not forms of abuse can predict PTSD, Depression or Anxiety among the study participants. It offers flexibility if the data violates the assumption of normality to test the relationship and the direction of the association. The regression model was selected in this study based on the nature of the studied variables, in which both the independent and dependent variables were continues. In real life situations many factors can predict the results, therefore, multiple regression model was performed to test how multiple independent variables (Negotiation, Psychological, Physical, Injury, Sexual, Economic Abuse) can influence one dependent variable (PTSD, Depression, and Anxiety level) in which was entered separately to predict the outcomes. Multiple assumptions for the studied covariate were satisfied and partially met for the Depression and PTSD data (Uyanık & Güler, 2013). The alternative nonparametric test for regression model efficiency is preferably conducted on a large sample size, however. The assumption of normality can sometimes be waived in the case of regression analysis such as linear regression (Li et al., 2012). The normality assumptions test for the PTSD and Depression covariates were violated as previously mentioned, however the anxiety covariate was normally distributed. Even with a non-normal distribution, regression models can still be valid measures (Castro & Ferreira, 2023; Ernst & Albers, 2017).

K. Al-Naama, *Domestic Abuse and Mental Health in Qatar*, Gulf Studies 23,
https://doi.org/10.1007/978-981-96-7392-6_4

Table 4.1 Variables studied in the primary and secondary objectives

Dependent Variable	Independent Variable
All forms of abuse that derived from two instruments. CTS-2 includes psychological, physical, sexual, and injury. Economic abuse scale	Derived from the following instruments. Danger assessment scale Attitude towards women scale Depression, anxiety, and PTSD scale.

Note. Model 1: This table provides a clear concise summary of studied variables examined in the primary and secondary objectives

Similarly was argued by Lumley et al. (2002). It is still possible to perform regression analysis regardless of data not being normally distributed since it is not considered a reason for data validity.

Qatari women are subject to a variety of types and patterns of abuse, and potential homicide risks are assessed in this chapter. Various forms of IPV are examined in this chapter to examine how they impact Qatari women's mental health. This will be done by assessing participants' anxiety, depression, and post-traumatic stress disorder levels. It is the objective of subcategories to explore factors that may be associated with domestic abuse victims. Victims' perspectives will also be examined concerning women's rights and roles in society.

The presentation of the qualitative findings comes right after the display of the numerical statistics. To provide an explanation for violence, both of these results will be addressed iteratively using feminist theory, social learning theory and gendered resource theory to get a deeper comprehension of the reasons behind why women continue to submit in abusive relationships. The following sections provide more specific information on the results of the primary, and secondary aims and subcategory objectives. The qualitative chapter will provide a different answer as to why women stay in abusive relationships.

In the current study, an ecological framework developed by Heise (1998) was used in an attempt to acquire a better understanding of the complexities of the numerous factors that influence domestic violence against women. Tables 4.1 and 4.2 present the variables studied in this study, the impact of the risk variables that enhance the possibility of women being subjected to domestic violence has been widely examined in prior systematic studies (Caicedo-Roa et al., 2020). As a result, the sociodemographic and sociocultural factors that are discussed in this research will assist in comprehending how women may become victims of the violent conduct of their husbands within the context of the male-dominated Arabic culture. As a result, the hypothesised risk factors have been classified, in a broad sense, into two models.

Table 4.2 Variables studied in the subcategory objectives

Dependent Variable	Independent Variable
All forms of abuse that derived from two instruments. CTS-2 includes psychological, physical, sexual, and injury Economic abuse scale	Independent variables have been split up into three different domains, which may be seen below: (A) Individual level risk factor. In this category, the risk factor is related to the victims or perpetrators. Age at marriage time and age difference between husband and wife Education level of husband and wife Employment status of husband and wife
	(B) Family-level risk factor. This category includes both marriage and socioeconomic-related factors. Number of children Financial factors Polygamous or monogamous partner Type of marriage Women married for the second or first time. Pregnancy and women's fertility status
	(C) Society-level risk factor. In this category, both the traditional gender role and cultural stereotype of masculinity have been examined through the following factors. Attitude towards women Polygamous father

Note. Model 2: This table provides a clear concise summary of studied variables examined in the subcategory objectives

4.1 Socio-Demographic Profiles of the Participants

The overall structure of the Quantitative chapter takes the form of six distinct sections: The first section of this chapter will present the socio-demographic profile of the participants. The remaining part of this chapter proceeds as follows: (1) This section will assess the pattern and prevalence of IPV by presenting a descriptive analysis of reported forms of abuse followed by a subsection about measuring the potential risk of homicide. (2) This section will attempt to examine the impact of IPV on women's mental health. (3) This section examines variables of the study which presumably increased risk factors for IPV victimization. (4) This section will analyse the attitude towards women's rights from victims' perspectives by presenting the descriptive analysis of the participant's responses and the key findings from statistical measures. This chapter concludes with a section summarizing and reporting the key findings.

Regarding the sociodemographic characteristics of 165 participant women who have experienced some form of abuse in their life, the minimum age of the participants was 20 years old, and the maximum age was 60 years old, while 35 years and 7.85 months was the average age. The participants' spouses' minimum age was 18 years old, and the maximum age was 60 years old, while 27.59 years and 6.59 months was the average age of the participants' spouses.

The participants aged ranged from 20 to 60 years, and the average age of the participants was 34.25 (SD = 7.86), and the age range of the victims' spouses at the time of marriage range from 18 to 60 years, and the average age of the victims' spouses at the time of marriage was 27.7 (SD = 6.56), and the majority of the women were married at the age of 23.58 (SD = 5.11). The mean age of the chosen sample of 165 Qatari adult women was 34.25 years (SD = 7.86), whereas the mean age of the victims' spouses was 27.7 years. There are 78.6% of participants whose age difference between husband and wife is less than 10 years, and 11.6% of participants whose age difference is more than 10 years (See Table 4.3).

Table 4.3 Descriptive statistics for female Qatari victims of abuse (n = 165)

Variable	%	M	SD
Age			
Age of participants	–	34.25	7.86
Age at marriage	–	23.58	5.11
Age difference between husband and wife (<10 years)	78.6	–	–
Age difference between husband and wife (>10 years)	11.6	–	–
Marital status			
Married	50	–	–
Never married	8.9	–	–
Divorced	40.2	–	–
Widowed	0.9	–	–
Type of marriage			
Arranged marriages	50	–	–
Love marriages	21.4	–	–
Forced marriages	4.5	–	–
Relative marriages	15.2	–	–
Education			
Bachelor's degree	53.6	–	–
High school diploma	20.5	–	–
Postgraduate degree	12.5	–	–
Not completed high school	4.5	–	–
Income			
< $25,000	>37.5	–	–
< $100,00	18.8	–	–
≥ $150,000	21.4	–	–
< $150,000	22.3	–	–

Around 50% of them were married, 8.9% had never been married, 40.2% were divorced, and 0.9% were widowed. The participants' marriages were classified into four groups. Fifty percent of the participants were in arranged marriages, 21.4% were in marriages based on love, 4.5% were in forced marriages, and 15.2% were in marriages with relatives. In terms of women's educational attainment, 53.6% had a bachelor's degree, 20.5% a high school diploma, 12.5% a postgraduate degree, and 4.5% had not completed high school. Forty point two percent of women's partners had a bachelor's degree, 37.5% had a high school diploma, 16.1% had less than a high school diploma, and 6.3% had a postgraduate degree. According to the yearly household family income of the participants, over 37.5% of the women survived on less than $25,000, 18.8% on less than $100,000, 21.4% on $150,000 or more, and 22.3% on less than $150,000.

According to their employment status, about 63.4% of the participants were employed, 14.3% were unemployed, 10.7% were self-employed, 10.7% were raising children at home, and 0.9% were retired (see Table 4.4). Seventy five percent of the partners of the victims were employed, 6.3% were jobless, 12.5% were self-employed, and 6.3% were retired, according to their employment status (see Table 4.5).

Sixty-six point one percent of married persons had children, with the mean number of children being 3.19 and the standard deviation being 1.89 children (see Table 4.6). Nonetheless, 25% of individuals did not have children (see Table 4.6).

Around 60% of the participants did not suffer any type of abuse throughout their pregnancy, whereas 39.3% of the participants did encounter abuse and 7.1% of the participants did not take their pregnancy to term due to partner abuse. Only 20.5% of people were engaged in polygamous partnerships, whereas 79.5% were monogamous.

Table 4.4 Descriptive statistics for female Qatari victims of abuse (n = 165)

Variable	%	M	SD
Employment			
Employed	63.4	–	–
Unemployed	14.3	–	–
Self-employed	10.7	–	–
Raising children at home	10.7	–	–
Retired	0.9	–	–
Abuse through pregnancy duration			
Did not suffer any abuse	60.7	–	–
Were abused	39.3	–	–
Loss pregnancy	7.1	–	–
Type of partnership			
Polygamous	20.5	–	–
Monogamous	79.5	–	–

Table 4.5 Descriptive statistics for spouses of female Qatari victims of abuse

Variable	%	M	SD
Age			
Age of spouse	–	27.7	6.56
Education			
Bachelor's degree	40.2	–	–
High school diploma	37.5	–	–
Postgraduate degree	16.1	–	–
Not completed high school	6.3	–	–
Employment			
Employed	75	–	–
Jobless	6.3	–	–
Self-employed	12.5	–	–
Retired	6.3	–	–

Table 4.6 Descriptive statistics for status of children of female Qatari victims of abuse

Children	%	M	SD
Have children	66.1	–	–
Number of children	–	3.19	1.89
Did not have children	25	–	–

The participants' ages at the time of their marriages 23.07 to (SD = 5.11) years, according to a categorization system that used intervals of 5 years. Seven point nine percent of all participants, or 13 out of the total, were married before reaching the age of 17 years old. Following closely after, 44.2% ($n = 73$) were married women who were between the ages of 23 and 27, followed by 8.5% ($n = 14$) who were between the ages of 28 and 32. Only 6.1% ($n = 10$) of those who were 33 or older were married at the time of their survey. When they were married, the husband was 27 years, 6 months, and 6 days old. Sixty-eight point five percent of the participants were women who were already mothers ($n = 113$), whereas only 31.5% of the participants were women who had never given birth before. The number of children that the individuals reported having ranged from 2.23 to 2.12. Thirty point three percent of respondents ($n = 50$) said that their husband had watched their fathers physically abusing their mothers when they were young, whereas 21.2% of respondents ($n = 35$) stated that their husband had not witnessed their fathers physically abusing their mothers. In contrast, more than half of the people who took part in the study (48.5%) were unaware of whether or not their spouse had seen their father physically abusing their mother when they were youngsters.

The participants who were the least likely to be married were those who had been divorced (35.2%; $n = 58$), those who were single (10.9%; $n = 18$), and those who had been widowed (0.6%; $n = 1$). More than half of the participants were married (53.2%; n = 88). The participants' marital statuses were divided into four distinct categories for the purpose of this study. Those who were from a consanguineous marriage category accounted for 15.2% ($n = 15.2$), those who were from an arranged marriage category accounted for 55.2% ($n = 91$), and those who were from a forced marriage category accounted for 4.2% ($n = 7$). The majority of participants were from arranged marriages, which accounted for $n = 91$ (55.2%), the second highest group reported that their marriage was classified as a love marriage, which accounted for 25.5% 88.5% of respondents, or 146 people, claimed that they were currently in their first marriage, while 11.5%, or 19 people, said that they were now in their second marriage. Fifty-five point two percent of respondents, or 91 individuals, had earned bachelor's degrees, while 28.5%, or 47 individuals, had just a high school diploma. While 4.2% ($n = 7$) of the total participants did not have a diploma of any kind, 12.1% ($n = 20$) of the participants had completed some level of postsecondary education. Intimate partner education level was also reported by respondents, who indicated that 37% ($n = 61$) had a high school diploma, 25.2% ($n = 58$) had a bachelor's degree, 18.2% ($n = 30$) had less than a high school diploma, and those with a postgraduate degree accounted for 9.7% ($n = 16$) of the least reported category. Respondents indicated that those with a postgraduate degree accounted for the least reported category.

The yearly revenue of the family was split into four categories. Thirty eight percent ($n = 63$) of the participants had an annual income of less than \$25,000, 25% ($n = 33$) of the participants had an annual income of less than \$100,000, 21.8% ($n = 36$) of the participants had an annual income of less than \$150,000, and 20% ($n = 33$) of the participants had an annual income of more than \$150,000. Significant numbers of participants had jobs, accounting for 75.2% of the total participants ($n = 124$), while those who were self-employed represented 9.1% of the total participants ($n = 15$), and those who were housewives represented 7.9% of the total participants ($n = 13$). In addition, unemployed persons made up 6.7% ($n = 11$) of the sample, while retired individuals made up 1.2% ($n = 1$) of the total. The job status of the abuser was reported by the respondents, who indicated that the majority were employed (73.3%; $n = 121$), 10.9% ($n = 18$) were self-employed, 9.1% ($n = 15$) were retired, and the smallest percentage were unemployed (6.7%; $n = 11$). The majority of the respondents were employed (73.3%; $n = 121$), 10.9% ($n = 18$) were self-employed, and 9.1% ($n = 15$) were retired. While 68.5% of the participants ($n = 113$) were not abused while they were pregnant, 31.5% of the people ($n = 52$) were mistreated at some point throughout their pregnancy. Only 5.5% of the participants ($n = 9$) stated that they had lost their pregnancy as a direct result of the abuse, while 94.5% ($n = 156$) of the participants claimed that they did not lose their pregnancy as a direct result of the abuse.

Women who did not see their father beat their mother when they were youngsters made up 71.5% ($n = 118$) of all participants, while women who did see their father beat their mother made up 28.5% ($n = 47$) of all participants. There were more than three-quarters of monogamous marriages among the participants, while 18.8% of the marriages ($n = 31$) were polygamous. Seventy seven percent of the participants ($n = 127$) claimed that their father had never been married to another woman, whereas 23% ($n = 38$) of the participants reported that their father had been married to more than one woman in the past. In this study, the age difference between a man and his wife was measured in 10-year intervals. The vast majority of people, 84.2% (n = 139), had an age difference that was less than 10 years, while just 15.8% (n = 26) of people had an age gap that was 10 years or greater.

4.2 Objective 1: Types, Patterns of Abuse, and Risk of Homicide

Different forms and patterns of domestic violence in intimate relationships will be examined, as well as their potential to escalate to murder. This objective will explore the various types of abuse, including physical, emotional, sexual, economic, and emotional injury, which victims in the current study have suffered. This will be done through descriptive analysis and parametric and non-parametric tests, depending on whether the data violate the normal distribution.

Regarding the descriptive analysis of forms of abuse that were indicated by the participant's responses, the number of the participants who met the study requirements were 165 female victims of domestic abuse, and through the descriptive statistics of the participants they were identified as experiencing negotiation violence, showing an overall mean score of 26.86 and (SD = 30.06). The mean score for negotiation emotion was 15.83 (SD = 17.67) and the mean score for negotiation cognitive was 11.04 (SD = 15.94).

The descriptive statistics for the participants showed that they can be identified as experiencing psychological aggression, revealing an overall mean score of 53.71 (SD = 48.54), while the mean score for minor psychological aggression was 35.06 (SD = 29.66), and for the severe psychological aggression, the mean score was 18.65 (SD = 23.99).

The descriptive statistics for physical assaults revealed an overall mean score of 30.49 (SD = 50.79), while the minor physical assaults scores mean was 19.09 (SD = 31.93), and for the severe physical assaults, the mean score was 11.40 (SD = 21.72).

The descriptive statistics for injury score among the participants mean to show their score was 9.60 (SD = 15.96), while for minor injury, the mean score was 4.67 (SD = 8.78) and for severe injury, the mean score was 4.93 (SD = 9.03).

The descriptive statistics for the sexual coercion score among the participants revealed an overall mean score of 15.80 (SD = 23.92), and those who were identified as experiencing minor sexual coercion revealed an overall mean score of 9.94 (SD = 15.28), while for severe sexual coercion, they showed an overall mean score of 5.86 (SD = 11.47). The Cronbach's alpha was equal to 86 for all 39 items in the survey. The Cronbach's alpha for the six items that make up the Negotiation subscale was 81, while the Cronbach's alpha for the eight items that make up the Psychological Aggression subscale was 85; the Cronbach's alpha for the 12 items that make up the Physical Assault subscale was 92; the Cronbach's alpha for the six items that make up the Injury subscale was 64; and the Cronbach's alpha. This research demonstrates that the CTS-2 scale has high levels of both internal consistency and dependability.

Regarding the descriptive analysis of the risk of economic abuse, the Scale of Economic Abuse (SEA-12) was used to analyse the descriptive data for economic abuse among the participants. The mean score for economic abuse was 32.34 (SD = 8.85), while the mean score for economic exploitation was 7.76 (SD = 3.50). In the group of victims, the average score for economic control was 15.12 (standard deviation = 4.78), whereas the average score for economic sabotage was 9.45 (standard deviation = 3.98). Economic Exploitation, where Cronbach's alpha coefficient was 52; (2) Economic Control, where Cronbach's alpha was 68; and (3) Employment Sabotage, where the Cronbach's alpha was 86. In this study, the scale overall scores showed good internal consistency and reliability, the Cronbach's alpha for the 12 items was 78.

This objective was to determine how many of the risk variables are present in people who have been victims of domestic violence and to quantify the murder risk factors that are associated with female victims who are living in violent relationships. The Danger Assessment Scale was utilised to achieve the second objective of the study, which was to determine the prevalence of the danger lethality level. The score was then classified into the following four categories: variable danger, increasing danger, severe danger, and extreme danger. The purpose of this step was to ensure that the study was successful in achieving both objectives.

Regarding the descriptive analysis for danger assessment scores among the participants, the results show that the overall mean score was 4.31 (SD = 3.40) and further show that 78.8% of the participants indicated experiencing variable danger, while 21.2% indicated experiencing increased danger. In this study's participant population, the scale exhibited good evidence of both internal consistency and validity. The Cronbach's alpha for the whole collection of 20 items was calculated to be 0.73.

The current sample scores do not indicate the other remaining danger and life-threatening categories: severe danger and/or extreme danger among the participants, where in this case, according to the scoring manual, the victims are required to engage in an assertive safety plan and high level of supervision should be applied on the perpetrator. However, the sample result scores below these categories of lethal violence. This means the current danger assessment scores are relatively low compared with the findings of other studies. Next, the rational justification will be presented.

Regarding the risk of homicide, an assessment was made of the amount of anticipated murder risk for individuals who had been subjected to a variety of kinds of abuse. To determine how deadly a threat was, a Danger Assessment Scale was used. This scale was split into four categories, which were as follows: variable danger, increasing danger, severe danger, and extreme danger. Because the results of the normality test indicated that the data did not follow a normal distribution, Mann-Whitney U tests were carried out. According to the research shown below, the findings for the lethality hazard vary solely between variable and elevated threats.

The test indicated that the difference was not statistically significant for the general negotiation abuse score and with the danger assessment category for assessing the risk of homicide. $U\ (N_{\text{incredible variable danger group}} = 130,\ N_{\text{increased danger group}} = 35) = 1895,\ z = -1.518,\ p = 0.129.$

A Mann-Whitney test indicated that the severe psychological aggression score was greater for those who experienced danger (*Mdn* = 12.00) than for victims who experienced incredible variable danger (*Mdn* = 5.00). *A Mann-Whitney U test for severe psychological aggression was statistically significant* $U\ (N_{\text{incredible variable danger group}} = 130,\ N_{\text{increased danger group}} = 35) = 1770.5,\ z = -2.019,\ p = 0.043$ *with a small effect size* $r = 0.16$.

A Mann-Whitney test indicated that the general physical assault score was greater for those who experienced danger (*Mdn* = 31.00) than for victims who experienced incredible variable danger (*Mdn* = 12.00). *A Mann-Whitney U test for general physical assault was statistically significant* $U(N_{\text{incredible variable danger group}} = 130,\ N_{\text{increased danger group}} = 35) = 1508,\ z = -3.071,\ p = 0.002$ *with a small effect size* $r = 0.24$.

A Mann-Whitney test indicated that the minor physical assault score was greater for those who experienced danger (*Mdn* = 21.00) than for victims who experienced incredible variable danger (*Mdn* = 5.00), *A Mann-Whitney U test for minor physical assault was statistically significant* $U(N_{\text{incredible variable danger group}} = 130,\ N_{\text{increased danger group}} = 35) = 1573.5,\ z = -2.822,\ p = 0.005$ *with a small effect size* $r = 0.22$.

A Mann-Whitney test indicated that the severe physical assault score was greater for those who experienced danger (*Mdn* = 8.00) than for victims who experienced incredible variable danger (*Mdn* = 3.00). *A Mann-Whitney U test for severe physical assault was statistically significant* $U(N_{\text{incredible variable danger group}} = 130,\ N_{\text{increased danger group}} = 35) = 1521,\ z = -3.058,\ p = 0.002$ *with a small effect size* $r = 0.24$.

A Mann-Whitney test indicated that the general injury score was greater for those who experienced danger (*Mdn* = 10.00) than for victims who experienced incredible variable danger (*Mdn* = 4.50). *A Mann-Whitney U test for the general injury score was statistically significant* $U(N_{\text{incredible variable danger group}} = 130,\ N_{\text{increased danger group}} = 35) = 1596.5,\ z = -2.756,\ p = 0.006$ *with a small effect size* $r = 0.21$.

A Mann-Whitney test indicated that the minor injury score was greater for those who experienced danger (*Mdn* = 4.00) than for victims who experienced incredible variable danger (*Mdn* = 2.00). *A Mann-Whitney U test for the minor injury score was statistically significant* $U(N_{\text{incredible variable danger group}} = 130,\ N_{\text{increased danger group}} = 35) = 1737.5,\ z = -2.230,\ p = 0.026$ *with a small effect size* $r = 0.17$.

A Mann-Whitney test indicated that the severe injury score was greater for those who experienced danger (*Mdn* = 4.00) than for victims who experienced incredible variable danger (*Mdn* = 2.00). *A Mann-Whitney U test for the severe injury score was statistically significant* $U(N_{\text{incredible variable danger group}} = 130,\ N_{\text{increased danger group}} = 35) = 1671,\ z = -2.50,\ p = 0.012$ *with a small effect size* $r = 0.19$.

A Mann-Whitney test indicated that the general score of sexual coercion was greater for those who experienced danger (Mdn = 15.00) than for victims who experienced incredible variable danger (Mdn = 7.00). *A Mann-Whitney U test for the general score of sexual coercion was statistically significant U(N incredible variable danger group* $= 130$, $N_{\text{increased danger group}} = 35) = 1675$, $z = -2.414$, $p = 0.016$ *with a small effect size* $r = 0.19$.

A Mann-Whitney test indicated that the minor sexual coercion score was greater for those who experienced danger (*Mdn* = 8.00) than for victims who experienced incredible variable danger (*Mdn* = 3.00). *A Mann-Whitney U test for the general score of sexual coercion was statistically significant* $U(N_{\text{incredible variable danger group}} = 130, N_{\text{increased danger group}} = 35) = 1778$, $z = -2.008$, $p = 0.045$ *with a small effect size* $r = 0.16$.

A Mann-Whitney test indicated that the severe sexual coercion score was greater for those who experienced danger (*Mdn* = 4.00) than for victims who experienced incredible variable danger (*Mdn* = 2.00). *A Mann-Whitney U test for severe sexual coercion was statistically significant* $U(N_{\text{incredible variable danger group}} = 130, N_{\text{increased danger group}} = 35) = 1607.5$, $z = -2.776$, $p = 0.005$ *with a small effect size* $r = 0.22$.

A Mann-Whitney test indicated that the general economic abuse score was greater for those who experienced increased danger (*Mdn* = 105.86) than for victims who experienced variable danger (*Mdn* = 76.85). *A Mann-Whitney U test for the general economic abuse score was statistically significant* $U(N_{\text{increased danger group}} = 35, N_{\text{variable danger group}} = 130) = 1475$, $z = -3.19$, $p = 0.001$ *with a small effect size* $r = 0.06$.

A Mann-Whitney test indicated that economic exploitation was greater for those who experienced increased danger (*Mdn* = 99.83) than for victims who experienced variable danger (*Mdn* = 78.42). *A Mann-Whitney U test for economic exploitation was statistically significant* $U(N_{\text{increase danger group}} = 35, N_{\text{variable danger group}} = 130) = 1686$, $z = -2.366$, $p = 0.018$ *with a small effect size* $r = 0.03$.

A Mann-Whitney test indicated that economic control was greater for those who experienced increased danger (*Mdn* = 100.2) than for victims who experienced variable danger (*Mdn* = 78.38). *A Mann-Whitney U test for economic control was statistically significant* $U(N_{\text{increase danger group}} = 35, N_{\text{variable danger group}} = 130) = 1674.5$, $z = -2.401$, $p = 0.016$ *with a small effect size* $r = 0.04$.

A Mann-Whitney test indicated that economic sabotage was greater for those who experienced increased danger (*Mdn* = 99.64) than for victims who experienced variable danger (*Mdn* = 78.52). *A Mann-Whitney U test for economic sabotage was statistically significant* $U(N_{\text{increase danger group}} = 35, N_{\text{variable danger group}} = 130) = 1692.5$, $z = -2.339$, $p = 0.019$ *with a small effect size* $r = 0.03$.

4.3 Objective 2: Impact of Intimate Partner Violence

A descriptive and statistical analysis of the effects of PTSD, depression, and anxiety on victims of intimate partner violence (IPV) is presented in this objective. An overview of the three mental health conditions is presented in the first part of the section, along with their symptoms and impacts. The second part of the section examines statistically the relationships between different types of IPV and PTSD, depression, and anxiety. Providing a comprehensive understanding of IPV's impact on mental health.

4.3.1 *An Overview of the Descriptive Analysis for PTSD, Depression, and Anxiety*

PTSD

Regarding PTSD results, to analyse the level of Post-Traumatic Stress symptoms among victims of domestic abuse, the PTSD checklist civilian version (PCL-C) was adapted to assess stressful events that occurred due to abuse. The scores were then categorized into four categories: A total score of 85 is calculated from the sum of the scores, and the interpretations of the sum scores are as follows: 28–29 represent some PTSD symptoms, 30–44 indicate moderate to moderately severe severity of PTSD symptoms, 45–85 indicates high severity, and 17–27 indicates little to no severity of PTSD symptoms. Cronbach's alpha for the 17 items of the PCL-C scale was 94 in this study, indicating high internal consistency and validity.

Regarding the descriptive analysis for PTSD level among the participants, the descriptive statistic for the PTSD score among the participants showed an overall mean score of 45.02 (SD = 18.88). The participant's response scores varied from little to no severity, accounting for 23.6%, and those who had experienced some PTSD symptoms accounted for 2.4% of the total participants. Meanwhile, those with moderate to moderately high severity of PTSD symptoms accounted for 25.5%, while most of the participants indicated having a high severity of PTSD symptoms, accounting for 48.5%. PCL-C scale has been widely studied in cross-cultural studies, including those conducted in Arabic societies.

Depression

Regarding the depression results, using the PHQ-9 depression severity scale, which indicated that a greater degree of depression corresponded to a higher score, the researcher was able to determine the prevalence of depression symptomology among individuals who had been victims of domestic violence. This scale is broken down into five different categories, which are as follows: An item's total score may range from 0 to 27, with a score of 5 indicating mild depression, 10 indicating moderate depression, 15 indicating moderately severe depression, and 16 or higher indicating severe depression. According to this study, the depression scale (PHQ-9) showed a high degree of reliability with all nine objects having a Cronbach's alpha of 0.92.

To accomplish the purpose of the research, descriptive analyses were carried out to determine the extent to which the individuals suffered from depression.

Regarding the descriptive analysis for depression levels among the participants, the descriptive statistics for the depression score for the participants showed that the overall mean score was 13.01 (SD = 5.75) and the level of depression varied among the participants. The established cutoff scores results showed that 49.7% had mild depression, and those who had moderate depression accounted for 33.3% of the total participants, moderate to severe depression accounted for 10.9%, and severe depression accounted for 6.1%.

Anxiety
Regarding the anxiety results, higher scores on the Taylor Manifest Anxiety Scales indicated higher levels of anxiety, which can be broken down into the following five categories: "No Anxiety" corresponds to scores ranging from 0 to 16, "Mild Anxiety" corresponds to scores between 21 and 26, "Moderate Anxiety" corresponds to scores between 27 and 29, and "Very Severe Anxiety" corresponds to scores between 30 and 50. All 50 items of the scale are valid for Cronbach's alpha, demonstrating strong internal consistency. It scores 85.

The purpose of this study was to determine the extent to which victims of domestic violence suffer from anxiety and to determine how to best treat it. To accomplish the goals of the research project, a descriptive analysis was performed to determine the extent to which individuals showed symptoms of anxiety.

Regarding the descriptive analysis of the state of anxiety among the participants, according to the descriptive data for the anxiety score, the total mean score for the participants was 27.80, and the standard deviation was 9.21. The participants' levels of anxiety ranged from mild to severe, with mild anxiety affecting 9.1% of the total participants, moderate anxiety affecting 18.8%, and severe anxiety affecting 9.7%. The results of the established cutoff scores show that 12.7% of the participants had no anxiety, 9.1% had mild anxiety, and 18.8% had moderate anxiety. The people who had the highest ratings overall indicated that they suffer from really severe anxiety. This group included 49.7% of the total participants.

4.3.2 *Output of the Statistical Analysis for PTSD, Depression, and Anxiety*

Regarding the key findings for the consequences of domestic abuse—State of Anxiety, a one-way ANOVA test was conducted to examine whether there are any differences between types of abuse and levels of anxiety. For those variables that differed significantly, post-hoc comparisons were carried out using the Tukey HSD test, after which an analysis followed. The test results showed an insignificant association between physical, sexual, injury, negotiation and economic abuse with the state and level of anxiety among the respondents.

There was a significant effect of severe psychological aggression on the anxiety levels of the victims at the $p < 0.05$ for the five conditions $F(4{,}160) = 3.62$, $p = 0.01$[. Post hoc comparisons using Tukey's HSD test indicated that the mean score for victims' severe anxiety ($M = 27.06$, $SD = 24.87$) was significantly different than for victims with moderate anxiety ($M = 24.87$, $SD = 28.86$), was significantly different than for very severe anxiety ($M = 20.24$, $SD = 24.84$), was significantly different for mild anxiety ($M = 7.06$, $SD = 9.75$), and was significantly different for no anxiety ($M = 5.66$, $SD = 7.04$).

There was a significant effect of minor physical assault on the anxiety levels of the victims at the $p < 0.05$ for the five conditions $F(4,160) = 3.16, p = 0.016$[. Post hoc comparisons using Tukey's HSD test indicated that the mean score for victims with severe anxiety ($M = 32.93$, $SD = 43.51$) was significantly different than for victims with very severe anxiety ($M = 22.51$, $SD = 32.44$), was significantly different than for moderate anxiety ($M = 20.38$, $SD = 36.57$), was significantly different for mild anxiety ($M = 4.0$, $SD = 4.40$), and mild anxiety did not differ significantly from no anxiety ($M = 4.04$, $SD = 6.74$). These results confirm that the risk of developing anxiety symptomology is high for those who experience forms of abuse.

Regarding the key findings for the consequences of domestic abuse—state of depression level, the study using the Kruskal-Wallis test was carried out to determine whether or not victims of domestic violence are at risk of acquiring symptoms of depression. Dunn's test was used to carry out a post-hoc test that included pairwise comparisons for the variables that exhibited significant differences.

The findings demonstrated that there was no discernible difference between the depression-level groups regarding the use of pecuniary coercion, sexual coercion, or abusive bargaining tactics. For instance, economic abuse scores demonstrated a statistically insignificant difference with the level of depression across the groups, the Kruskal Wallis test was not significant $H(3) = 1.38$, $P = 0.711$, the effect size by eta squared was = 0.0084 which considered a small effect size. For the mild depression group (Mean Rank = 86.43, n = 82), the moderate depression group (Mean Rank = 77.95, n = 55), the moderate to severe depression group (Mean Rank = 86.81, n = 18), and the severe depression group (Mean Rank = 75.85, $n = 10$).

Given that this contradicts the results of previous studies, it was rather unexpected that economic abuse did not have a significant influence on the participants' levels of depression, anxiety, or PTSD.

A Kruskal Wallis test showed that there was a statistically significant difference in psychological aggression score between the different depression level groups: $H(3) = 8.97$, $P = 0.030$, the effect size was medium, eta—squared = 0.056 for mild depression group (Mean Rank = 78.01, $n = 82$), moderate depression group (Mean Rank = 89.80, $n = 55$), for moderate to severe depression (Mean Rank = 102, $n = 18$), and severe depression (Mean Rank = 52.35, $n = 10$).

A post-hoc test using pairwise comparisons of Dunn's test indicated that the null hypothesis is rejected at $P = 0.030$, showing significant differences between victims who have severe depression ($Mdn = 19.50$) and between the moderate depression group ($Mdn = 53.00$) $p = 0.023$. The same significant difference was observed between the severe depression group ($Mdn = 19.50$) with victims in moderate to severe depression group ($Mdn = 52.00$) $p = 0.008$, whereas no other difference was statistically different.

The same results revealed that the Kruskal Wallis test showed that there was a statistically significant difference in minor psychological aggression score between the different depression level groups: $H(3) = 11.95$, $P = 0.008$, the effect size was medium, eta-squared = 0.074 for mild depression group (Mean Rank = 79.66, $n = 82$), moderate depression group (Mean Rank = 89.03, $n = 55$), for moderate to severe depression (Mean Rank = 102.86, n = 18), and for severe depression (Mean Rank = 41.50, n = 10).

A post hoc test using pairwise comparisons Dunn's test indicated that the null hypothesis is rejected at $p = 0.008$, showing significant differences between victims in the severe depression group (*Mdn* = 5.50) with victims with mild depression (*Mdn* = 28.00) $p = 0.01$. The same can be observed among those with severe depression (*Mdn* = 5.50) and those in the moderate depression group (*Mdn* = 36.00) $p = 0.004$, while the same significant difference is also observed between the severe depression group (*Mdn* = 5.50) and with victims in the moderate to severe depression group (*Mdn* = 42.50) $p = 0.001$, while no other difference was statistically different.

The same results revealed that the Kruskal Wallis test showed that there was a statistically significant difference in severe psychological aggression score between the different depression level groups: H(3) = 8.23, P = 0.041, the effect size was medium, eta-squared = 0.0513 for mild depression group (Mean Rank = 73.40, n = 82), moderate depression group (Mean Rank = 94.29, n = 55), for moderate to severe depression (Mean Rank = 96.75, n = 18), and for severe depression (Mean Rank = 74.85, n = 10).

A post-hoc test using pairwise comparisons Dunn's test indicated that the null hypothesis is rejected at $p = 0.041$, showing significant differences between victims with mild depression (*Mdn* = 4.00) and with victims with moderate depression (*Mdn* = 12.00) $p = 0.012$, whereas no other difference was statistically different. There is a direct correlation between different kinds of IPV and depression among victims who have been traumatised.

A Kruskal Wallis test showed that there was a statistically significant difference in physical assault scores between the different depression level groups. H(3) = 8.65, P = 0.034, the effect size was medium, eta-squared = 0.0539.For mild depression group (Mean Rank = 73.11, n = 82), moderate depression group (Mean Rank = 90.63, n = 55), moderate to severe depression (Mean Rank = 104.56, n = 18), and for severe depression (Mean Rank = 83.35, n = 10). A post-hoc test using pairwise comparisons Dunn's test indicated that the null hypothesis is rejected at $p = 0.034$, showing significant differences between victims with mild depression (*Mdn* = 8.00) and victims with moderate depression (*Mdn* = 12.00) P = 0.035. The same was also observed between those with mild depression (*Mdn* = 8.00) and victims who have moderate to severe depression (*Mdn* = 12.00) $p = 0.11$, while no other difference was statistically different.

The same results demonstrated that the Kruskal Wallis test showed there was a statistically significant difference in minor physical assault score between the different depression level groups. H(3) = 8.06, P = 0.045, the effect size was medium, eta-squared = 0.050. For the mild depression group (Mean Rank = 74.38, n = 82), moderate depression group (Mean Rank = 91.23, n = 55), for moderate to severe depression (Mean Rank = 102.94, n = 18), and for severe depression (Mean Rank = 72.55, n = 10).

A post-hoc test using pairwise comparisons Dunn's test indicated that the null hypothesis is rejected at P = 0.045, showing significant differences between victims with mild depression (*Mdn* = 5.00) and victims with moderate depression (*Mdn* =

6.00) P = 0.041, while the same was observed among those with mild depression (*Mdn* = 5.00) and victims with moderate to severe depression (*Mdn* = 8.50) P = 0.020, whereas no other difference was statistically different.

The Kruskal Wallis test showed that there was a statistically significant difference in severe physical assault score between the different depression level groups: H(3) = 10.7, P = 0.013, the effect size was medium, eta—squared = 0.0674 for mild depression group (Mean Rank = 72.05, *n* = 82), moderate depression group (Mean Rank = 89.5, *n* = 55), for moderate to severe depression (Mean Rank = 106.81, *n* = 18), and for severe depression (Mean Rank = 94.15, *n* = 10).

A post-hoc test using pairwise comparisons Dunn's test indicated that the null hypothesis is rejected at $p = 0.013$, showing significant differences between victims with mild depression (*Mdn* = 2.00) and victims who have moderate depression (*Mdn* = 6.00) $p = 0.033$, while the same was observed among victims with mild depression (*Mdn* = 2.00) and victims who have moderate to severe depression (*Mdn* = 7.00) $p = 0.004$, whereas no other difference was statistically different.

A Kruskal Wallis test showed that there was a statistically significant difference in injury general score between the different depression level groups: H(3) = 13.2, P = 0.004, the effect size was medium, eta-squared = 0.084. The score for mild depression group (Mean Rank = 70.73, *n* = 82), moderate depression group (Mean Rank = 89.91, *n* = 55), for moderate to severe depression (Mean Rank = 107.06, *n* = 18), and for severe depression (Mean Rank = 102.35, *n* = 10).

A post-hoc test using pairwise comparisons Dunn's test indicated that the null hypothesis is rejected at $p = 0.004$, showing significant differences between victims with mild depression (*Mdn* = 2.50) and victims with moderate depression (*Mdn* = 6.00) $p = 0.019$. The same can be observed among victims with mild depression (*Mdn* = 2.00) and victims who have severe depression (*Mdn* = 6.00) $p = 0.044$, while the same observation can also be made of victims with mild depression (*Mdn* = 2.50) and victims with moderate to severe depression (*Mdn* = 7.50) $p = 0.003$, whereas no other difference was statistically different. Similarly, as shown by Esie et al. (2019), major depression episodes increase when the frequency and severity of abuse increases. They also observed that physical assault and injuries caused by an intimate partner increases the odds of meeting the criteria of major depression symptomology.

A Kruskal Wallis test showed that there was a statistically significant difference in severe injury score between the different depression level groups: H(3) = 16.8, P = 0.001, the effect size was medium, eta—squared = 0.107. The score for mild depression group (Mean Rank = 69.19, *n* = 82), moderate depression group (Mean Rank = 91.74, *n* = 55), for moderate to severe depression (Mean Rank = 109.78, *n* = 18), and for severe depression (Mean Rank = 1020, *n* = 10).

A post-hoc test using pairwise comparisons Dunn's test indicated that the null hypothesis is rejected at $p = 0.004$, showing significant differences between victims with mild depression (*Mdn* = 0.00) and victims with moderate depression (*Mdn* = 4.00) $p = 0.005$, while the same can be observed among victims with mild depression (*Mdn* = 0.00) and victims with severe depression (*Mdn* = 4.00) $p = 0.046$. Moreover, the same observation can be made among victims with mild depression (*Mdn* = 0.00) and victims with moderate to severe depression (*Mdn* = 4.00) $p = 0.001$, whereas no other difference was statistically different. The data presented here provide more evidence that there is a link between depressive and anxious states and the types of abuse that a person has been subjected to.

Regarding the key findings for the consequences of domestic abuse—PTSD, to assess whether domestic abuse victims are at risk of developing PTSD symptoms, Kruskal Wallis tests were conducted for variables that differ significantly. A post hoc test was conducted using pairwise comparisons of Dunn's test. Below is an analysis of the significant variables.

The results of this study show no significant differences between groups when it comes to negotiation abuse, injury, sexual pressure, economic abuse, and PTSD symptoms. For example, the economic abuse scores show a statistically insignificant difference with the level of PTSD symptoms manifest in the groups: H(3) = 5.93, P = 0.115, the effect size was small and insignificant, eta- squared = 0.0377. The score for the little to no severity group (Mean Rank = 74.54, $n = 39$), for some PTSD symptoms group (Mean Rank = 92.13, $n = 4$), for moderate to moderately high severity of PTSD symptoms (Mean Rank = 73.11, $n = 42$), for victims with high severity of PTSD symptoms (Mean Rank = 91.86, $n = 80$).

The current finding does not show a significant effect of sexual coercion on the development of PTSD among the participants, which partially contradicts a study that was conducted on 162 female victims of domestic abuse by examining factors associated with depression and PTSD.

A Kruskal Wallis test showed that there was a statistically significant difference in psychological aggression score between the different PTSD symptoms level groups: H(3) = 14.7, $p = 0.002$, the effect size was medium, eta-squared = 0.0933. The score for little to no severity group (Mean Rank = 62.08, $n = 39$), for some PTSD symptoms group (Mean Rank = 55.5, $n = 4$), for moderate to moderately high severity of PTSD symptoms (Mean Rank = 80.58, $n = 42$), and for victims with high severity of PTSD symptoms (Mean Rank = 95.84, n = 80). A post-hoc test using pairwise comparisons Dunn's test indicated that the null hypothesis is rejected at $p = 0.002$, showing significant differences between the little to no severity symptoms group (*Mdn* = 15.00) and with victims who exhibit high severity PTSD symptoms (*Mdn* = 53.00) $p < 0.01$, whereas no other difference was found to be statistically different.

A Kruskal Wallis test showed that there was a statistically significant difference in minor psychological aggression scores between the different PTSD symptoms level groups: H(3) = 13.4, P = 0.004, the effect size was medium, eta—squared = 0.086. The score for little to no severity group (Mean Rank = 62.90, $n = 39$), for some PTSD symptoms group (Mean Rank = 65.75, $n = 4$), for moderate to moderately high severity of PTSD symptoms (Mean Rank = 79.04, $n = 42$), and for victims with high severity of PTSD symptoms (Mean Rank = 95.74, $n = 80$). A post-hoc test using pairwise comparisons of Dunn's test indicated that the null hypothesis is rejected at $p = 0.004$, showing a significant difference between the little to no severity symptoms group (*Mdn* = 12.00) and with victims who exhibit high severity

PTSD symptoms (*Mdn* = 42.00) $p < 0.01$, whereas no other difference was found to be statistically different.

A Kruskal Wallis test showed that there was a statistically significant difference in severe psychological aggression score between the different PTSD symptoms level groups: H(3) = 11.9, P = 0.007, the effect size was medium, eta-squared = 0.077. The score for little to no severity group (Mean Rank = 66.53, *n* = 39), for some PTSD symptoms group (Mean Rank = 37.75, *n* = 4), for moderate to moderately high severity of PTSD symptoms (Mean Rank = 83.19, *n* = 42), and for victims with high severity of PTSD symptoms (Mean Rank = 93.19, *n* = 80).

A post hoc test using a pairwise comparison Dunn's test indicated that the null hypothesis is rejected at P = 0.007, showing significant differences between some PTSD symptoms group (*Mdn* = 2.50) with victims who exhibit high severity PTSD symptoms (*Mdn* = 12.00) P = 0.023, while the same was observed in the little to no severity symptoms group (*Mdn* = 4.00) and with victims who exhibit high severity PTSD symptoms (*Mdn* = 12.00) $p = 0.004$, whereas no other difference was found to be statistically different.

A Kruskal Wallis test showed that there was a statistically significant difference in physical assault score between the different PTSD symptoms level groups: H(3) = 8.82, P = 0.032, the effect size was small, eta-squared = 0.058. The score for little to no severity group (Mean Rank = 67.72, *n* = 39), for some PTSD symptoms group (Mean Rank = 64.88, *n* = 4), for moderate to moderately high severity of PTSD symptoms (Mean Rank = 78.89, *n* = 42), and for victims with high severity of PTSD symptoms (Mean Rank = 93.51, *n* = 80).

A post-hoc test using pairwise comparisons Dunn's test indicated that the null hypothesis is rejected at $p = 0.032$, showing significant differences between victims who exhibit high severity PTSD symptoms (*Mdn* = 13.50) and between little to no severity symptoms group (*Mdn* = 12.00) $p = 0.005$, while no other difference was statistically different.

A Kruskal Wallis test showed that there was a statistically significant difference in minor physical assault score between the different PTSD symptoms level groups: H(3) = 11.19, P = 0.011, the effect size was medium, eta-squared = 0.073. The score for little to no severity group (Mean Rank = 66.49, *n* = 39), for some PTSD symptoms group (Mean Rank = 64.13, *n* = 4), for moderate to moderately high severity of PTSD symptoms (Mean Rank = 77.19, *n* = 42), and for victims with high severity of PTSD symptoms (Mean Rank = 95.04, *n* = 80).

A post-hoc test using a pairwise comparisons Dunn's test indicated that the null hypothesis is rejected at $p = 0.011$, showing significant differences between victims who exhibit high severity PTSD symptoms (Mdn = 7.00) and between the little to no severity symptoms group (*Mdn* = 5.00) $p = 0.002$. Meanwhile, the same significant difference was observed between moderate to moderately high severity of PTSD symptoms (*Mdn* = 5.00) and with victims with high severity of PTSD symptoms (*Mdn* = 7.00), whereas no other difference was statistically different.

Multiple regression analysis was performed to predict the dependent outcomes (PTSD, Depression, Anxiety) for women how have experience different forms of intimate partner violence (Negotiation, Psychological, Physical, Sexual, Injury, Economic Abuse) as independent covariate in this model.

4.3.3 Model One

Multiple regression (Table 4.7) was conducted to examine the relationship between PTSD (dependent variable) and set of predictor variables (Negotiation, Psychological, Physical, Sexual, Injury, Economic Abuse). The regression model (Table 4.7) provided an excellent fit to the data, as indicated by an R-squared value of 0.118, suggesting that approximately 12% of the variance in the dependent variable was accounted by the predictors.

Results for the multiple linear regression (Table 4.7) indicated that there was a collective significant effect psychological aggression, economic abuse on predicting the level of PTSD among participants. The results of the regression the two predictors explained 12% of the variance, and the significant regression equation was found (F(6,158) = 3.507, $p < 0.003$), *The results showed that the Psychological Aggression and Economic Abuse were significant positive predictors of PTSD level* ($\beta = 0.180$, $t = 2.32$, $p < 0.001$, and $\beta = 0.272$, $t = 2.625$, $p < 0.001$, respectively). The results showed that other forms of abuse such as Negotiation, Physical, Injury and Sexual coercion were not significant predictor of PTSD level among the participants (Table 4.7).

4.3.4 Model Two

Multiple regression (Table 4.8) was conducted to examine the relationship between Depression (dependent variable) and set of predictor variables (Negotiation, Psychological, Physical, Sexual, Injury, Economic Abuse). The regression model (Table 4.8) provided an excellent fit to the data, as indicated by an R-squared value of 0.075, suggesting that approximately 7.5% of the variance in the dependent variable was accounted by the predictors.

The results of multiple linear regression analyses indicate that there was a significant effect of the economic abuse on Depression level. The significant regression equation was found (F(6,158) = 2.146, p < 0.001). Whereas other forms of abuse were not a significant predictor of depression level (Table 4.8).

Table 4.7 Summary of model one

Model	R	R Square	Adjusted R Square	Std. Error of the Estimate
1	343[a]	0.118	0.084	18.07130

ANOVA[b]

Model		Sum of squares	df	Mean square	F	Sig.
1	Regression	6871.537	6	1145.256	3.507	0.003[c]
	Residual	51598.366	158	326.572		
	Total	58469.903	164			

Coefficients[d]

Model		Unstandardized coefficients		Standardized coefficients	t	Sig.	Collinearity statistics	
		B	Std. error	Beta			Tolerance	VIF
1	(Constant)	27.864	5.631		4.948	0.000		
	Negotiation abuse total score within past 12 months	−0.032	0.048	−0.052	−0.674	0.501	0.956	1.046
	Psychological aggression total score within past 12 months	0.106	0.040	0.272	2.625	0.010	0.520	1.922
	Physical assault total score within past 12 months	−0.028	0.054	−0.075	−0.512	0.610	0.263	3.803
	Injury total score within past 12 months	0.105	0.158	0.088	0.663	0.508	0.314	3.185

(continued)

Table 4.7 (continued)

Coefficients[d]

Model		Unstandardized coefficients		Standardized coefficients	t	Sig.	Collinearity statistics	
		B	Std. error	Beta			Tolerance	VIF
	Sexual coercion total score within past 12 months	−0.015	0.071	−0.019	−0.210	0.834	0.689	1.452
	Mean of economic abuse	0.384	0.165	0.180	2.324	0.021	0.929	1.076

[a]Predictors: (constant), mean of economic abuse, negotiation abuse total score within past 12 months, physical assault total score within past 12 months, sexual coercion total score within past 12 months, psychological aggression total score within past 12 months, injury total score within past 12 months
[b]Dependent variable: PTSD score
[c]Predictors: (constant), mean of economic abuse, negotiation abuse total score within past 12 months, physical assault total score within past 12 months, sexual coercion total score within past 12 months, psychological aggression total score within past 12 months, injury total score within past 12 months
[d]Dependent variable: PTSD score

Table 4.8 Summary of model two

Model	R	R Square	Adjusted R Square	Std. Error of the Estimate
2	274[a]	0.075	0.040	5.63923

ANOVA[b]

Model		Sum of squares	df	Mean square	F	Sig.
2	Regression	409.427	6	68.238	2.146	0.051[c]
	Residual	5024.548	158	31.801		
	Total	5433.976	164			

Coefficients[d]

Model		Unstandardized coefficients		Standardized coefficients	t	Sig.	Collinearity statistics	
		B	Std. error	Beta			Tolerance	VIF
2	(Constant)	17.162	1.757		9.767	0.000		
	Negotiation abuse total score within past 12 months	0.013	0.015	0.065	0.835	0.405	956	1.046
	Psychological aggression total score within past 12 months	−0.013	0.013	−0.107	−1.013	0.313	0.520	1.922
	Physical assault total score within past 12 months	−0.001	0.017	−0.013	−0.087	0.931	0.263	3.803

(continued)

Table 4.8 (continued)

Coefficients[d]

Model		Unstandardized coefficients		Standardized coefficients	t	Sig.	Collinearity statistics	
		B	Std. error	Beta			Tolerance	VIF
	Injury total score within past 12 months	0.063	0.049	0.174	1.274	0.204	0.314	3.185
	Sexual coercion total score within past 12 months	0.012	0.022	0.049	0.529	0.597	0.689	1.452
	Mean of economic abuse	−0.141	0.052	−0.216	−2.724	0.007	0.929	1.076

[a]Predictors: (Constant), Mean of Economic Abuse, Negotiation Abuse total score within past 12 months, Physical Assault total score within past 12 months, Sexual Coercion total score within past 12 months, Psychological Aggression total score within past 12 months, Injury total score within past 12 months
[b]Dependent Variable: Depression Score
[c]Predictors: (Constant), Mean of Economic Abuse, Negotiation Abuse total score within past 12 months, Physical Assault total score within past 12 months, Sexual Coercion total score within past 12 months, Psychological Aggression total score within past 12 months, Injury total score within past 12 months
[d]Dependent Variable: Depression Score

4.3.5 Model Three

Multiple regression (Table 4.9) was conducted to examine the relationship between level of Anxiety (dependent variable) and set of predictor variables (Negotiation, Psychological, Physical, Sexual, Injury, Economic Abuse). The regression model (Table 4.9) provided an excellent fit to the data, as indicated by an R-squared value of 0.086, suggesting that approximately 8.6% of the variance in the dependent variable was accounted by the predictors.

Results for the multiple linear regression indicated that there was a significant effect Negotiation Abuse on predicting the level of Anxiety among participants. The results of the regression the one predictors explained 8.6% of the variance, and the significant regression equation was found ($F(6,158) = 2.488$, $p < 0.001$), *The results showed that the Negotiation Aggression were significant predictors of Anxiety level* ($\beta = 0.167$, $t = 2.146$, $p < 0.001$, The results showed that other forms of abuse such as Psychological, Physical, Injury and Sexual coercion were not significant predictor of Anxiety level among the participants (Table 4.9).

4.4 Objective 3: Risk Factor for Victimization

This objective investigates the impact of various factors that are likely to be associated with victims of IPV. It draws upon an ecological framework by running a descriptive and statistical analysis considering the individual, family and societal level variables. The results will help to explain the complex relationships between the proposed variables in IPV occurrence. These relationships will be discussed and explained in depth in the qualitative chapter.

4.4.1 Age Disparity Between Husband and Wife

To examine factors associated with the likelihood of domestic abuse occurrence, several factors were analysed such as the age difference between husband and wife. For this, first, we need to investigate whether there is a correlation between an age gap of more than 10 years between a husband and wife with an increased risk of physical or sexual abuse. Mann-Whitney u test Because the results of the normality tests indicated that the data did not follow a normal distribution, U tests were carried out to account for this anomaly.

The effect size is calculated from the difference between the participants' average scores and those of their control counterparts (Lakens, 2013). Cohen's interpretation of the effect size indicated that 0.2 and below is a small effect, 0.5 is a medium effect, and 0.8 and above is a large effect (McLeod, 2019). The procedure for carrying out an analysis of the findings is outlined in the following. A Mann-Whitney U test was

Table 4.9 Summary of model three

Model	R	R Square	Adjusted R Square	Std. Error of the Estimate
3	294[a]	0.086	0.052	8.97574

ANOVA[b]

Model		Sum of squares	df	Mean square	F	Sig.
3	Regression	1202.710	6	200.452	2.488	0.025[c]
	Residual	12729.084	158	80.564		
	Total	13931.794	164			

Coefficients[d]

Model		Unstandardized coefficients		Standardized coefficients	t	Sig.	Collinearity statistics	
		B	Std. error	Beta			Tolerance	VIF
3	(Constant)	23.634	2.797		8.450	000		
	Negotiation abuse total score within past 12 months	0.051	0.024	0.167	2.146	033	0.956	1.046
	Psychological aggression total score within past 12 months	0.035	0.020	0.185	1.753	082	0.520	1.922
	Physical assault total score within past 12 months	−0.007	0.027	−0.040	0.271	787	0.263	3.803

(continued)

Table 4.9 (continued)

Coefficients[d]

Model		Unstandardized coefficients		Standardized coefficients	t	Sig.	Collinearity statistics	
		B	Std. error	Beta			Tolerance	VIF
	Injury total score within past 12 months	0.057	0.078	0.099	729	467	0.314	3.185
	Sexual coercion total score within past 12 months	0.010	0.035	0.025	270	787	0.689	1.452
	Mean of economic abuse	0.013	0.082	0.013	164	70	0.929	1.076

[a]Predictors: (Constant), Mean of Economic Abuse, Negotiation Abuse total score within past 12 months, Physical Assault total score within past 12 months, Sexual Coercion total score within past 12 months, Psychological Aggression total score within past 12 months, Injury total score within past 12 months
[b]Dependent Variable: Anxiety Score
[c]Predictors: (Constant), Mean of Economic Abuse, Negotiation Abuse total score within past 12 months, Physical Assault total score within past 12 months, Sexual Coercion total score within past 12 months, Psychological Aggression total score within past 12 months, Injury total score within past 12 months
[d]Dependent Variable: Anxiety Score

conducted on the data ($n = 165$) to see if age difference (with a cutoff of 10 years above or below) differed in the negotiation abuse score.

The test indicated that the difference was not statistically significant for the negotiation abuse score in general, along with emotional abuse, and cognitive abuse in association with the age difference between husband and wife. For example, negotiation abuse (in general) was not significantly associated with the age difference between husband and wife [$U(N_{below\ 10\ years} = 139, N_{10\ years\ and\ above} = 29) = 1690$, $z = -0.525$, $p = 0.600$].

The test indicated that the difference was not statistically significant for the psychological aggression score in general, minor psychological aggression, and severe psychological abuse in association with the age difference between husband and wife. For example, psychological aggression, in general, was not significantly associated with the age difference between husband and wife $U(N_{below\ 10\ years} = 139, N_{10\ years\ and\ above} = 29) = 1715.5$, $z = -0.409$, $p = 0.682$.

The test indicated that the difference was not statistically significant for the physical assault score in general, minor physical assault, and severe physical assault in association with the age difference between husband and wife. For example, the physical assault score, in general, was not significantly associated with the age difference between husband and wife $U(N_{below\ 10\ years} = 139, N_{10\ years\ and\ above} = 29) = 1576$, $z = -1.038$, $p = 0.299$.

The test indicated that the difference was not statistically significant for the minor injury score in general and assault in association with age difference between husband and wife, $U(N_{below\ 10\ years} = 139, N_{10\ years\ and\ above} = 29) = 1442.5$, $z = -1.697$, $p = 0.090$.

A Mann-Whitney U test for injury score in general in association with age difference between husband and wife indicated that this difference was statistically significant $U(N_{below\ 10\ years} = 139, N_{10\ years\ and\ above} = 29) = 1353.5$, $z = -2.067$, $p = 0.039$, and had a small effect size $r = 0.16$. A Mann-Whitney U test for severe injury score in general in association with age difference between husband and wife indicated that this difference was also statistically significant $U(N_{below\ 10\ years} = 139, N_{10\ years\ and\ above} = 29) = 1327$, $z = -2.22$, $p = 0.029$, with a small effect size $r = 0.17$.

The test indicated that the difference was not statistically significant for the general sexual coercion score, minor sexual coercion, and severe sexual coercion in association with age difference between husband and wife. For example, general sexual coercion $U(N_{below\ 10\ years} = 139, N_{10\ years\ and\ above} = 29) = 1636$, $z = -0.772$, $p = 0.440$.

The test indicated that the difference was not statistically significant for the general economic abuse score, economic exploitation, economic control, and economic sabotage in association with age difference between husband and wife; the general economic abuse score was $U(N_{below\ 10\ years} = 139, N_{10\ years\ and\ above} = 29) = 1659.5$, $z = -0.660$, $p = 0.509$.

4.4.2 Age at Marriage

Regarding the age at marriage, to examine whether participants' age at marriage time increases the likelihood of abuse, Kruskal Wallis tests were conducted, since the data are not normally distributed. For those cases where there are significant differences, a post hoc test pairwise comparison Dunn's test was conducted, and the results are described in the next section.

A Kruskal Wallis test was conducted on the data ($n = 165$) to examine if age at marriage time may increase the risk of being victimized. The result showed there was no statistically significant difference between negotiation abuse, sexual coercion, and the participants' age group at the time of marriage. For example, the participant age group had no influence on the sexual coercion score, H(4) = 5.25, P = 0.263, the effect size was small, eta-squared = 0.033 victims who married before the age of 17 years old (Mean Rank = 108.88, n = 13), those who married between 18–22 years (Mean Rank = 76.92, $n = 73$), those who married between 23–27 (Mean Rank = 84.07, $n = 55$), those who married between 28–32 (Mean Rank = 87.39, $n = 14$, and those who married at age of 33 years and above (Mean Rank = 81.70, $n = 10$).

A Kruskal-Wallis H test was performed, and the results showed that the general severe psychological aggression score was statically significantly different between the severe psychological aggression scores and the influence of age group at marriage time, H(4) = 10.5, P = 0.03, the effect size was small to medium, eta-squared = 0.067 victims who married before the age of 17 years old (Mean Rank = 95.23, $n = 13$), those who married between 18–22 years (Mean Rank = 88.93, $n = 73$), those who married between 23–27 (Mean Rank = 67.18, $n = 55$), those who married between 28–32 (Mean Rank = 86.50, $n = 14$), and those who married at age of 33 years and above (Mean Rank = 105.9, $n = 10$).

A post hoc test using a pairwise comparison of Dunn's test indicated that the null hypothesis is rejected at $p = 0.033$, showing significant differences between those who married between the age of 23–27 years (*Mdn* = 4.00) and those who married between the age of 18–22 years (*Mdn* = 9.00) P = 0.010. Moreover, the same significant difference can be observed among those who married between the age of 23–27 years (*Mdn* = 4.00) and with those who married at the age of 33 years and above (*Mdn* = 19.00) $p = 0.018$, whereas no other difference was statistical.

A Kruskal-Wallis H test was performed and the results showed that for the general physical assault scores there was a statically significant difference between the physical assault scores and the influence of age group at marriage time, H(4) = 13.3, P = 0.010, the effect size was small to medium, eta-squared = 0.084 victims who married before the age of 17 years old (Mean Rank = 110.12, $n = 13$), those who married between 18–22 years (Mean Rank = 87.84, $n = 73$), those who married between 23–27 (Mean Rank = 66.56, $n = 55$), those who married between 28–32 (Mean Rank = 82.86, $n = 14$), and those who married at age of 33 years and above (Mean Rank = 103.0, $n = 10$).

A post hoc test using a pairwise comparison of Dunn's test indicated that the null hypothesis is rejected at $p = 0.010$, showing significant differences between those who married between the age of 23–27 years (*Mdn* = 5.00) and those who married between the age of 18–22 years (*Mdn* = 12.00) $p = 0.012$. Moreover, the same significant difference was observed between those who married between the age of 23–27 years (*Mdn* = 5.00) and with those who married at or before the age of 17 years (*Mdn* = 31.00) $p = 0.003$, while no other difference was statistically different.

A Kruskal-Wallis H test results showed that the minor physical assault score revealed a statistically significant difference between the physical assault scores and the influence of age group at marriage time, H(4) = 10.85, P = 0.028, the effect size was small, eta-squared = 0.069 victims who married before the age of 17 years old (Mean Rank = 106.3, $n = 13$), those who married between 18–22 years (Mean Rank = 86.55, $n = 73$), those who married between 23–27 (Mean Rank = 68.78, $n = 55$), those who married between 28–32 (Mean Rank = 82.39, $n = 14$), and those who married at age of 33 years and above (Mean Rank = 105.85, $n = 10$).

A post-hoc test using pairwise comparisons Dunn's test indicated that the null hypothesis is rejected at P = 0.028, showing significant differences between those who married between the age of 23–27 years (*Mdn* = 5.00) and those who married between the age of 18–22 years (*Mdn* = 5.00) P = 0.036. Furthermore, the same significant difference was observed among those who married between the age of 23–27 years (*Mdn* = 5.00) and with those who married at age of 33 and above (*Mdn* = 6.50) P = 0.023, those who married between the age of 23–27 years (*Mdn* = 5.00), and with those who married when their age are 17 years or less (*Mdn* = 17.00) $p = 0.010$, while no other difference was statistically different.

Further Kruskal-Wallis H test results revealed that the severe physical assault score showed a statistically significant difference between the physical assault scores and the influence of age group at marriage time, H(4) = 18.02, P = 0.001, the effect size is medium, eta-squared = 0.113, the score with victims who married before the age of 17 years old (Mean Rank = 112, $n = 13$), those who married between 18–22 years (Mean Rank = 90.19, $n = 73$), those who married between 23–27 (Mean Rank = 62.87, $n = 55$), those who married between 28–32 (Mean Rank = 86.11, $n = 14$), and those who married at age of 33 years and above (Mean Rank = 99.15, $n = 10$).

A post-hoc test using a pairwise comparisons Dunn's test indicated that the null hypothesis is rejected at $p = 0.001$, showing significant differences between those who married between the age of 23–27 years (*Mdn* = 2.00) and those who married between the age of 18–22 years (*Mdn* = 7.00) $p = 0.001$. Moreover, the same significant difference was observed among those who married between the age of 23–27 years (*Mdn* = 2.00) and with those who married at age of 33 and above (*Mdn* = 7.00) $p = 0.025$, those who married between the age of 23–27 years (*Mdn* = 2.00), and with those who married when their age are 17 years or less (*Mdn* = 14.00) $p = 0.001$, whereas no other difference was statistically different.

A further Kruskal-Wallis H test was performed and the results showed that the general injury score revealed a statistically significant difference between the injury scores and the influence of age group at marriage time, H(4) = 15.10, P = 0.004, the effect size is medium, eta-squared = 0.094, the scores with victims who married before the age of 17 years old (Mean Rank = 110.6, $n = 13$), those who married between 18–22 years (Mean Rank = 84.5, n = 73), those who married between 23–27 (Mean Rank = 67.1, n = 55), those who married between 28–32 (Mean Rank = 91.3, n = 14), and those who married at the age of 33 years and above (Mean Rank = 111.8, n = 10).

A post-hoc test using a pairwise comparisons Dunn's test indicated that the null hypothesis is rejected at P = 0.004, showing significant differences between those who married between the age of 23–27 years (*Mdn* = 2.00) and those who married between the age of 18–22 years (*Mdn* = 6.00) $p = 0.038$. Furthermore, the same significant difference was observed among those who married between the age of 23–27 years (*Mdn* = 2.00), those who married when their age was 17 years or less (*Mdn* = 8.00) $p = 0.003$, with those who married between the age of 23–27 years (*Mdn* = 2.00), and with those who married at age of 33 and above (*Mdn* = 7.00) $p = 0.006$, while no other difference was statistically different.

A Kruskal-Wallis H test was performed and the results showed that minor injury scores revealed a statistically significant difference between injury scores and the influence of age group at marriage time, H(4) = 10.37, P = 0.035, it has a small effect size, eta-squared = 0.058 and with victims who married before the age of 17 years old (Mean Rank = 99.81, n = 13), those who married between 18–22 years (Mean Rank = 88.08, n = 73), those who married between 23–27 (Mean Rank = 67.45, n = 55), those who married between 28–32 (Mean Rank = 92.71, n = 14), and those who married at age of 33 years and above (Mean Rank = 96.0, n = 10).

A post-hoc test using a pairwise comparisons Dunn's test indicated that the null hypothesis is rejected at $p = 0.035$, showing a significant difference between those who married between the age of 23–27 years (*Mdn* = 0.00) and those who married between the age of 18–22 years (*Mdn* = 2.00) $p = 0.012$. Moreover, the same significant difference was observed among those who married between the age of 23–27 years (*Mdn* = 0.00), and those who married when they were 17 years or less (Mdn = 3.00) $p = 0.022$, while no other difference was statistically different.

A Kruskal-Wallis H test was performed and the results showed that severe injury score revealed a statistically significant difference between injury scores and the influence of age group at marriage time, H(4) = 20.19, P < 0.001, the effect size is large, eta-squared = 0.198 and victims who married before the age of 17 (Mean Rank = 114.69, n = 13), those who married between 18–22 years (Mean Rank = 82.42, n = 73), those who married between 23–27 (Mean Rank = 66.6, n = 55), those who married between 28–32 (Mean Rank = 94.9, n = 14), and those who married at age of 33 years and above (Mean Rank = 119.0, n = 10).

A post-hoc test using a pairwise comparisons Dunn's test indicated that the null hypothesis is rejected at P < 0.01, showing significant differences between those who married between the age of 23–27 years (*Mdn* = 0.00) and those who married between the age of 28–32 years (*Mdn* = 4.00) $p = 0.04$. Furthermore, the same significant difference was observed among those who married between the age of 23–27 years (*Mdn* = 0.00), those who married when they were 17 years or less (*Mdn* = 5.00) $p = 0.001$, and with those who married between the age of 23–27 years (*Mdn* = 0.00), with those who married at age of 33 and above (*Mdn* = 6.00) $p = 0.001$, those who married between the age of 18–22 years (*Mdn* = 3.00), those who married before the age of 17 years (*Mdn* = 5.00) $p = 0.02$, those who married between the age of 18–22 years (*Mdn* = 3.00), and with those who married when they were 30 years old and above (*Mdn* = 6.00), while no other difference was statistically different.

A Kruskal-Wallis H test results showed that the economic abuse score was revealed to have a statistically significant difference between the economic abuse score and the influence of age group at marriage time, H(4) = 10.53, P = 0.032, the effect size was small, eta-squared = 0.023 and on victims who married before the age of 17 years old (Mean Rank = 86.42, $n = 13$), those who married between 18–22 years (Mean Rank = 76, $n = 73$), those who married between 23–27 (Mean Rank = 97.17, $n = 55$), those who married between 28–32 (Mean Rank = 57.61, $n = 14$), and those who married at the age of 33 years and above (Mean Rank = 87.25, $n = 10$).

A post-hoc test using a pairwise comparisons Dunn's test indicated that the null hypothesis is rejected at $p = 0.03$, showing significant differences between those who were married between the ages 28–32 years (*Mdn* = 13.50), with those who married between the age of 23–27 years (*Mdn* = 17) $p = 0.008$, those who married between the age of 18–22 years (*Mdn* = 14), and with those who married between the age of 23–27 years (*Mdn* = 17) $p = 0.006$, whereas no other difference was statistically different.

Further Kruskal-Wallis H test results showed that the economic sabotage scores revealed a statistically significant difference between economic abuse score and the influence of age group at marriage time, H(4) = 9.99, P = 0.041, the effect size was small, eta-squared = 0.021. The score with victims who married before the age of 17 years old (Mean Rank = 91.88, $n = 13$), those who married between 18–22 years (Mean Rank = 80.20, $n = 73$), those who married between 23–27 (Mean Rank = 93.09, $n = 55$), those who married between 28–32 (Mean Rank = 49.96, $n = 14$), and those who married at the age of 33 years and above (Mean Rank = 82.65, $n =$ 10).

A post-hoc test using a pairwise comparisons Dunn's test indicated that the null hypothesis is rejected at $p = 0.04$, showing significant differences between those who married between the age 28–32 years (*Mdn* = 6.5) and those who married between the age of 18–22 years (*Mdn* = 9) P = 0.03, and between those who married between the age of 28–32 years (*Mdn* = 6.5), and with those who married before the age of 17 years old (Mdn = 11) $p = 0.02$. Furthermore, it also showed significant differences between those who married between the age of 28–32 years (*Mdn* = 6.5), with those who married between the age of 23–27 years (*Mdn* = 10) $p = 0.002$, while no other difference was statistically different.

4.4.3 Number of Children

Regarding the number of children, Spearman's rho correlation was carried out in order to investigate how the number of children may result in an increased risk of domestic violence. Due to the fact that the data are not regularly distributed, as shown by the results of the normality test, this analysis was carried out. In the following, you will find a description of the analysis.

The results of Spearman's rank correlation revealed no significant difference between negotiation abuse, psychological aggression, and economic abuse with the number of children. For example, the results revealed no significant difference between economic abuse in general and the number of children, $r_s(163) = -0.005$, $p = 0.947$. The effect size was very small, 0.0003 Additionally, the results of Spearman's rank correlation indicated that there is a positive significant correlation between severe sexual coercion and the number of children, $r_s(163) = 0.165$, $p = 0.034$, the effect size was a small but significant relationship ($p = 0.034$).

4.4.4 Pregnancy Loss and Infertility

Regarding women's fertility, in order to investigate if a woman's fertility was a basic risk factor that increased the likelihood of abuse, Mann-Whitney U tests were carried out. The results of the normality test indicated that the data did not follow a normal distribution, thus these tests were carried out. The next parts are going to offer a description of the data analysis that was done.

A Mann-Whitney U test was conducted on the data (N = 165) to see if fertile or infertile women score differently on the abuse scale. The test indicated that the difference was not statistically significant for negotiation abuse, psychological abuse, sexual coercion, physical abuse, injury, economic abuse, and with fertile or infertile women. For example, the general economic abuse score was $U(N_{\text{fertile women}} = 113, N_{\text{infertile women}} = 52) = 2844.50$, $z = -0.328$, $p = 0.743$, The Mann-Whitney U test revealed a moderate effect size = 0.567.

The data infers that childless women are less likely to experience domestic abuse, however, there are several key factors that have a greater influence on spouse violence, other than the wife's fertility condition.

Regarding pregnancy as a risk factor for abuse, to determine whether a pregnancy was a risk factor that increases the chance of abuse, Mann-Whitney U tests were conducted, since the data were not normally distributed based on normality test results. Below, an analysis is provided.

The test indicated that the difference was not statistically significant for negotiation abuse, injury, sexual coercion, and physical assault scores with victims who were pregnant or not. For example, the physical assault general score was $U(N_{\text{pregnant victims}} = 52, N_{\text{non-pregnant victims}} = 113) = 2497$, $z = -1.554$, $p = 0.120$. The Mann-Whitney U test showed a small to moderate effect size = 0.358.

A Mann-Whitney test indicated that the general score of psychological aggression was greater for those who were abused during pregnancy (*Mdn* = 60.00) than for victims who were not pregnant when the abuse occurred (*Mdn* = 31.00), while *A Mann-Whitney U test for the general score of psychological aggression was statistically significant,* $U(N_{\text{pregnant victims}} = 52, N_{\text{non-pregnant victims}} = 113) = 2079$, $z = -3.014$, $p = 0.003$ *with a small effect size* $r = 0.06$.

A further Mann-Whitney test indicated that minor psychological aggression was greater for those who were abused during pregnancy (*Mdn* = 41.50) than for victims who were not pregnant when the abuse occurred (*Mdn* = 23.00), while the same *test for minor psychological aggression was statistically significant* $U(N_{\text{pregnant victims}} = 52, N_{\text{non-pregnant victims}} = 113) = 2088.5, z = -2.983, p = 0.003$, *with a small effect size* $r = 0.05$.

A Mann-Whitney test indicated that the economic control score was greater for those who were abused during pregnancy (*Mdn* = 17.5) than for victims who were not pregnant when the abuse occurred (*Mdn* = 15), while the same test *for economic control score was statistically significant* $U(N_{\text{pregnant victims}} = 52, N_{\text{non-pregnant victims}} = 113) = 2269.5, z = -2.352, p = 0.019$, *with a small effect size* $r = 0.03$. The study's results underlined the fact that women with lower levels of educational attainment are more likely to be abused when they are pregnant. Furthermore, the study found that having an abusive parent as a child increased the likelihood of becoming a victim of emotional violence as an adult.

Regarding pregnancy loss, to determine if domestic abuse results in pregnancy loss, as a result of the non-normal distribution of data, Mann-Whitney U tests were conducted; below is an analysis of that data. *The test indicated that the difference was not statistically significant for negotiation abuse, sexual coercion, physical abuse, injury, and economic abuse with victims who lost their pregnancies. For example, the general economic abuse score was* $U(N_{\text{lost pregnancy}} = 9, N_{\text{did not lose pregnancy}} = 156) = 599, z = -.740, p = 0.459$, *and the effect size was small* $r = 0.056$.

A Mann-Whitney test indicated that the severe psychological aggression score was greater for victims who lost their pregnancy (*Mdn* = 29.00) than for victims who did not lose their pregnancy (*Mdn* = 6.00) while regarding the same test *for severe psychological aggression and the pregnancy loss status, this difference was statistically significant* $U(N_{\text{lost pregnancy}} = 9, N_{\text{did not loss pregnancy}} = 156) = 417, z = -2.054, p = 0.040$, *with a small effect size* $r = 0.16$.

4.4.5 Family of Origin Violence

Regarding the family of origin violence victim, to examine if a history of abuse in the victim's family of origin increases the chance of abuse they might experience when they are married, Mann-Whitney U tests were conducted since the data are not normally distributed. Below is an analysis of the results.

A Mann-Whitney U test was conducted on the data ($N = 165$) *to determine if victims who witnessed their father abusing their mother or not scored differently on the form of abuse scale. The test indicated that the difference was not statistically significant for psychological abuse, sexual coercion, physical abuse, injury, and economic abuse in connection with victims who had witnessed their fathers abusing their mothers in their childhood versus those who had not. For example, the general economic abuse score was* $U\ (N_{\text{witnessed parent abuse}} = 47, N_{\text{did not witness parent abuse}} =$

118) = 2532.5, z = −.869, p = 0.385. The effect size was small to moderate, r = 0.376.

A Mann-Whitney test indicated that the negotiation cognitive abuse score was greater for victims who witnessed their father beating their mother (*Mdn* = 6.00) than for victims who did not witness their father abusing their mother (*Mdn* = 3.00), *while A Mann-Whitney U test for the negotiation cognitive abuse score with victims who had witnessed a parent abuse their wife and those who had not witnessed the same showed that the difference was statistically significant* $U(N_{witnessed\ parent\ abuse} = 47, N_{did\ not\ witness\ parent\ abuse} = 118) = 2241, z = -1.948, p = 0.05$, *with a small effect size r = 0.15.*

Regarding the husbands who witnessed their fathers abusing their mothers, a Kruskal-Walli's test was carried out since the data did not fall into a normal distribution. The purpose of this test was to determine whether the fact that the husbands had seen their fathers assaulting their mothers when they were youngsters had any effect on them when they are adults. Dunn's test for pairwise comparisons was used in a post-hoc analysis to look for statistically significant differences. The analysis is broken down into the following paragraphs.

Based on the data (n = 165), a Kruskal Wallis test was carried out to determine whether or not the abuser's exposure to violence in his own family of origin enhances the likelihood that he would abuse his spouse. The findings revealed that there was no statistically significant difference between the scores of negotiation abuse, psychological abuse, physical assault, injury, and sexual abuse in connection with a partner witnessing violence in their family of origin. This was the case for all five types of abuse. In the case of physical assault, for instance, there is no statistically significant difference between abusers who saw violence in their own families of origin and those who did not experience such violence: H(2) = 0.508, P = 0.776, with a small effect size = 0.0031, the score with the abuser/partner witnessing their fathers beating their mother (Mean Rank = 84.27, *n* = 50), partners who did not witness their fathers beating their mothers (Mean Rank = 77.91, *n* = 35), and with those victims who did not know if their partner had witnessed their father beating their mother (Mean Rank = 84.43, *n* = 80).

Furthermore, a Kruskal Wallis test for economic abuse shows a statistically significant difference in the abuser witnessing his father beating his mother, H(2) = 6.65, P = 0.036, showed small to medium effect size = 0.040 and on those who witnessed their father beating their mother (Mean Rank = 31.88, *n* = 50), those who did not witness their father beating their mother (Mean Rank = 29.40, *n* = 35), as well as those who did not know if their partners had witnessed their father beating their mother (Mean Rank = 33.92, *n* = 80).

A post hoc test using a pairwise comparison of Dunn's test indicated that the null hypothesis is rejected at $p = 0.034$, showing significant differences between those abusers who did not witness their father beating their mother in their childhood (*Mdn* = 30) and those who did not know if their abuser has witnessed their father abusing their mother in childhood (*Mdn* = 35) $p = 0.013$, while no other difference was statistically significant.

A Kruskal Wallis test for economic sabotage showed a statistically significant difference for the abuser witnessing his father beating his mother, H(2) = 6.39, P = 0.041, showed a small to medium effect size = 0.039, the score for those who witnessed their father beating their mother (Mean Rank = 82.43, *n* = 50), for those who had not witnessed their father beating their mother (Mean Rank = 66.36, *n* = 35), and for those who did not know if their partner had witnessed their farther beating their mother (Mean Rank = 90.64, *n* = 80).

A post-hoc test using a pairwise comparisons Dunn's test indicated that the null hypothesis is rejected at $p = 0.041$, showing significant differences between abusers who did not witness their father beating their mother in their childhood (*Mdn* = 7) and those who did not know if their abuser had witnessed their father abusing their mother in their childhood (*Mdn* = 9, $p = 0.012$), whereas no other difference was statistically significant.

These results are consistent with the findings of the investigation stated before. Domestic violence and other types of IPV are more prevalent when women are more prepared to accept punishment and men are more likely to administer it. This is the result of a societal paradigm that legitimises the act of spanking women for failing to satisfy their husbands' expectations or for refusing to comply with them. This occurs because of a sociocultural paradigm that legitimises the spanking of women. A lower level of education among women and the existence of domestic violence in either the husband's or wife's family of origin have both been demonstrated to increase the risk that a woman may become a victim. According to research, the existence of these two variables raises the probability of becoming a victim.

4.4.6 Marriage Type

Regarding the victims with a polygamist father, since the data do not follow a normal distribution, a Mann-Whitney U test was performed to find out whether or not women whose fathers were polygamists were more likely to experience domestic abuse than women whose fathers were monogamists. This was done because the results of normality tests indicated that the data did not follow a normal distribution. Below is an analysis of the same.

The test indicated that the difference was not statistically significant for negotiation abuse, physical assault, psychological aggression, sexual coercion, injury, and economic abuse with victims who have polygamist or monogamist fathers. For example, the general economic abuse score was U *(*$N_{\text{polygamist father}}=38$, $N_{\text{monogamist father}} = 127$*)* $= 2334$, $z = -.308$, $p = 0.758$ *showed a very small effect size* $r = 0.019$.

Regarding the victims with a polygamist partner, since the data did not follow a normal distribution, Mann-Whitney U tests were carried out to determine whether women who were married to polygamists were more likely to be the victims of domestic violence than women who were married to monogamists. An examination of the same may be found farther down.

The test indicated that the difference was not statistically significant for negotiation abuse, physical assault, psychological abuse, injury, and economic abuse with victims who have a polygamist or monogamist partner. For example, the economic abuse score was $U\ (N_{monogamist\ partner} = 134,\ N_{polygamist\ partner} = 31) = 1965.5,\ z = -.469,\ p = 0.639$ *showed a very small effect size* $r = 0.057$.

A Mann-Whitney test indicated that the sexual coercion general score was greater for those who married a polygamist partner (*Mdn* = 14.00) than for victims who married a monogamist partner (*Mdn* = 7.00), while *A Mann-Whitney U test for sexual coercion was statistically significant,* $U(N_{monogamist\ partner} = 134,\ N_{polygamist\ partner} = 31) = 1534,\ z = -2.287,\ p = 0.022$, *with a small effect size* $r = 0.18$.

A Mann-Whitney test indicated that the minor sexual coercion score was greater for those who married a polygamist partner (Mdn = 8.00) than for victims who married a monogamist partner (Mdn = 3.00), while *A Mann-Whitney U test for* minor *sexual coercion was statistically significant,* $U(N_{monogamist\ partner} = 134,\ N_{polygamist\ partner} = 31) = 1544.5,\ z = -2.252,\ p = 0.024$, *with a small effect size* $r = 0.18$.

Regarding married for the second time, to examine whether women who were married for the second time were more likely to experience domestic abuse than those who had only married once, Mann-Whitney U tests were conducted, since the data were not normally distributed based on normality tests. An analysis of the same is presented below.

The test indicated that the difference was not statistically significant for negotiation abuse, physical assault, psychological abuse, injury, and sexual coercion with victims who have been married either for the first or second time. For example, the physical assault score was $U(N_{first\ marriage} = 146,\ N_{second\ marriage} = 19) = 1171,\ z = -1.105,\ p = 0.269$ *showed very small effect size* $r = 0.07$.

A Mann-Whitney test indicated that the economic abuse score was greater for those who married for a second time (*Mdn* = 9) than for victims who married once (*Mdn* = 8), while *A Mann-Whitney U test for economic abuse was statistically significant,* $U(N_{first\ marriage} = 146,\ N_{second\ marriage} = 19) = 783.5,\ z = -3.08,\ p = 0.002$, *with a small effect size* $r = 0.06$.

A further Mann-Whitney test indicated that the economic sabotage score was greater for those who married for a second time (*Mdn* = 13) than for victims who married once (*Mdn* = 8), while *A Mann-Whitney U test for economic sabotage was statistically significant,* $U(N_{first\ marriage} = 146,\ N_{second\ marriage} = 19) = 800.0,\ z = -3.019,\ p = 0.003$, *with a small effect size* $r = 0.06$.

Regarding the marriage type, to determine whether marriage type increases the chance of abuse, Kruskal Wallis tests were performed, since the data are not normally distributed. For those examples where there was a significant difference, a post hoc comparison of Dunn's test was conducted; details of the results can be found below.

A Kruskal-Wallis H test was performed to explore if marriage type influences the forms of abuse experienced by the victims. A Kruskal Wallis H test showed that there are no statistically significant differences between negotiation abuse, psychological abuse, physical abuse, sexual coercion, and economic abuse in the marriage type group. For example, the economic abuse scores show an insignificant difference with marriage type group H(3) = 3.31, P = 0.345 the effect size nu et squared = 0.024, the score for the arranged marriage group (Mean Rank = 78.66, $n = 91$), the love marriage group (Mean Rank = 82.17, $n = 42$), forced marriage group (Mean Rank = 94, $n = 7$), and consanguineous marriage (Mean Rank = 97.10, $n = 25$).

A further Kruskal walls H test showed a statistically significant difference between a minor injury and marriage type group, H(3) = 13.27, P = 0.004 showed a moderate effect size, eta-squared = 0.232, the scores for the arranged marriage group (Mean Rank = 85.91, $n = 91$), the love marriage group (Mean Rank = 91.94, $n = 42$), the forced marriage group (Mean Rank = 98.07, $n = 7$), and also for consanguineous marriage (Mean Rank = 53.16, $n = 25$).

A post-hoc test using a pairwise comparisons Dunn's test indicated that the null hypothesis is rejected at $p = 0.004$, showing significant differences between the consanguineous marriages group (*Mdn* = 0.00) and with the arranged marriage group (*Mdn* = 2.00) $p = 0.002$. It also showed a significant difference between consanguineous marriage group (*Mdn* = 0.00) and those in love marriage group (*Mdn* = 2.00) $p = 0.001$. Similarly, it showed that there is a significant difference between the consanguineous marriage group (*Mdn* = 0.00) and forced marriage group (*Mdn* = 4.00) $p = 0.002$, while no other statistical difference was found.

4.4.7 Employment, Educational Status and Household Income

Regarding the abuser's employment status, to determine whether the abuser's work situation plays a role in increasing the risk of abuse because the results of the normality tests did not point to the fact that the data follow a normal distribution, Kruskal Wallis tests were carried out. A comprehensive investigation is presented in the following text.

The data (n = 165) were put through a Kruskal Wallis test to investigate the role that the work level of the abuser plays in determining the likelihood of a woman becoming a victim of domestic violence. The findings demonstrated that there was no statistically significant difference between the employment status of the abuser and any of the following forms of abuse: psychological aggression in general, physical assault in general, injury in general, sexual coercion in general, or economic abuse in general. For instance, negotiation abuse in general and the employment status of the abuser on employed (Mean Rank = 84.68, n = 121), unemployed (Mean Rank = 88.23, n = 11), retired (Mean Rank = 57.80, n = 15), and self-employed (Mean Rank = 89.53, n = 18), H (3) = 4.86, $p = 0.182$ showed a very small effect size r = 0.03.

There was no discernible difference between the occupational level of the abuser and any of the following forms of abuse: negotiation abuse, psychological aggression, physical assault, injury, sexual coercion, economic abuse, and economic abuse.

Regarding the victim's employment status, to determine whether victims' employment status is associated with a higher risk of domestic abuse, Kruskal Wallis tests were conducted, since the data are not normally distributed, an analysis of the same is provided below.

A Kruskal Wallis test was conducted on the data ($n = 165$) to examine the influence of the victim's employment status on increasing the likelihood of being abused. The results showed that there was no statistical difference between negotiation abuse, psychological aggression, physical assault, injury, sexual coercion, or economic abuse and the employment status of the victim. For example, the results showed that there was no statistical difference between economic abuse score and victims' employment status, employed (Mean Rank = 85.04, $n = 124$), unemployed (Mean Rank = 78.86, $n = 11$), self-employed (Mean Rank = 91.33, $n = 15$), for being a housewife (Mean Rank = 65.81, $n = 13$), and for the retired (Mean Rank = 28.50, n = 2), H(4) = 5.13, $p = 0.274$ showed a very small effect size r = 0.03.

Regarding the victim's education level, since this data did not follow a normal distribution, Kruskal-Wallis tests were carried out to determine whether the victim's degree of education had any bearing on the risk that they would be abused. In this part, we will examine the same.

An investigation of the relationship between the educational level of the victim and the likelihood that they were abused was carried out using the Kruskal Wallis test, and the sample size was 165. According to the findings, there was not a statistically significant correlation between the educational level of the victims and negotiation abuse, psychological abuse, injury, sexual abuse, or economic abuse. Similarly, there was no correlation between the educational level of the victims and sexual abuse. For example, economic abuse H(3) = 2.07, P = 0.556 showed a very small effect size = 0.01 and education level (high school degree (Mean Rank = 75.37, n = 47), higher education degree (Mean Rank = 82.23, n = 20), Bachelor's degree (Mean Rank = 87.44, n = 91), and less than a high school diploma (Mean Rank = 78.71, n = 7) all had significantly different results.

The findings, when compared with those of other research, demonstrate a correlation between a person's degree of education and their tendency to mistreat their wives.

Regarding the abuser's education level, to find out whether the level of education of the abuser increases the likelihood of domestic abuse, a Kruskal Wallis test was adopted, since the data do not follow normal distribution based on normality test results. For those that showed significant differences, a post hoc test using a pairwise comparison of Dunn's test was carried out. Below is an analysis of the same.

A Kruskal Wallis test was conducted on the data ($n = 165$) to examine the influence of the abuser's educational level on increasing the risk of abusing their life partner. The results showed that there was no statistical difference between negotiation abuse and economic abuse with the educational level of the abuser. For example, economic abuse showed no statistical difference between the abuser's level of education, H(3) = 4.74, P = 0.191 showed a small effect size = 0.03 higher education degree (Mean Rank = 62.84, $n = 16$) and less than a high school diploma (Mean Rank = 78.45, n

= 30), high school degree (Mean Rank = 90.62, $n = 61$), and a Bachelor's degree (Mean Rank = 82.90, $n = 58$).

On the other hand, a Kruskal Wallis test showed that there was a statistically significant difference in severe psychological aggression score between different education levels of the abuser, H(3) = 8.29, P = 0.040 showed a small effect size, with an eta -squared = 0.05 and with high school degree (Mean Rank = 70.60, $n = 61$), higher education degree (Mean Rank = 85.19, $n = 16$), Bachelor's degree (Mean Rank = 86.72, $n = 58$), and with less than a high school diploma (Mean Rank = 99.85, $n = 30$).

A post hoc test using a pairwise comparison of Dunn's test indicated that the null hypothesis is rejected at $p = 0.04$, showing significant differences between the abuser having less than a high school diploma (*Mdn* = 10.00) and those who had completed their high school degree (*Mdn* = 4.00), $p = 0.006$. No other differences were found to be statistically significant.

A Kruskal Wallis test showed that there was a statistically significant difference in General physical assault score, which was affected by the educational level of the abuser, H(3) = 8.94, p = 0.030, the effect was a small, with an eta-squared = 0.057 with a high school degree (Mean Rank = 73.13, $n = 61$), Bachelor's degree (Mean Rank = 80.23, $n = 58$), higher education degree (Mean Rank = 92.53, $n = 16$), and less than a high school diploma (Mean Rank = 103.3, $n = 30$). A post-hoc test using a pairwise comparisons Dunn's test indicated that the null hypothesis is rejected at $p = 0.03$, showing significant differences between abusers who have less than a high school diploma (*Mdn* = 19.50) and those who have completed their high school degree (*Mdn* = 8.00), P = 0.004. No other differences were statistically significant.

There was also a statistically significant difference in the minor physical assault score, which was affected by the educational level of the abuser, H(3) = 8.83, p = 0.032 showed small effect size = 0.077, the score for those with a high school degree (Mean Rank = 73.87, $n = 61$), Bachelor's degree (Mean Rank = 79.40, $n = 58$), higher education degree (Mean Rank = 92.63, $n = 16$), and less than a high school diploma (Mean Rank = 103.4, $n = 30$). A post-hoc test using a pairwise comparisons Dunn's test indicated that the null hypothesis is rejected at P = 0.032, showing significant differences between abusers who have less than a high school diploma (*Mdn* = 13.00) and those who have completed their high school degree (*Mdn* = 5.00), $p = 0.005$. No other differences were statistically significant.

There was also a statistically significant difference in severe physical assault score, which was affected by the educational level of the abuser, H(3) = 7.89, P = 0.048, the effect was small = 0.034, the score for those with high school degree (Mean Rank = 75.34, $n = 61$), Bachelor's degree (Mean Rank = 78.22, $n = 58$), higher education degree (Mean Rank = 94.81, $n = 16$), and less than a high school diploma (Mean Rank = 101.5, $n = 30$). A post-hoc test using a pairwise comparison of Dunn's test showed insignificant differences between abusers who have less than a high school diploma (control group) and those who have completed their high school degree, $p = 0.094$.

A post-hoc test using a pairwise comparisons Dunn's test indicated that the null hypothesis is rejected at $p = 0.048$, showing significant differences between abusers who have less than a high school diploma (*Mdn* = 7.00) and those who have completed their high school degree (*Mdn* = 3.00), $p = 0.012$, as well as between those with less than a high school diploma (*Mdn* = 7.00) and those who completed their bachelor's degree (*Mdn* = 3.00) at $p = 0.028$, while no other differences were statistically significant.

A Kruskal Wallis test showed that there was a statistically significant difference in injury minor score, which was affected by the educational level of the abuser, H(3) = 8.37, P = 0.039, with a significant effect size r = 0.049, the score for those with high school degree (Mean Rank = 72.20, $n = 61$), Bachelor's degree (Mean Rank = 82.60, $n = 58$), higher education degree (Mean Rank = 93.75, $n = 16$), and less than a high school diploma (Mean Rank = 100, $n = 30$).

A post-hoc test using a pairwise comparisons Dunn's test indicated that the null hypothesis is rejected at $p = 0.039$, showing significant differences between abusers who have less than a high school diploma (*Mdn* = 2.00) and those who have completed their high school degree (*Mdn* = 1.00), $p = 0.007$.

A Kruskal Wallis test showed that there was a statistically significant difference in severe sexual coercion score, which is affected by the educational level of the abuser, H(3) = 7.85, P = 0.049, showed small effect size r = 0.210, the score for those with a Bachelor's degree (Mean Rank = 76.70, $n = 58$), with a high school degree (Mean Rank = 77.19, n = 61), higher education degree (Mean Rank = 92.84, $n = 16$), and less than a high school diploma (Mean Rank = 101.75, $n = 30$). A post-hoc test using a pairwise comparisons Dunn's test indicated that the null hypothesis is rejected at P = 0.049, showing significant differences between abusers who have completed their bachelor's degree (*Mdn* = 1.00) and those who have less than a high school diploma (*Mdn* = 4.00) $p = 0.015$, and also for those who have a high school degree (*Mdn* = 2.00) with those who have less than high school diploma (*Mdn* = 4.00), at $p = 0.016$.

Regarding household income, to determine whether income level per year increases the chance of abuse victims may experience, a Kruskal-Wallis test was conducted since the data are not normally distributed. For those that showed some statistical significance, pairwise comparisons of Dunn's tests were performed. An analysis of the same is provided below.

A Kruskal-Wallis H test was performed to explore if household income influences the risk of being abused by a life partner. A Kruskal Wallis H test showed that there was no statistically significant difference between negotiation abuse, psychological abuse, physical abuse, injury, and sexual coercion with the level of household income. For example, physical abuse shows an insignificant difference between the groups of household income per annum, H(3) = 6.08, P = 0.107 showed a small effect size r = 0.035, the score for those with less than 25 k$ household income per annum (Mean Rank = 81.79, $n = 63$), those with less than 100 k$ (Mean Rank = 96.21, $n = 33$), those with less than 150 k$ (Mean Rank = 86.75, $n = 36$), and for those who earn 150 k$ and above (Mean Rank = 68.02, $n = 33$).

Furthermore, a Kruskal Wallis test revealed a significant difference among the level of household income per annum groups affecting the score of economic exploitation, H(3) = 11.3, P = 0.010 showed a small effect size r = 0.069, the score for those with less than 25 k$ household income per annum (Mean Rank = 97.60, $n = 63$), for those with less than 100 k$ (Mean Rank = 80.48, $n = 33$), for those with less than 150 k$ (Mean Rank = 65.99, $n = 36$), and for those who earn 150 k$ and above (Mean Rank = 76.21, $n = 33$).

A post-hoc test using a pairwise comparison of Dunn's test indicated that the null hypothesis is rejected at $p = 0.01$, showing significant differences between those who less than 150 k$ per annum (*Mdn* = 7), with those who earn less than 25 k$ per annum (*Mdn* = 9) $p < 0.01$. Moreover, it also showed a significant difference between those who earn 150 k$ and above and less than 100 k$ respectively (*Mdn* = 8) with those who earn less than 25 k$ per annum (*Mdn* = 9) $p = 0.04$, whereas no other statistical difference was found.

4.4.8 Women's Rights and Roles in Society

Regarding women's belief system, the Attitude Against Women Scale was used to investigate whether or not liberal or conservative ideas are associated with an increased risk of abusive behaviour towards women. If you have a higher score, this shows that your views are more progressive and supportive of feminist causes, whilst a lower score indicates that your views are more conventional and conservative.

The Attitude Towards Women Scale was used to measure victims' beliefs about women's roles in society and how it can lead to a greater risk of being victims of domestic abuse. The scale was administered, and the scores were classified into two categories: high scores indicate pro-feminism and egalitarianism, whereas low scores indicate more traditional attitudes. The purpose of this study was to measure how victims' beliefs about women's roles in society and how it can lead to a greater risk of being victims of domestic abuse. Because the data did not follow the assumptions of normality that are made for data distribution and because the data did not follow the normal distribution, a non-parametric test was explored to accomplish this goal. Therefore, a Spearman rho correlation was carried out to accomplish this goal and to ascertain whether or not the views held by women enhanced their likelihood of being victims of domestic violence. An examination may be found below.

Regarding the descriptive analysis for attitude towards women scale score, the present participants had an average score of 38.55 (standard deviation of 7.44), and 50.9% of them stated that they are more egalitarian and pro-feminist, while 49.1% said that they are conventional and conservative. The total Cronbach's alpha for this experiment including 25 distinct goods was 0.72. Consequently, a high overall score indicates that a person supports equality and liberal thought, while a low total score indicates that a person has more traditional and conservative views.

Regarding the statistical analysis for the attitude towards women scale, Spearman's rank correlation results revealed no significant difference between negotiation abuse and attitude towards women, $r_s(163) = 0.026, p = 0.742$ showed a very small effect size r = 0.974 while the same insignificance was shown between injury, sexual coercion and attitude towards women from victims with a traditional or liberal belief system. However, the results regarding the relationship between psychological aggression and attitude towards women showed a negative and statistically very weak correlation with psychological aggression in general, $r_s(163) = -0.272$, $p < 0.001$ showed a large effect size -0.690 while the same negative and very weak correlation was indicated between minor aggression and attitude towards women $r_s(163) = -0.316$, $p < 0.001$ shows a weak, and negative correlation between the two variables, indicating medium effect size = 0.316.

Results of Spearman's rank correlation indicated that there was a very weak positive and statistical association between severe physical assault and attitude towards women, $r_s(163) = 0.197$, $p = 0.011$ with the effect size = 0.199 while another indicator of Spearman's rank correlation indicated that there was a significant positive association between injury in general and attitude towards women, $r_s(163) = 0.172$, $p = 0.027$ showed a small to moderate effect size = 0.153 Additionally, there was a positive correlation between severe injury and attitude towards women, $r_s(163) = 0.280$, $p < 0.001$showed large effect size = 0.290 Furthermore, the results of the Spearman's rank correlation indicated that there was a positive and very weak association between severe sexual coercion and attitude towards women, $r_s(163) = 0.186$, $p = 0.01$ shows moderate effect size = 0.186.

To account for the fact that the data do not follow a normal distribution, Mann-Whitney U tests were carried out. A comprehensive investigation is presented in the following.

A Mann-Whitney U test *indicated that the difference was not statistically significant for negotiation abuse, physical assault, and economic abuse with victims who scored having more liberal or conservative attitudes and beliefs. For example, the general economic abuse score was* $U(N_{\text{egalitarian and more liberal}} = 84, N_{\text{traditional and conservative}} = 81) = 3391.5$, $z = -.03$, $p = 0.972$, *with a small effect size* $r = 0.0017$.

A Mann-Whitney test indicated that the severe sexual coercion score was greater for victims who held traditional and conservative beliefs (Mdn = 4.00) than for victims who held more egalitarian and liberal beliefs (Mdn = 0.500), *while A Mann-Whitney U test for severe sexual coercion was statistically significant,* $U(N_{\text{egalitarian and more liberal}} = 84, N_{\text{traditional and conservative}} = 81) = 2821$, $z = -1.976$, $p = 0.040$, *with a small effect size* $r = 0.15$.

A Mann-Whitney test indicated that the severe injury score was greater for victims who held traditional and conservative beliefs (*Mdn* = 4.00) than for victims who held more egalitarian and liberal beliefs (*Mdn* = 0.00), while *A Mann-Whitney U test for severe injury was statistically significant,* $U(N_{\text{egalitarian and more liberal}} = 84, N_{\text{traditional and conservative}} = 81) = 2599$, $z = -2.718$, $p = 0.007$, *with a small effect size* $r = 0.20$.

A Mann-Whitney test indicated that the psychological aggression general score was greater for those who held more egalitarian and liberal beliefs (*Mdn* = 53.00) than for victims who held traditional and conservative beliefs (*Mdn* = 31.00), while *A Mann-Whitney U test for psychological aggression general score was statistically significant,* $U(N_{\text{egalitarian and more liberal}} = 84, N_{\text{traditional and conservative}} = 81) = 2543$, $z = -2.801$, $p = 0.005$, *with a small effect size* $r = 0.22$.

A further Mann-Whitney test indicated that the minor psychological aggression score was greater for those who held more egalitarian and liberal beliefs (*Mdn* = 39.00) than for victims who held traditional and conservative beliefs (*Mdn* = 19.00), *while A Mann-Whitney U test for psychological aggression general score was statistically significant,* $U(N_{\text{egalitarian and more liberal}} = 84, N_{\text{traditional and conservative}} = 81) = 2537$, $z = -2.82$, $p = 0.005$, *with a small effect size* $r = 0.22$.

The results of the tests in this chapter provide several important findings which will be interpreted and explained at a later stage in the discussion chapter. As a follow-up to these quantitative results, the next chapter presents a qualitative analysis of the collected data. This will offer a more in-depth understanding of the participant experience and will help illuminate the research questions.

The correlation and differences between the sociodemographic parameters and the results were analysed in light of the sociodemographic characteristics of the study population that are significantly associated with different types of domestic abuse. Based on the analysis, the following key findings emerged: Age differences between husband and wife, with a 10-year cutoff, age at the time of marriage, pregnant women, pregnancy loss, the family of origin violence among female victims, husbands who witness their father abusing their mother, victims with a polygamous partner, women who are married for a second time, husbands' educational level, annual household income, and marriage type were found to be significantly associated with various forms of abuse. The current results indicate that an increase in the number of children is related to an increase in sexual coercion. Fertility, the abuser's job position, the abuser's employment status, and victim's employment status and the victim's education level were not significantly associated with types of abuse in the sample group.

References

Caicedo-Roa, M., Da Veiga Pereira, T., & Carlos Cordeiro, R. (2020). PROTOCOL: Risk factors for femicide. *Campbell Systematic Reviews, 16*(4), e1123, 1–12. https://doi.org/10.1002/cl2.1123

Castro, H. M., & Ferreira, J. C. (2023). Linear and logistic regression models: When to use and how to interpret them? *Jornal Brasileiro De Pneumologia: publicacao oficial da Sociedade Brasileira de Pneumologia e Tisilogia, 48*(6), e20220439. https://doi.org/10.36416/1806-3756/e20220439

Chan, Y. H. (2003). Biostatistics 102: Quantitative data - Parametric & non-parametric tests. *Singapore Medical Journal, 44*(8), 391–396. http://www.smj.org.sg/sites/default/files/4408/4408bs1.pdf

Ernst, A. F., & Albers, C. J. (2017). Regression assumptions in clinical psychology research practice - A systematic review of common misconceptions. *PeerJ, 2017*(5), 1–16. https://doi.org/10.7717/peerj.3323

Esie, P., Osypuk, T. L., Schuler, S. R., & Bates, L. M. (2019). SSM - population health intimate partner violence and depression in rural Bangladesh: Accounting for violence severity in a high prevalence setting. *SSM – Population Health, 7*(August 2018), 100368. https://doi.org/10.1016/j.ssmph.2019.100368

Heise, L. L. (1998). Violence against women: An integrated, ecological framework. *Violence Against Women, 4*(3), 262–290. https://doi.org/10.1177/1077801298004003002

Lakens, D. (2013). Calculating and reporting effect sizes to facilitate cumulative science: A practical primer for t-tests and ANOVAs. *Frontiers in Psychology, 4*, 863. https://doi.org/10.3389/fpsyg.2013.00863

Li, X., Wong, W., Lamoureux, E. L., & Wong, T. Y. (2012). Are linear regression techniques appropriate for analysis when the dependent (outcome) variable is not normally distributed? *Investigative Ophthalmology & Visual Science, 53*(6), 3082–3083. https://doi.org/10.1167/iovs.12-9967

Lumley, T., Diehr, P., Emerson, S., & Chen, L. (2002). The importance of the normality assumption in large public health data sets. *Annual Review of Public Health, 23*, 151–169. https://doi.org/10.1146/annurev.publhealth.23.100901.140546

McLeod, S. (2019). *What does effect size tell you?*. Simply Psychology https://www.simplypsychology.org/effect-size.html

Siegel, S. Y. (2012). Non parimetric tests statistics. *The American Statistician, 11*(3), 13–19. http://www.jstor.org/stable/2685679

Song, Y. Y., & Lu, Y. (2015). Decision tree methods: Applications for classification and prediction. *Shanghai Archives of Psychiatry, 27*(2), 130–135. https://doi.org/10.11919/j.issn.1002-0829.215044

Uyanık, G. K., & Güler, N. (2013). A study on multiple linear regression analysis. *Procedia - Social and Behavioral Sciences, 106*, 234–240. https://doi.org/10.1016/j.sbspro.2013.12.027

Chapter 5
Narratives of Domestic Abuse Against Women

This chapter follows on from the previous quantitative chapter which examined the prevalence of different forms of domestic abuse and how it affects their mental health and how might put them at risk of homicide, and other risk factors that influence their victimization. The previous chapter has also outlined how the attitude towards women emerged from the victims' perspective. The primary purpose of this chapter was to gain a deeper comprehension of the findings by making use of quantitative data, to provide an explanation for the findings, and to offer support for the findings by increasing understanding of the forms of domestic violence that are experienced by women in Qatar and why they are not leaving the abusive relationship. Determine whether social context and societal aspects influence participants' decisions to remain passive in an abusive relationship.

Qatari women were voluntarily recruited from the quantitative phase who have experienced or have been exposed to a variety of kinds of abuse took part in the research study. Participants in the qualitative study were twenty Qatari women ranging in age from 24 to 55 years old and have either a married or divorced status at the time of the interview. In addition, they disclosed whether or not they were now employed, unemployed, housewives, or married to a partner who was either monogamous or polygamous.

The present chapter presents the findings from thematic analysis which was employed on participants' narratives who experienced intimate partner violence. To produce a more accurate transcription and remove repetition, the Intelligent Verbatim Transcription method was employed (Preece & Williams, 2017).

From the thematic analysis, four themes were identified for further analysis about the research questions which were represented with underpinning codes supported by participants' quotations. In this analysis, step-by-step thematic approaches by Braun and Clarke (2006) were employed in which the participants' narratives were openly coded (Table 5.1).

Patterns were identified in the data, codes were developed to capture these patterns, and then themes were grouped based on the codes. The themes were reviewed and

K. Al-Naama, *Domestic Abuse and Mental Health in Qatar*, Gulf Studies 23,
https://doi.org/10.1007/978-981-96-7392-6_5

Table 5.1 Description of Analytical steps as per

Steps	
Familiarizing yourself with your data	In this stage, intelligent verbatim was employed equally to all transcripts and read several times to get a deeper understanding of the content.
Generating initial codes	Repetitive patterns concerning meaningful themes were identified as an initial reflection by developing an initial label or code.
Searching for themes	Cods were divided into themes and sub-themes to find patterns and relevance to the topic of investigation and group them into one theme as fit.
Reviewing themes	Critically reviewing all themes against each excerpt, those with similarities were identified as core themes, and a final review was conducted to ensure all codes were captured and adjusted to make them fit.
Defining and naming themes	Core themes were identified and represented using relevant and representative names that define each theme clearly to give meaningful information about the research questions.
Producing the report	Coherent and engaging themes were created for the analysis phase.

Sources: Braun and Clarke (2006)

refined to make sure they accurately reflected the data (see Table 5.1 for more description), even a single statement was reviewed it considered a common opinion across all participants or if it represents a self-opinion. Data analysis was based on these emerging themes and the significance of these statements was closely examined. Participants' views were represented by unique numbers representing each participant's views to protect their identity (participant 1). Five themes were identified for further analysis as it seems relevant to the study objectives: (1) Types and Pattern of Abuse, (2) Impact of Intimate Partner violence on mental and physical health, (3) Risk factor for victimization, (4) leaving an abusive relationship, (5) Bureaucracy and Post Separation abuse (Table 5.2).

The interview protocol and guide were pre-defined by semi-structured open questions, which helped enrich the discussion about the proposed questions and gave the researcher control over the discussion process (Kvale & Brinkmann, 2009). In this questionnaire, introductory questions focused on intimate partner violence in general and how respondents felt about it, probing questions were asked of them, and they were encouraged to expound on those topics further and asked them to illustrate what they meant by their response (See Appendix 10).

By asking the responder, "Can you tell me some of the things you remember about this situation?" the second question enabled the participant to recollect some information about their own experience with an abusive spouse. Could you please explain? The questions that followed were designed to get an understanding of how a person reacts when their spouse displays an aggressive attitude towards them and how it makes a person feel.

Table 5.2 Thematic Analysis

Themes	Underlying Cods	Participants Quotes
1. Types and Patterns of Abuse	Psychological, Physical, neglect, injuries, and emotional Abuse. Economic abuse during marriage and post marriage	He is a very aggressive person; he shows no respect to me in front of my children and sometimes when he gets upset, he damages the TV and anything in front of him. He beat me and threw things at me, trying to hurt me, he does not leave marks on me and when I talk to his family, they said I complain too much. (Participant 2) In addition to physically and psychologically abusing me, he failed to keep his promise that he would treat both of [co-wives] us equally. (Participant 6)
2. Impact of Intimate Partner violence on mental and physical health	PTSD, depression, anxiety, hopelessness, sad, lonely	My stress level is unbearable. I am so anxious and in deep pain. I still cannot believe what happened, and I was shocked when I found out he married a second wife one week after our divorce took place. (Participant 8)
3. Risk factors for victimization	Husband and wife socioeconomic status, age at marriage, age disparity between husband and wife	I am almost alone. He barely talks to me and does not pay me anything. I stay with him because he is a good father but a bad husband. My brother and mother support me financially. (Participant 11)
4. Leaving an abusive relationship	Divorce types, husband manipulation, social stigma, Personal Autonomy, family and social, rights,	I was told by my parents that the divorce condition is unbearable in our family. I must save my marriages regardless of the sacrifices that I have to make. (Participant 11) When a divorced mother wants to remarry again her child custody rights by default will shift to her ex-husbands. That's why most women will prefer to remain single and preserve their child custody rights. (Participant 1)
5. Bureaucracy and Post Separation abuse	Financial settlement, child custody, Family law, Welfare Bureaucracy Court prolongs procedure	I think the current child custody procedure is another limitation of personal freedom. I always I must chase my husband in the court to maintain the post-divorce payments. (Participant 17) I think the court procedure is very long, especially when it involves child custody arrangements. (Participant 11)

Due to the delicate nature of the subject matter, these questions were posed in a way that included probes and warnings to reduce the likelihood that the interviewee might have a traumatic flashback while it was still ongoing. Following the introductory questions. The second format of questions was presented to discuss the research questions and to make comments whenever possible. To grasp the source of the abusive behaviours and to obtain the victim's perceptions: "What do you think caused you to suffer this kind of abuse? Please elaborate". When confronted with the question, "Are there any particular reasons why you have not acted to stop or leave the abuser?" I have made the argument that some women may choose to stay inactive in response to the inquiry. After that, the participants were questioned on social and economic hurdles by having them answer the following question: "What were some difficulties, if any, that you have encountered?" If the response did not make itself clear, an investigation into the financial element of the matter was carried out by asking the following question: "To clarify: do you mean that you have financial links that prohibit you from being independent?". They were asked about the effect of IPV on them by asking the following question: What physical or emotional symptoms have you experienced since the violent incident? Furthermore, they were asked if their partner's behaviour during pregnancy had negatively impacted their emotional or physical well-being. In addition, Participants were commenting on the quantitative findings and provided better insight and explanations of the situation of IPV in Qatar.

The final questions were designed to summarize the topics discussed with the participants and to allow them to add additional information before the interview was concluded (Krueger & Casey, 2009). To get further information from them about the primary concern that made them feel uneasy. "Is there anything else you would want to add?" was the last question directed at the participants in order to guarantee that all research topics were covered. Participants were invited to remark on some of the results from the qualitative research. During the concluding comments, the researcher briefed them on the last step that was required before their screenplay could be approved. They were told that the researcher would analyse the information that they supplied, and if they were interested, they were allowed to have a copy of the analysis sent to them through email (see Appendix 10).

5.1 Findings from Thematic Analyses

5.1.1 Theme 1: Types, Patterns of Abuse, and Risk of Homicide

Throughout the course of the investigation, broad themes emerged and were then connected straightforwardly to the theoretical underpinnings of the research questions. This was supported by the findings from the quantitative questionnaire, which dealt with the types of abuse experienced by female victims and how their experience influences their decision to leave or stay in an abusive relationship. The findings of the questionnaire provided evidence for this assertion. The following themes emerged across all of the participants: Table 5.3 illustrates how the analysis has been carried over to these themes. The identified themes have been supported by some quotations from excerpts. (1) Types and Patterns of Abuse, (2) Impact of Intimate Partner Violence on mental and physical health, (3) Risk factor for victimization, (4) leaving an abusive relationship and (5) Bureaucracy and Post Separation abuse.

These findings arguably provide us with a more comprehensive understanding of the nature of domestic abuse that occurs in Qatari culture. According to responses from 50% of the people surveyed, psychological aggression is the kind of domestic violence that occurs most often against women. The findings from the quantitative research point to a wide range of abusive conduct in the home. There was a mean score of 29.86 for abusive negotiation, a mean score of 53.71 for psychological aggression, a mean score of 30.49 for abusive physical assault, and a mean score of 15.80 for abusive sexual coercion. The mean score on the economic abuse sub-scale is 32.34, which indicates that there are significant instances of economic exploitation.

The participants were made aware of these statistics, but they did not seem to be astonished by the idea that psychological abuse is the most common kind of domestic violence. This is because psychological abuse may present itself in ways that are not audible. Take, for instance, what one of the participants had Described her experiences with abuse, stating that "I was cut off from everyone. He limited my social network, was jealous and beat me up if I talk to any man. I was forced to leave my house when he got married to a second wife" (Participant 1).

Another participant had an alternative viewpoint of the many types of physical violence, which may take covert manifestations, which makes it very challenging to report this form of violence since it does not leave any traces. There is a tendency for abusers to limit their wives' access to social networks to ensure they are incapable of getting adequate help to resolve or end abuse. Another participant outlined how social isolation was a common practice that she endured while living with her abusive husband. According to her, evaluating the cause of the divorce, which could be related to psychological abuse, is crucial.

Table 5.3 Emergent Theme and Research Questions

Research Questions	Themes addressing the question
Is there anything you can tell me about the types of abuse you have suffered?	Theme (1): Types and Pattern of Abuse
What impact has abuse had on your physical and mental health?	Theme (2): Consequences of intimate partner violence
Why do these factors make victims more likely to be victimized, and how do they contribute?	Theme (3): Risk factor for victimization
Why would women remain passive in an abusive relationship?	Theme (4): leaving an abusive relationship.

> I still do not find it shocking that women are psychologically abused by their partners, due to the high divorce rate. My husband used to intimidate and call me names. He leaves me alone most of the time and he is very stingy. (Participant 3)

When analysing responses to this kind of abuse in marriage, it is essential to have a solid understanding of the complexities of psychological aggression and its effects on the health and wellness of women. One of the participants draw attention to comprehending how psychological abuse emerged in marriage based on her personal experience with an abusive spouse, she said,

> I think it is all a form of unpleasant behaviour that controls women's freedom. For example, he [her husband] always puts me down, he does not want me to dress well and does not go outside with me. I just have to stay at home, serve his needs and take care of the children. He only talks to me in front of our kids, but whenever we are alone, he never talks to me and avoids eye contact. If he needs something he calls the housemaid and he asks me to live in a separate room. (Participant 4)

Most participants claimed that psychological abuse was the most prevalent kind of domestic violence they had experienced or heard about. Moreover, there was a sense of concern amongst the interviewees about their autonomy which was an issue that broaden the discussion.

> He was abusing me psychologically, trying to control everything I do since he admitted his impotence. He follows me everywhere, embarrasses me in front of my colleagues at work, questions my faithfulness and loyalty to him, and always makes fun of me. He is very jealous and suspicious of everyone, and he became violent whenever I asked him if we should separate. (Participant 5)

Another participant concurred that limiting social life is another form of psychological abuse exerted by men. Arguably, some might be hesitant to share their experience because people tend to undermine emotional abuse, consider them less serious and sometimes might be neglectful:

> It depends on what you determine to be psychological abuse. My husband said I don't want you to work, I just want to see you staying at home, but it turns out he intentionally limited my social life, and I was even prevented from visiting my friends and relatives. In my opinion, this goes beyond psychological abuse as you describe. (Participant 7)

In another interview, when asked about why domestic abuse is pervasive and goes unreported like many other forms of abuse, said:

> In our culture, they don't acknowledge this form of abuse [emotional abuse], therefore no one questions men about this attitude and the simple response to those who complain would be this is all because you [victim's attitude] don't know how to talk to your husband in a good manner. (Participant 1)

Similar accounts were shared by several respondents about psychological abuse and other forms of violence that disrupt family members. Economic abuse extends beyond the norms and traditions of breadwinner duty. This is incredibly difficult to define and defies the concept that the primary breadwinner in the family should handle the family's spending. The following excerpt is extracted from one participant's narrative that shared her experience with domestic abuse.

> Can you imagine that? My husband used to give me only 100 QR per month but he pays for all the house and children's expenses. Bear in mind, I am an unemployed wife. My mother is the one who supports me financially and pays for my children's education fees. (Participant 10)

When asked to elaborate more on psychological abuse and how or when it occurs, one participant indicated that males in Arabic culture dislike being questioned about their financial choices. The stability of the family was of particular concern to her, even if it might provoke an angry reaction from him, said:

> He does not like anyone to question his decisions, he always has to be right. I cannot let him do that because he spends our money on infeasible investments, which always come to a loss. Then he controls what is left of our money to close his debts. (Participant 2)

There was a recurring theme in the interviews that showed half of the participants felt financial abuse manifested in a variety of situations. This was probably culturally influenced. Moreover, the Kruskal Wallis test revealed a significant difference between family income per year groups in terms of economic exploitation. This involves a wife using credit cards or spending frivolous money. This finding is echoed in the study's questionnaire results. For example, one interviewee commented on economic abuse and how it may influence other forms of aggressive action as it surfaced mainly in relation to the importance of looking rich. She states:

> My husband wants to show off and pretend that he is rich, especially when it comes to his social image. As I told you, I used to pay for his hunting trips [hunting by falcon]. I stopped doing that because I cannot afford it anymore and he got married to another wealthy wife. (Participant 9)

The most significant challenge for another respondent is to maintain and meet the needs of her children. Stating that:

> He's very stingy with his money. He never gives me money or spends it on our children. I always have to buy things with my salary until I have nothing left. I must chase him down for groceries. It's so hard to live that way. (Participant 8)

The theme of economic and psychological abuse recurred repeatedly throughout the dataset and respondents' narratives. Abusers' main concern to continue this relationship with their partner was to maintain full control over financial assets, bank accounts and property. The following excerpt illustrates how she was struggling to gain her legitimate rights over her inheritance. She asked about the various forms of domestic abuse that she had been through., stated:

> I was forced to give him an authorized bank order, so when I felt unsafe and a substantial amount was missing from my bank account, I deactivate the authorization [authorization to approve any financial transaction without getting the accounts owner's approval]. He yelled and shouted at me and when I reminded him that it is my right to keep my inheritance, he beat me up till he broke one of my ribs and I lost consciousness. (Participant 19)

Regarding the risk of femicide, this conversation sheds light on the fact that some women face physical danger at the hands of their husbands when the two of them get into heated disagreements. This brings attention to the results of the assessment of the possible risk of harm that is present inside an abusive relationship. The present findings from the danger assessment scale results had a somewhat lower score, which does not elicit worries that they are at a larger risk of femicide. In the interview data, even if the minority mentioned injuries carefully and barely touched the subject, issues regarding murder risk were not overwhelmingly prevalent.

Participants were asked to remark on whether they believe there is a possibility that they may be killed by their spouse, talking about this issue an interviewee said, "Certainly not. He knows [her husband] that my family would not tolerate any form of physical abuse, so imagine what would happen if he threatened to murder me" (Participant 13).

Another participant highlighted that Arabic culture disparages husbands who use their physical ability to displace their wives and stated that Arabic culture does not consider physical violence to be a masculine measure. In another interview, when asked if the risk of homicide is relatively low based on the quantitative findings, an interviewee said, "I don't think he dares to physically beat me. He knows that legal measures are taken seriously regarding any physical violence, especially when it comes to women and children" (Participant 4).

The data presented here provide credence to research of this kind that evaluates the participants' possible exposure to the risk of murder. The current investigation illustrates how the reported scale suggests that the risk of murder is low according to the scoring manual, which goes from feeling danger to terrible danger.

The next section of the qualitative findings will elaborate on the mental and physical lifelong consequences of IPV. This theme was a major concern of investigation in the present study. This theme was evident throughout the participants' narratives.

5.1.2 Theme (2): Consequences of Intimate Partner Violence

This theme was derived from a qualitative analysis of the impact of domestic violence on women's mental health. This analysis shows a broad range of devastating impacts on women's mental and physical well-being, particularly pregnancy complications. As victims' experiences are explored, it becomes clear that many had elevated symptoms of PTSD, depression, and anxiety. The participants discussed the potentially stressful circumstances that could arise for women if they decided to report the abuse to healthcare providers. Regarding the mental health and form of abuse, as a victim of intimate partner abuse, women feel frightened, stressed, and sad while deciding whether to remain or leave. Participants noted this. They say this might cause unpleasant sentiments and harm their health.

In one interview, one interviewee was asked what physical or emotional symptoms she had experienced since the violent incident. According to her:

> I don't have confidence anymore. When he just divorced me without even stating his opinion, I feel a pain in my chest [depressed], afraid that no one would like me anymore [no one would marry her again]. I don't want to stay alone I am so depressed. (Participant 14)

Many issues were identified in this theme. One of the study participants shared her perspective on intimate partner violence's consequences, shedding light on the multi-faceted nature of this issue. She said:

> It's so hard to understand how painful the divorce experience is. It drains your energy and your soul. My family tried hard to fix this situation [he left her and never called her back or answered her phone calls]. I am confused and I cry when I used to be alone. I don't want to show this weakness to my children. (Participant 4)

Several findings from the interviews indicate that depression and anxiety were common among victims of intimate partner violence, with many reporting persistent symptoms and a negative effect on the quality of life. According to one participant, she was trying to scarify and save her marriage, which was considered painful psychologically. She said:

> I tried to reconcile with him to save our marriage, but he refused because I stopped him from abusing me emotionally by having an affair with someone else many times over the years. It's so hard to stay alone after so many years of marriage, I think nobody can understand how depressed I am. Even my parents always say to me that I have to adapt to this situation [live with him] but they cannot understand what it is like to be trapped with someone whom you are not allowed to have a normal conversation with. (Participant 4)

All things considered; participants' perspectives indicate that victims of intimate partner violence are significantly more likely to suffer from psychological complications as a result of their experiences. A number of issues were identified in one of the interviews about her concern even when the abuse end, she said:

> I want to save my marriage, even if he is married to another woman, I am so sad and desperate, but I want to raise my kids with their fathers. I don't feel safe, and I cannot go back to my parents' house as there is not enough space for us. (Participant 8)

The trauma of post-divorce has affected women's self-sense of reality among those who did not want to get divorced. Women encounter fears of family rejection, and the community ostracizes them, which complicates the leaving process since staying with an abusive husband is psychologically and physically extremely destructive. Among the participants, one further supported this theme by sharing their own experience of feeling hopeless, she said:

> I received a text message saying that you are divorced. I fainted, and I don't know why, it was a shock for everyone. Our life was quite normal, with no heated arguments at all. I cried so much, and I don't feel I am well anymore. I tried to remember what I did to deserve this punishment; he disappeared suddenly. (Participant 14)

In light of the emergence of this theme, which was supported by several excerpts, it is imperative to recognize IPV's systemic nature and its effect on women's mental health. One of the participants also commented on how mentally distressful they become when no one understands their complaints about not being able to talk to their husband and have a normal couple conversation.

> Sometimes even you cannot explain it well, it is deep sadness. For example, if he needs anything he ignores me and makes requests from our housemaid. He never requests anything from me. We live like two strangers. I am depressed and disappointed that he does not want to sort this situation out. I mean, he is my husband by name only. (Participant 17).

As part of the current theme, there is also considerable concern concerning the profound effects of intimate partner violence on the lives of victims. This is particularly in the context of newly formed marriages. Some felt that they cannot continue this marriage anymore while others became mentally unwell, they stated:

> I am overthinking at night; it's like being trapped in a nightmare. I cannot fall asleep easily, I am anxious and worried about my future. I don't want to stay alone, and I cannot imagine that he [her husband] is living with his new wife. (Participant 18)

> I cannot continue with him anymore. I am deeply injured from inside [emotionally]. For six years I prayed every day that he is going to change and treat us equally [herself and his new wife]. I am on medication now to treat my symptoms [depression and anxiety] and this has developed when I was shocked by knowing that he married a second wife and I saw how my mother struggled when my dad did it [polygamous father]. (Participant 16)

> We decided to marry, and I became his second wife, but things started to fall apart when he was not able to balance both of our rights and he was not able to manage the needs of both of our families [his first wife and I] I feel so sad. (Participant 20)

She reported that her husband's use of reproductive control to exert control over her while having intimate relationship may undermine their capacity to be future mothers. She felt undermined and anxious, which was consistent with the current theme. She said:

> I cannot forget him; he was everything in my life. We married for two years only, and it seems to me he was already planning [to divorce her]. He used protection during intimate relationship, and now I understand that he did not want to get me pregnant because it is easy for him to divorce me, I am so depressed. (Participant 22)

Another participant held high hope that these violent acts are temporary, and things might get better. Recurring issues emerged from the participants' narratives interplay between being unable to act to stop violence and how they are mentally suffering and being deeply concerned which is in line with the majority of the participants, One participant commented on why she was feeling down and worried about the negative experience of being trapped with an abusive partner, she said, "I feel down most of the time, but still, I love him so much and I believe that he is going to change in the future" (Participant 12).

A significant and distressing theme emerged from the current analysis of the interview data concerning the impact of intimate partner violence on mental health. A wide range of uncomfortable feelings, including depression, anxiety, PTSD, and insomnia, were reported by most participants, general trends and patterns were identified across participants' narratives that may provide an important insight into the prevalence impact of domestic abuse on women's mental health and the complex nature of experiences that have been shared by the participants. The following are two examples of different excerpts from different participants:

> Out of the blue, he decided to divorce me and to leave as a bachelor for no apparent reason, travelling around the word, leaving us [herself and her kids] alone. I am so depressed and emotionally confused, I picture him everywhere in our house. I tried everything to change his mind to save our marriage. (Participant 10)

> I still cannot get his voice out of my head, after intimate relationship, he always said 'I don't know how you are going to mother my children' [he undermined her capacity as a mother

> sarcastically]. I asked him to divorce me. I cannot bear his negative remarks about the way I look or what I wear, I lose confidence in myself. I am scared to get married again. (Participant 5)

Participants offered insight into the psychological and emotional impact of domestic violence by sharing their experiences. Another revealing observation emerging from this theme is that several informants shared their experiences of domestic abuse during pregnancy. They were asked if their partner's behaviour during pregnancy had negatively impacted their emotional or physical well-being. A variety of perspectives were discussed.

> I cannot believe I lost my pregnancy to him. Three years have passed since the incident, and I still cannot forgive him. I feel deeply hurt and very shaken. (Participant 20)

> Can you imagine that? I had lost my pregnancy when he attacked me physically. Instead of showing regret or even giving a simple apology for what he has done, he threatened to divorce me if I told the truth to the hospital staff. I kept quiet to save my marriage. (Participant 7)

> As a mother with two kids and an employee, I have asked him if he can hire a housemaid to help me. I am currently pregnant. Rather than helping me, he divorced me; this was not the first time. (Participant 8)

The findings of the current study provide crucial new insights into how the husbands of a very tiny percentage of women who had had a miscarriage abused their wives. These adverse health outcomes include pregnancy miscarriages, low childbirth rates, and premature delivery. When asked about her experience with abuse during pregnancy, an interviewee shared:

> I was in my second month of pregnancy, and I had argued with my husband on the street. He shouted at me as we stood next to our car. When he locked the passenger door, I couldn't open it. Then he drove the car as I ran after him, and he stopped at the traffic light and opened the door to let me in. After we arrived at our house, I started bleeding; he called the ambulance, but it was too late [I lost the foetus]. (Participant 6)

Consequently, the replies of the participants were compatible and supported the present theme, which was supported by the quantitative data, namely that there is a strong connection between pregnancy loss and severe psychological hostility. In addition, recent research revealed that psychological aggressiveness and economic control were the frequent risk factors throughout pregnancy. The findings may offer meaningful insights into the factors involved in pregnancy loss. A handful of the people who took part in the study expressed concern that if they told healthcare providers about their experiences with miscarriage, it may make their marriage more difficult or perhaps end it altogether.

Through their stories and experiences, participants provide insight into the often-hidden impact of domestic abuse on women's mental and physical health. Various risk factors associated with domestic violence victimization emerged as a major focus of the third theme. As a result, the researcher was able to explore and understand the factors that contribute to domestic violence victimisation.

5.1.3 Theme 3: Risk Factor for Victimization

A broader discussion of the various factors associated with victimization was generated by this theme. The questionnaire data suggests that a high number of women are at increased risk of IPV victimization based on their husband's socioeconomic status. This in turn highlights the level of understanding among the participants, who observed that the abuser's education level has an impact on influencing forms of abuse against women. When asked about the socioeconomic status of the husbands and how it may contribute to the risk of victimization, an interviewee said :

> My husband depends on me financially. I take care of our living expenses; his salary cannot cover our life expenses since he did not complete his high school degree. He decided to get a second wife to meet his financial needs, which are mainly his leisure activities, such as hunting trips. (Participant 9)

On the other hand, the assumption was made that the victims' employment status increased their risk factor of being abused, which is not a condition among the participants. The excerpt below suggests that the study has identified specific contexts or situations that are particularly relevant to the experiences and perspectives of participants. In turn, this may provide meaningful insight into the contributors to IPV. Family structure in Arabic culture might play a significant role in victims' lives, thereby changing how these factors are addressed. Families support their daughters after marriage in order to save their marriage when it does not fulfil the financial needs of their husbands.

> Many times, I tried to remind him about the good moments, but still, after 15 years of marriage, my husband insisted on the divorce and threatened to cut me off Nafaqa [financial support paid after divorce for a certain period] whenever I asked him to visit his children. He does not want to see them anymore. My mother is taking care of mine and my children's living expenses. (Participant 10)

The participant quotations above are corroborated by a larger spectrum of financial abuse that is substantially linked to economic exploitation and annual family income. Participants shared the belief that, following divorce, men do not always fulfil their parental responsibilities. In most situations, men seek custody of their children as an emotional retaliation against their spouses which will be covered by the next theme.

According to the current findings, earlier research has revealed that socioeconomic status differences between husband and wife might have a detrimental impact on domestic violence. Another response to this question was made by another participant highlighting the importance of the educational factor between couples, stated that:

> I think that education variance between husband and wife has a huge impact on communication style. My husband only has a secondary school degree. I cannot discuss any topic with him without having a big fight. If he does not like anything, he will simply start to yell at me or leaves the room. (Participant 1)

The issue of husband-wife social status was determined by the many perspectives expressed by the participants about the causes of abuse and the way cultural norms and traditions may impact marital status. According to the findings of the survey, the victim's degree of education does not influence whether they would become a victim of domestic abuse. On the other side, the husband's degree of education significantly influences whether he would use domestic violence as a kind of coercive control to reprimand his wife or behave violently towards them.

One of the participants, for instance, discussed the logic of why a person's social position may have an impact on the relationship between a husband and wife. This comment suggests that some husbands have reservations about their wives' competence to operate and manage the family's financial commitments and assets.

> I know for sure that he loves me, but he always undermines my capacity as a productive woman whenever it comes to a major decision in the family. He simply says that I know nothing about life, and he knows everything, even though I have a higher degree and he does not, but I think it is all about being threatened by the possibility that I could be independent. (Participant 1)

Another participant also noted that some husbands might feel insecure when their wife pursues higher education, this statement highlights the importance of identifying them. One informant explicitly refers to feeling insecure as a reason for her husband's aggressive attitude. Stating that:

> To be honest with you, I am so disappointed. Whenever it comes to pursuing my higher education he always [her husband] tries to put me down and reminds me about my duties as a wife towards him and my children. (Participant 7)

In line with other participants' experiences, when the spouse has a lesser level of education, these remarks illustrate the stress that women may have while attempting to become more independent by gaining additional credentials. One participant described:

> He is an uneducated person [secondary school], very hostile and manipulative and so jealous that I have a well-paid job. One day in the middle of the night, my baby woke up crying for milk. He started [her husband] to yell at me and threw things. I ran out of the room with my baby to try to protect him; he was going crazy almost going to hit him [baby]. (Participant 2)

Another element that emerged from the narratives of the participants included in this theme (and was corroborated by the results of the questionnaire) was that second-time-married women are more likely to suffer economic abuse and economic sabotage. Participants were invited to expound on this result, and their responses are consistent with prior studies on second marriages. Many participants described how they have to hide their feelings due to family pressure and other complications associated with being married for the second time, for example:

> I don't want to get a negative influence from my parents, especially as this was my second marriage. I proceeded with a divorce without telling my family because they would force me to continue with him no matter how bad he is, because of the shame associated with a second marriage divorce. (Participant 13)
>
> In a second marriage, the woman has to give away a lot of her right to have a normal life. I have to settle for less to survive in my marriage. My chances of better opportunities at this age are nearly non-existent. My family's original reputation and my self-identity will be damaged if I asked for a divorce again. (Participant 9)

The participants in this environment saw, and the findings of the survey verified, that the classification of marriage, especially forced marriage, may enhance the likelihood of a person being a victim of physical or sexual violence. Across multiple narratives, a common thread was the financial domain. This was reported frequently by many themes in this study. It was asked whether the type of marriage increases the risk of IPV, she stated, "I was forced by my family to marry him [my rich husband]. We were too poor; my family were no longer able to take care of us financially and we lived on my dad's retirement pension" (Participant 12).

This was seen among individuals with an annual income of less than $25,000 Dunn's post hoc comparisons demonstrated that these women are more susceptible to exploitation. In response to the question of whether household income influences the risk of abuse, one person disagreed and provided an alternative explanation, stating:

> Maybe the situation is quite different in our culture since most parents continue to support their daughters after marriage. In my case, I am an unemployed wife, forced to stay with him according to his terms because I don't have sufficient financial support. However, many women are lucky enough to have their parents' financial support, but my family are poor. (Participant 7)

The findings of the current study show a significant association between marrying a polygamous partner and minor sexual coercion. Further, those who were married for a second time had a higher chance of being economically abused by their partner. In the quantitative questionnaire, the statistical analysis shows (via the Mann-Whitney test) that sexual coercion was the most predominant form of abuse that women married to polygamist partners faced. This was reflected by another participant, who preferred to keep their sexual life history confidential, and a range of responses was elicited. For example, one informant felt that:

> I think that sexual coercion is a very sensitive issue. We cannot disclose this information to anyone, especially our family, it is taboo [a woman's sexual life]. However, I think they [polygamist partners] want to prove that they still can maintain and meet the intimate desire their senior wife and believe that this is a sign of apology and love that the wife would forgive and simply accept the new life arrangements [splitting time and family resources with new wife]. (Participant 14)

The aforementioned conclusions are reinforced by data from the quantitative chapter, in which it was hypothesised that polygamist wives' experiences with domestic violence varied considerably. Participants held a wide variety of views about polygamy, according to a thematic analysis of the interview data in response to these results, participants presented fundamental reasons backed by prior research. In a polygamous union, the ladies must equally share everything. Incongruously, this presents a difficulty since connected aspects influence the character of the interaction. The statistical analysis supports the victims' statements and their explanations about the association between the kind of abuse and polygamist-married women. Participants were asked to clarify the relationship between polygamist marriage and any forms of abuse that might occur, One participant stated:

> When I married my husband [polygamist partner], I challenged my family to marry him, and I was taking accountability for my decision. They would blame me if I asked them to do something [stop the abusive husband], and I cannot be in this situation [tolerate my family pressure and blame]. (Participant 15)

Another reported problem that emerged under this theme was the marriage type and risk of abuse. women whose marriage was based on love or was coerced are more likely to have minor injuries as a result of physical violence, according to the present data. During the discussion, participants were asked to elaborate on how the type of marriage could increase the risk of IPV, several patterns emerged and captured the rich and complex nature of marriage institutes in Qatar which was supporting the key theme of this section. One participant said, "I always have to show my family that everything is going well. I must deal with the abuse silently. My family will divorce me from him, and I don't want that [divorce] because they don't like him [my husband]" (Participant 1).

Participants shared their perspectives and experiences when asked about marriage types and the potential risk of abuse. This led to the identification of several interconnected themes. The abuse situation was rationally explained by several reasons that highlight multifactor risks. According to them:

> I am not quite sure, but I guess the challenge might be way more complicated for those who go against their parents [arranged marriage] and marry someone whom they choose and love. (Participant 1)
>
> I am a second wife, and our marriage can be classified as a love marriage. I was surprised that he was acting aggressively after marriage to resolve any conflict and sometimes I get injured, and he caused a few bruises. I don't understand him anymore. He used to be very romantic and then he changed. (Participant 15)
>
> Our marriage is arranged. I don't think he loves me; he yells and screams at me for every little detail, and the other day he slapped me because I gave my child chocolate bars. I try to defend myself. He says, 'it's your fault for not obeying me'. (Participant 8)

In response to sexual coercion, most surveyed participants said their husbands might feel challenged or threatened by their manhood ideology. Therefore, sexual coercion and violence escalated. This data analysis provides several reasons that support the current theme.

> It does not happen in my situation, but when he got married to a second wife, he tried a couple of times to have intimate relationship with me, but I rejected his request stating that I don't want to have intimate relationship with him anymore. Some men might act aggressively because they might think their manhood has been challenged. (Participant 16)

Another participant emphasised the significance of gaining an awareness of the motivations behind entering a polygamous marriage and the factors that may contribute to instances of sexual abuse:

> Women understand that if she falls in love with or marries a polygamist partner, she always has to fulfil her husband's inimate desire because this is the main reason for getting another wife. So, if the wives are unable to meet their husband's inimate desire, she might end up the victim of spousal rape or sexual coercion. (Participant 15)

According to the data analysis, several reasons supported the discussion regarding the number of children. Participants were aware of the findings of a recent statistical investigation. This showed that many moms who have many children were at an increased risk of sexual coercion. Their reasons include life arrangements for newly born babies and issues with life balance. According to them:

> I think this is because mothers are so busy with their children, especially if they have a new-born baby crying all night and there is no time for him [to meet his sexual needs]. (Participant 4)

> I think that physical intimacy becomes violent because the mother is no longer able to form a balance between her life as a mother and wife, especially if she has a new baby. For example, I am so exhausted, and I have a poor sleep routine because my son always cries at night. This disturbs him [husband] and he tries to finish it up so quickly [orgasm] that I don't feel comfortable with him anymore [during intimacy]. (Participant 9)

Regarding fertility, the participants were asked for their opinions on reproductive concerns that arise between married couples, specifically about whether this raises the chance of domestic violence. The outcomes of the study indicate that a woman's fertility is not linked to their likelihood of becoming a victim, as shown by the results of the Mann-Whitney U test. These results are rather unexpected when considered with the findings of previous studies that revealed that factors leading to infertility increase the probability of being victimised. The participants explained this link between those factors, which was found to be negligible:

> I think husbands in our culture are influenced by religious beliefs when it comes to accepting this reality [wife infertility condition]. They might not commit abuse, but they may proceed to file for a divorce. (Participant 2)

> I think infertile women become emotionally isolated and try to avoid any heated arguments or conversations with their husbands. (Participant 7)

> My husband feels sorry for me but will always be under family pressure to marry other women and have normal marriage life [have kids]. (Participant 18)

According to the opinions expressed by the participants, the cultural factor that addresses problems related to reproduction is often resolved, and it is a perfectly acceptable excuse for males to marry more than one woman. Consequently, there is a possibility that this will not lead to the lady being subjected to physical or other types of violence. On the other hand, this might lead to women suffering and embracing being co-wives if they are willing to do so. Therefore, they will transition from a monogamous to a polygamous marriage state.

> They keep themselves [husbands] busy to distance themselves from the reality [wife's infertility condition] by travelling and enjoying their life as a bachelor. They usually think of keeping their wife but marrying other women to have kids. (Participant 18)

The present research has shown a connection between sexual coercion, economic abuse, and polygamy as a social practice. Nevertheless, the participants' own words helped us get a deeper comprehension of the dynamics at play when co-wives engage in abusive behaviour against one another. Many direct quotations from the participants illustrate yet another significant facet of the issue of abuse in polygamous marriages and the extent to which women are required to compromise to preserve their relationships. The findings that a major change in the wife's lifestyle, sharing financial resources, and splitting unequal time with co-wives are associated with emotional, physical, and sexual abuse, which is a consequence of a husband's unjust treatment, and this is not practised in compliance with Islamic principles have been supported by other researchers who have examined the impact of polygamous marriages among Muslim.

The panellists were unanimous in their support of the notion that males in Arabic culture keep their distance from women and accept their sterility. As mentioned by one of the participants, this situation is what inspires some men to get remarried.

> I think the rationale behind their attitude towards female infertility is manifested in a second wife life because ordinarily men already have established their family with their first wife and prefer not to have children in their second marriage to reduce responsibility and to enjoy their life but in infertility condition, men are culturally justified to married another woman not to act aggressively because this is a god decision. (Participant 7)

These ideas and perceptions stand in contrast to the results of another study, which demonstrate that an infertile woman may be at a higher risk of being mistreated in the home. On the other hand, the results so far do not necessarily raise any concerns. These statements give the impression that infertile women could strive to avoid having any dialogue that might place them in a position where they would have to address their anxieties and discuss them with their spouses.

Regarding the decision to leave, according to research, a woman's choice to quit or remain in a relationship involves facing her fear. The complexity of ending a relationship with a violent spouse is unique to each woman, according to several research.

One participant noted that her rights as a wife alter when her husband marries another woman, with housing rights being her primary worry:

> We used to love each other so much and when he married a second wife, I asked him that we should be treated equally [me and his new wife]. He does not want to do it and hurt me with his response when he said that [her husband]. I have spent whole my life with you and now I need my time [stay with his new wife]. I am so scared that I could lose my current house because of his marriage. (Participant 16)

> Even if he marries another woman, I still want my children to be raised by their father. I don't feel safe, and I can't go back to my parents' home because there is not enough room for us. (Participant 8)

The most typical repercussion of polygamous marriages is the treatment of the first wife as somewhat unjustly, which is seen as a significant and more debilitating kind of emotional abuse:

> He does not listen to me, and I don't feel secure anymore. He threatens to divorce me if I don't follow exactly his role model of wifely duty. I am completely broke, and I cannot afford the cost of divorce. (Participant 2)

When the participants were asked about the violence in the family of origin and how it may influence their chances to become victims of domestic abuse. Several remarks made by the participants give a variety of potential reasons for this. One of the participants speculated that the fact that their spouse had an abusive upbringing would affect how they matured as adults, and this was a recurring remark underpinning this theme. For example:

> I remember that my mother-in-law used to treat her husband in a very unpleasant and aggressive way. My husband does not like his father because he was weak, but he is unconsciously replicating his mother's behaviour. (Participant 1)

> My father-in-law was very rich, but he was very stingy. He even brought poor-quality food and screamed at us whenever we brought food from outside. When we moved to our new house my husband started to do the same [become stingy]. I guess the entire family are used to this violent environment. (Participant 7)

Several questions were asked about family-of-origin violence such as, what role does family-of-origin violence play such as witnessing violence in the family of origin with other forms of violence in adulthood such as intimate partner violence? Many rational responses were given by the participants for example, one participant said that their spouse could be under the assumption that their behaviour was perfectly typical in the sense that they need complete authority over the money that their family spent on their day-to-day activities. According to other participants, exposure to family-of-origin violence promotes unhealthy attitudes towards wives on a long-term basis:

> My husband told me that his dad barely gives them any money. Whenever I remind my husband that he is doing the same we end up in a heated argument. (Participant 4)

> My husband had an unpleasant childhood experience. His father used to be very aggressive towards him and his mother. He would see his father continually mocking his mother. (Participant 20)

This theme is underpinned by these explanations and draws attention to the societal and family factors that govern marriages which were explored in the quantitative phases, such as age at marriage time, age disparity between couples, mindset type of the wife and attitude towards women were examined and significantly contribute to forms of domestic violence. The researcher explored the participants' narratives at this level of analysis for remarkable comments about family and societal factors. A notable observation emerged from a number of participants, about How husbands are influenced by their father's economic status which leads to unfair comparisons between the family of the husband and the economic status of the wife. Another participant spoke about the role that the manhood principle and Arabic culture might play in victimization.

> His dad always undermined his wife, and he always had the final word in our life as a couple. If I don't obey him, he started to remind me about how poor I was and how I become lucky that he accepted his son to marry me. (Participant 19)

> Some parents have a misconception about the notion of manhood. They believe acting aggressively and controlling your spouse's life is a sign of a strong personality, no matter how action manifests or in which form. (Participant 19)

> I am not sure about that, it appears my husband has a good relationship with his parents, but he does not love me and that's why we have an ongoing dispute and heated argument. However, sometimes his mum encourages him to play his traditional gender role as a husband

> and keep the values of his family tradition, which always ends up in aggression as he wants to possess me. (Participant 3)

Within the theme of increasing risk of victimization, there were some differences within the perception of women's belief system when the participants were asked to remark on the mentality and mental attitude of women who have conventional and liberal belief systems regarding women's rights.

The rational answers given by participants do vary depending on the circumstances and nature of the domestic abuse they were exposed to, even though blaming them for their beliefs is unjustifiable. One of the participants had the opinion that questioning the conventional gender roles of husbands may have an impact on the relationship between a husband and his wife:

> Since I started to confront him, saying that I deserve to be treated respectfully and that he should listen to me when making a major decision in the family, he has started to keep me out of any decision-making and repeatedly suggests that I know nothing about life, even when he built our house, he did not take my opinion on anything at all. (Participant 17)

Another interesting aspect of the notion of roles of women obeying their husbands fully concerned with meeting their expectations and needs, however still it has been identified by the participants that her understanding of being docile and submissive might be questionable.

> No, I always obey him and I try to accommodate his needs but he seems to become more aggressive and sometimes I believe he wants to suppress me and weaken my personality. (Participant 8)

A further participant offered another explanation by stating that their husband feels threatened, especially when their wife's education level potentially outweighs the husband's qualifications. The incompetence associated with being uneducated or having poor educational attainment was evident, as participants struggled when initiating conversation with their partner to discuss her ambitions to pursue higher education or to be involved actively in family decision-making.

> He always puts me down whenever I talk to him about my intention to pursue higher education, he makes fun of me, and always says that my wifely duty is above everything and he told me look at me, I have a normal degree [secondary school degree] and I have a decent job. (Participant 1)

The comments below illustrate that whenever women stand up for their rights, they might be called stubborn women and might be punished for that said that:

> My husband and his dad went crazy when I told them it is my legitimate right to have control over my financial accounts and study the major that I love [law]. My husband strangled me and said you never use legal language in my house while talking to me or my dad. (Participant 19)

Several quotations demonstrate how the husband was intimidated by his wife's financial independence; Elements of this theme have been repeatedly mentioned by participants in the discussion of the previous themes. As a result of this theme, important insights are gained regarding how the education level of a husband affects domestic violence and its effect on the spouse. Men feel uneasy when their wives become more independent, said another participant; "I feel that my husband became more threatened after I earned my degree and got a decent job. He became so jealous and aggressive. He knows that I don't need to beg him anymore asking for money" (Participant 17).

Another participant expanded on the reasons why traditional women could have a more stable lifestyle and less heated disagreements with their spouses due to the fact that they are more likely to be married. A lot of the participants agreed with the statement that women may have a conventional worldview and yet be able to accept abuse.

> I think that those women who have traditional belief systems are less likely to argue with their husbands since other women who have liberal belief systems are more likely to decontextualise traditional norms and the traditional husband's role within the family. (Participant 14).

The participants felt that people who accept or tolerate traditional gender roles are culturally safe from abuse in the sense that they will not challenge their family's model of dealing with their husbands, once this model is breached, women are suppressed by their own families. For example; one interviewee said, "I don't think I have heard any one of my relatives being physically abused by her husband because our family is always emphasizing that decent women should bow to her husband's wishes" (Participant 17).

Many findings from this theme point to the contribution of traditional gender roles of husbands and wives to domestic violence. Regarding the age at the time of marriage, another line of reasoning was presented to the participants regarding their age at the time of marriage, in terms of whether it affects becoming a victim of domestic abuse or not. Conflict of opinion in many participants' narratives about the age at which they got married, the age disparity between husband and wife and the associated risk of abuse when they were asked to comment on these questions. One interviewee said, "I think being married at a young age could somehow cause tension in the marital relationship. Both husband and wife have a different agenda, and everyone wants to prove that they are right" (Participant 13).

Another participant thought that the financial life of the married couple could result in a mismatch between their expectations: "I want to enjoy my life. He cannot afford the financial life that my parents used to offer. He does not accept any financial support from my family. He considers this as weakening his manhood principle" (Participant 21).

There was a sense of undeveloped understating of family life responsibility that emerged across participants' quotations. One participant commented that the responsibility concept of forming a new family is not highly developed among young couples when it comes to family commitment:

> I think, at a young age, couples have a different sense of reality. Many women during the first year of their marriage do not want to get pregnant. In this case, husbands face pressure from relatives, because it's quite normal to be asked if your wife is pregnant or not. (Participant 4)

Another participant further clarified certain issues surrounding marrying young and how misconceptions are manifested among young couples: "I think many men prefer to marry a young woman because it's so easy to get along with her [easy to raise her]. However, nowadays, they [young women] are not quite so docile because they are educated" (Participant 2).

When it comes to the second set of findings underpinning this theme, another line of reasoning suggests that the observations of the participants vary since getting married later in life might have its own set of triggers, such as difficulties with fertility and feelings of insecurity while living under such a great deal of pressure, a range of response was elicited.

> I think those who got married late suffer more from social and relative pressure, that women should get pregnant quickly to prove that they are still young and can have kids. (Participant 18)

> Yes indeed, it might have some influence on marriage life stability. In my situation, I got married quite late and I think at this age it's normal to challenge your husband because you are mature enough and you have been through a lot in your life [good and bad experiences]. You don't want anyone simply to take the steering wheel from you because he became your partner. (Participant 1)

> In my opinion, when women get married late, it's hard to exercise the traditional husband role on her, because she most likely manages her personal life individually and has become more independent. She cannot accept that suddenly someone will control and dictate her life. (Participant 13)

One participant commented on marrying later in life which seems problematic among the current sample, several participants reported that late marriage can be stressful for their marriage because spouses have differing priorities and perceptions of life.

> Women at a young age like to enjoy their life they don't want a serious commitment that restricts their joy while men in my opinion they more likely to think about the future of their family especially if age gap is huge. (Participant 13)

Stating factors associated with the risk of abuse was paired with narratives that focus on breaking the cycle of abuse. In this way, the next theme about ending or leaving abusive relationships was developed. Various challenges were recurrent and underpin this theme which will focus on challenges that alter women's decision to seek professional help or end an abusive relationship.

5.1.4 Theme 4: Leaving an Abusive Relationship

The most frequent variant of leaving an abusive relationship was child custody rights and post-divorce arrangements, which underpin this emerging theme. Participants reported family pressure and social stigma are two other reasons women consider before leaving an abusive partner? All of these elements were analysed deeply to understand how difficult the leaving process is.

One of the participants in her response to the question about why women stay or remain passive in an abusive relationship. As her family does not accept divorce, she felt disappointed. Consequently, she had no chance to end this abusive relationship but held high hope that he would be willing to change. Become hopeless as no one cares about how she should resolve her issue. She stated:

> My family does not accept the idea of being a divorced woman, and I tend to believe that I will not be able to find a better person than him. So, I prefer to continue with him until he changes instead of facing family pressure. I am so sad, no one cares anymore. (Participant 11)

When discussing the idea of being unable to confront fears that are associated with family pressure in terms of deciding to leave or stay in the relationship. The participant's mom doesn't accept the shame associated with divorce, and she was forced to normalize her feelings: "My mum told me that marriage life is quite a challenge. you go in a white dress, and you are allowed to come back only in a white shroud. Simply, my parents cannot accept it [being divorced]" (Participant 11).

In circumstances where a marriage may be dissolved, the caste attitudes of divorced women significantly declined and became less stigmatised to shield the victims from future negative repercussions of unsatisfactory marriages. Several participants mentioned the importance of understanding how stigma and social pressure hinder them from seeking the right help or letting go of their abusive husbands. Several narratives underpin this theme, suggesting that this is a crucial factor to consider when exploring why women remain passive and do not break the abuse cycle. As evidenced by the following quotes

> He knows that I cannot talk to my family about his attitude because they will blame me for my decision; they gave me the freedom to marry him. I don't want to be under family pressure, I will sort it out. (Participant 15)

In addition to the social stigma associated with abuse, another participant in response to the same question thought that post-divorced family pressure and control measures might be worse than continuing to live with an abusive partner due to relative gossip and blame: "It's very hard in my family for a divorced woman to live a normal life. The gossip and blame from relatives are unbearable" (Participant 3).

This social pressure was narrated by the majority of the current participants, who suggested that they should remain in their bonds with their abusive husbands for the sake of their children. This topic emphasises how the participants considered their perspectives were sensible, given their knowledge and reasons for why abused women remain passive in relationships. After analysing the data, the topic of seeking professional advice was further discussed.

Participants were asked if they had considered involving family, friends, or professionals in their journey to break the cycle of abuse. A recurring sentiment among participants or not seeking professional help was centred on losing their post-marriage settlements such as children's education assistance. Other participant concerns were about the image and reputation of the husband which might be misperceived and complicate the marriage.

> I cannot ask for professional help because I know it is a very sensitive subject that may worsen my post-marriage financial life by cutting Nafaqa or even cause problems by changing

> my children's school from private to public or withdrawing the housemaid and the driver. (Participant 10)

> No, I cannot ask for professional help because I know it is a very sensitive subject that may worsen my marriage and my husband might divorce me for that because he does not want anything to damage his reputation. (Participant 7)

One notable finding from the data was the emergence of elements associated with the divorce process such as the high cost of attorney fees, long court proceedings and post-divorce abuse that underpin a new theme: Bureaucracy and Post Separation Abuse, which adds nuance to understanding how post-divorce dimension interplay with women's decision to seek freedom.

5.1.5 Theme 5: Bureaucracy and Post Separation Abuse

Regarding the post-divorce settlements, the subsequent sections will go through many restrictions and arrangements that women must put up with in order to put a stop to the abuse. One of the participants expressed her concern that most divorced mothers will stay single due to the limitations of the current child custody law. This is because her child custody rights entitlement will subsequently change once she gets married again. With one saying:

> I am a divorced mother and remarrying is not an option. I want to raise my children and save my child custody rights. I rejected a couple of marriage proposals after my divorce. That's the reason why many divorced women are unable to remarry. (Participant 14)

As one participant pointed out, leftover rooms are limited in their grandparents' houses, so understanding the stress arising from residential mobility is imperative. Current child custody laws limit the chances of divorced mothers remarrying. According to her:

> Remarrying is not an option in most cases because once a woman decides to marry again, the child custody by default will shift to the husband. Mothers sometimes asked to leave their houses and stay with their own families. Do you think there is enough room to accommodate the children, mother and her housemaid? In most cases, this is a burden, which divorced women encounter. (Participant 3)

This theme emerged as a key finding in the analysis. They cited it as a significant factor in understanding how forms of domestic abuse continue. These forms of abuse can deter them from making their decision or force them to form unhealthy attachments with their abuser. A participant emphasized this when she explained how her ex-husband used children as a weapon to punish her for the divorce by holding the original copy of their children's identification papers, which requires her to assert her rights for minor things through the court system.

> As a divorced mother, I struggle to obtain my children's identification documents to enrol them in school and struggle when I decide to travel with them. I have to seek court permission because my ex-husband does not give me the document. Thus, I have to seek court permission

> to authorize the existing permit or must get a passport to complete school registration. (Participant 2)

Another participant, during a discussion of the question, why would a divorced woman find it difficult to accept leaving her home or receiving financial assistance as part of her post-divorce entitlements? Her answer clearly shows that their basic right to remain in the same house with their kids was undermined or misunderstood, especially since that house is most likely to be offered to the new wife, as stated:

> I think it's quite common for husbands to ask their ex-wives to leave their home when they are divorced. I cannot accept the idea of leaving my children's house for someone else [his new wife] even if he offers another accommodation as an option. (Participant 19)

In the data, bureaucracy and post-divorce themes are prominent, suggesting it is one of the most significant factors for women to consider when ending abusive relationships. According to one participant, her post-divorce financial entitlement left her unable to afford a house in the city due to high rental costs. Since affordable housing is located outside of the city, she will have to deal with another challenge related to commuting to school. Drop-off and pick-up times are generally the same at most schools. She said:

> My lawyer shocked me when he told me that the court ordered my ex-husband to pay me 8000 QR a month to find a new home. They do not seem to understand that for this amount of money I will only be able to find a small house approximately an hour's drive from Doha. How can I get to work and how can I drop my 4 kids at school, they relatively finish at the same time? (Participant 17)

These elements are pervasive in several interviews and underpin this theme among different participants. According to other participants, divorce mothers continue to be concerned about new living arrangements and associated financial burdens. One participant worried about her divorce and leaving the home is pricey for women with several children which underpin this. According to her:

> The current family law permits the husband to keep one housemaid and one driver, which is good for a small family. I have six kids in different schools. One driver cannot drop them off and take them from the school at the same time. This increases the financial burden on mothers who have a big family to take care of. (Participant 10)

On participants in her comments on post-divorce abuse, add another line of thought that warrants further investigation. She was unable to restore their normal life after the divorce. As a result, she was unable to claim her financial contribution to property that she left in previous divorces. Her lack of adequate knowledge of court proceedings makes her suffer, which she finds unjust. Stating:

> It is so unfair that I don't have proof or evidence to claim the money that I have invested in our house for furniture and other items. I lost everything when I got divorced because he was going to marry other women due to my condition [infertility]. (Participant 18)

The current theme of bureaucracy and post-divorce abuse led the discussion to explore the issue of high attorney fees when women are actively considering leaving an abusive relationship. Women's hesitation to file a case or seek professional assistance, settle their disputes or end abuse sparked a new line of thought about the court process and how it can be difficult to afford an attorney. As one interviewee said, "I cannot afford to pay the attorney's fees. I am financially broke and depend on him [her husband] to pay my financial expenses" (Participant 11).

The participants also thought that the procedure to file a case in court might be too complicated and further believed that the procedure might deplete them financially if substantial time was required to resolve the conflict. Other participants highlighted that their husbands might push them to surrender their financial rights by forcing them indirectly to file a khula case. She stats:

> 'I was psychologically abused by him. He does not talk to me at all [my husband]. I tried many solutions, but nothing works out. I asked him to divorce me, but he refused. He said if you want [a divorce] go and file a khula [Islamic divorce where the woman has to give up her financial rights]. (Participant 17)

Another participant revealed similar concerns about the forms of divorce they were subjected to once they wanted to seek their freedom. She emphasised, on the other hand, that filing a khula action would result in the loss of a significant portion of her pecuniary rights. For example, one interview said:

> I cannot afford the divorce cost. I cannot stay with him anymore [my husband]. He does not perform his husband's duty [physical relationship]. He asked me to file a *khula* if I want to get divorced, which means I have to give away all my financial rights. (Participant 4)

Several participants' narratives were interlinked with other themes as well. In the following narratives, several issues have been identified that demonstrate her entitlement to fail a divorce case. These statements demonstrate that women have challenges resolving marital issues. She said:

> After few days after my wedding night, my husband requested that I undergo surgery to do IVF. I was shocked by his request and when he justified his request by saying that he had suffered from impotence, he abused me psychologically when I reject his request and started to act violently towards me. Following receiving family support, I filed for divorce on a fault-based basis. (Participant 5)

Many quotes provided valuable insight into their experiences and perspectives on bureaucracy and the post-divorce theme. An essential aspect of understanding how to end abuse in Arabic culture has to do with understanding the cultural complexity of the divorce situation in Qatar.

5.2 Summary

The analysis of participant narratives revealed several key themes in this chapter. The following themes are presented in the data, including Theme (1) Types and Pattern of Abuse, Theme (2) Impact of Intimate Partner violence on mental and physical health, Theme (3) Risk factor for victimisation, Theme (4) leaving an abusive relationship, Theme (5) Bureaucracy and Post Separation abuse. A nuanced understanding of the research questions was provided, as well as an expansion of the quantitative findings. Based on these findings, it is necessary to critically re-evaluate the current family policy law and the courts' process for divorce. In addition, there is a need to develop awareness programs. Awareness programs educate couples about the risk of abuse on mental and physical health and when it is most likely to increase. In the next chapter, findings from both quantitative and qualitative chapters will be integrated and discussed in detail, as well as recommendations for future research.

References

Braun, V., & Clarke, V. (2006). Using thematic analysis in psychology. *Qualitative Research in Psychology, 3*(2), 77–101. https://doi.org/10.1191/1478088706qp063oa

Krueger, R. A., & Casey, M. A. (2009). *Focus groups: A practical guide for applied research.* Sage Publications.

Kvale, S., & Brinkmann, S. (2009). *Interviews: Learning the craft of qualitative research interviewing* (2nd ed.). Sage Publications.

Preece, D., & Williams, K. (2017). Transcription: A review of the literature and implications for psychotherapy research. *Psychology and Psychotherapy: Theory, Research and Practice, 90*(3), 406–423. https://doi.org/10.1111/papt.12126

Chapter 6
The Sounds of Silence: Making Sense of the Domestic Abuse

Literature reviews on domestic abuse against women have devoted considerable attention to this critical topic. This study was undertaken with the aim of assessing the prevalence of Intimate Partner Victimization (IPV), the risk of homicide, and their adverse effects on Qatari women's mental health. Depression, anxiety, and PTSD were measured. The secondary objective was to explore factors associated with IPV among women and why women remain passive in abusive relationships.

The discussion chapter is organized in alignment with the study's objectives and aims. Each point is discussed, analysed, and interpreted to summarize the findings of the study and provide a conclusion.

6.1 Types, Patterns of Abuse, and Risk of Homicide

The first set of questions aimed at examining the prevalence of IPV among Qataris women, while the second set examines homicide risk. The findings from quantitative phases indicated that psychological abuse was the most common kind of abuse that the participants reported experiencing with (M = 53.71; SD = 48.54). While the most surprising aspect of the data is that the least form of abuse was injuries, with (M = 9.60; SD = 23.92). The current findings shows that psychological and economic abuse were pervasive all age group and specifically among young those who get married at aged 22 or below, and 33 years and above are experiencing a wide range of IPV including psychological aggression, physical assault, injury, and economic abuse.

Another important finding reported by the current study was economic abuse, which emerged as the second most predominant form of violence reported by the participants, with a mean score of 32.34 and a standard deviation of 8.85. These results were consistent with the frequent narratives reported by participants during the qualitative phase of the study. Economic abuse is relevant to the concept of

K. Al-Naama, *Domestic Abuse and Mental Health in Qatar*, Gulf Studies 23,
https://doi.org/10.1007/978-981-96-7392-6_6

manhood ideology (emphasize power and control as core aspects of dominance, men may feel entitled to maintain a privileged level of control over their partners, viewing them as subordinate and less capable in decision-making processes (Usta et al., 2013).

This belief system often positions manhood as synonymous with authority and dominance, which can normalize intimate partner violence (IPV) by reinforcing the idea that men have the right to assert control in their relationships. Such ideologies can become more pronounced during times of financial instability or when traditional gender roles are challenged, leading men to intensify their efforts to reassert their dominance and authority (Mshweshwe, 2020) as some husbands expressed reservations about their wives' competence in managing the family's financial commitments and assets. Another recurring explanation provided by participants was the divergence in financial priorities between husbands and wives in managing married life and forming families. This mismatch could escalate tension between couples, especially among those with differing life perceptions, as narrated by them.

This finding aligns with the qualitative data collected from study participants who had experienced various forms of domestic abuse. Among these, psychological abuse patterns included social isolation, poor communication styles, and exclusion from major family decisions. As one participant stated, "psychological abuse may present in silent", manifesting in various ways, including neglect. Another narrative quoted an extreme context: "My husband used to intimidate and call me names". It does not leave any traces and is considered less serious sometimes by relatives or professionals which makes getting adequate help challenging. Therefore, these forms of actions can occur as a daily routine among couple life conversations or attitude, that usually undermine by others as it might perceived as normal arguments between husband and wife, which is not. These results are consistent with the findings that were reported before (Al-Ghanim, 2009).

As expected in previous research, the prevalence of IPV in the current study was in line with Ali et al.'s (2011) research which examined the risk variables linked to IPV victims and produced the most fascinating findings. It was shown that physical abuse accounted for 56.3% in the previous 12 months. Sexual assault accounted for 54.4%. However, the most prevalent kind of abuse was psychological aggression, which was reported by 83.6% of the participants. According to the findings of the multivariate analysis, the risk factor of the study was that physical abuse tends to be greater among men who have informal education credentials.

These results emerged from assessing the prevalence of domestic abuse in the current study was reported in several previous studies. For example, building on existing evidence gathered from a systematic review which included a meta-analysis of 29 studies from ten Arab countries with 19,101 female victims of domestic abuse to assess patterns of domestic violence against women (Hawcroft et al., 2019). The majority of studies reported exclusively on married or formerly married women. Physical assault was experienced by 35.6% of victims, sexual coercion by 22%, and psychological aggression by 49.8%.

These results are consistent with previous studies that have also found similar results regarding IPV prevalence. In a cross-sectional study conducted on 1883 Saudi married women, we sought to determine the prevalence of domestic abuse. The study revealed that psychological abuse among the participants accounted for 22%, sexual coercion and assault accounted for 12.7%, and physical assault was the least reported form of abuse, which accounted for 9% of the total participants (Alquaiz et al., 2021).

Similar findings were reported in a systematic review that was conducted in the Middle East between the years 1995 and 2020 to measure the prevalence of domestic abuse against women found that economic abuse accounted for 19% of participants, sexual coercion accounted for 18.5% of participants, and injuries accounted for 18.4% of participants (Moshtagh et al., 2021). These findings are also consistent with the findings of the current study.

Similar findings were match those observed in earlier studies, that was conducted in the United States on a total of 130 participants found that psychological violence was the most reported form of abuse, making up 92.3% of the study participants, while physical assault made up 80.8% of the participants, and sexual violence made up 64.4% of the participants (King et al., 2017). This study's findings are similar to those that were previously published (Tashkandi & Rasheed, 2009). There was a total of 689 female participants in the research, whose ages varied from 16 to 60 years. The participants were assessed using the Modified Conflict Tactics scale; however, the perpetrator questionnaire was omitted from the study. The study findings revealed that 25.7% of respondents had been victims of physical violence, while 32.8% had been victims of both physical and psychological abuse. In addition, the physical abuse data revealed that 63.3% of the victims had severe injuries, while 36.7% of the victims sustained light injuries. The effects of physical abuse were unrelated to the age of the women, although the effects of psychological aggressiveness were. The findings demonstrated that psychological violence occurred more often among women aged 20 and older (35%) than among younger female victims (12.5%).

Consistent with the current findings, in a previous study in Qatar that measured the prevalence of forms of domestic abuse against women among students, the findings of the study revealed that 64% were physically abused and it was concluded that victims maintained their relationship in fear and were hesitant to file for divorce. Moreover, history of domestic violence in the family of origin during childhood was confirmed by 27% of female students who were currently continuing to be abused (Al-Ghanim, 2009).

In comparison to findings from similar region, previous research that has focused on Arabic society and the most common forms of domestic abuse against women has come to conclusions that are relatively similar to the findings of the current study. These studies have found that the nature of domestic abuse against women differs from culture to culture. Specifically, in Kuwait, the most common form of violence was physical assault committed by a husband against his wife, which accounted for 30% of cases. Psychological aggression accounted for 25.3% of cases, and nearly 71% of respondents believed that the cause of the violence was the husband's behavioural problems. On the other hand, financial insufficiency on the part of the husband accounted for 34% of violent incidents (Decima Research Inc., 2002).

Another systematic and meta-analysis review on the prevalence of domestic violence against women and the associated health consequences was carried out by Hawcroft et al. (2019) in a clinical setting within the Arab region. They found that the most prevalent form of abuse was emotional and psychological violence (49.8%), while physical violence represented 35.6%, and sexual abuse accounted for 22%. In addition, those who didn't get enough sleep were more likely to suffer from health issues such as depression and hypertension.

The results of this study confirm that economic abuse takes on various forms, contributing to and intensifying marital tension between intimate partners. It emerged as the second most prevalent type of abuse that's extended beyond post-divorce phase. These results are in accord with a recent study conducted by Kutin et al. (2017) indicating that of intimate partners experiencing some form of economic abuse 9.6% of the victims indicated that their property was damaged, and 5.8% of the participants reported having problems obtaining information about their family finances. A woman's likelihood of being economically abused by her spouse increases if she is unemployed, divorced, and lives in a poor home. Another plausible explanation for the existence of economic abuse was found in a study conducted by Al-Ekri et al. (1994), who found that economic abuse in cultures with Arabic roots can appear in a variety of ways.

For example, in a cross-sectional study, 602 Bahraini women who had attended primary care clinics were assessed for domestic abuse and other risk factors. Only 32% of the people had been physically beaten, while 60% had suffered mental abuse. The majority of participants reported difficulty obtaining employment, and 21.3% reported being financially abused. Sexual compulsion was reported the least often, accounting for 13.4% of all abuse reports. The current findings are in line with those of previous research that found that economic control was the form of economic abuse that was reported the most often (Davila et al., 2021).

Continuing with the second set of questions posed at the beginning of this study, this study's sub-objective included evaluating the homicidal risk associated with the IPV, which could lead to murder. The current research findings show approximately 78.8% of the total participants indicated insignificant risk of homicide. The majority of the scores were relatively low. Among the remaining 21.2%, there was an increased danger, which also implies a low homicide risk; the other two categories, severe and extreme danger, indicate a high homicide risk, but were not reported by participants.

There is no indication for a life-threatening category which indicate a high risk of homicide among the current participants. Findings were supported by the narrative from the qualitative phase that justified why risk of homicide are relatively low. As reported by the majority of the participants, the murder risk was not overwhelmingly prevalent. Arabic culture disparages husbands who use their physical ability to displace their wives and states that Arabic culture does not consider physical violence to be a masculine measure. Strict measures imposed by the authorities act as a preventive action. According to one participant, "legal measures are taken seriously regarding any physical violence". The weak association between forms of abuse and the risk of homicide in this study is interesting but not surprising. Several participants reported feeling vulnerable and fearful after experiencing domestic abuse, as revealed in the qualitative analysis. There was, however, no express or implicit mention of the risk of homicide among participants. It could be argued that the positive outcome can be attributed to social and firm security measures taken by the government. The current results contradict with findings reached by Campbell et al. (2008) study who found victims were 20-fold more likely to suffer abuse. Among abused women, only 40% are murdered. Half of those killed in the experiment did not take their spouse's threats seriously. Thus, violence may also increase the risk of murder. Violence, psychological intimidation, and suicide threats are the main reasons for this.

Another study's findings yield a similar conclusion to that reached by Campbell (2017), showing that a sample population was screened for a more serious form of domestic abuse: the risk of femicide. Here, the Danger Assessment Scale was administered to two groups of participants. The first group included 310 women involved in intimate partner femicide cases, and the control group consisted of 324 victims of domestic abuse from 11 cities in the United States (Collins et al., 2017). The findings revealed that the mean and median scores for attempted femicide and actual femicide were rated similar on the Danger Assessment Scale, but the scores were more than double in comparison to the abused group (control group). The findings for the attempted femicide group showed that 54.5% of the participants group were under the extreme danger category, 1.3% fell under the increased danger category, while in contrast to the control group, only 3.5% were under extreme danger and 53.1% were under a level of danger.

Similarly, An African population in Vhembe reported high scores on the Danger Assessment Scale, in a study that measured the consequences of domestic abuse. The lethality aspect of serious forms of abuse was evaluated through the Danger Assessment Scale (Peltzer et al., 2013). Two hundred and sixty eight victims of domestic abuse who had received a protective order and whose age was between 18 and 65 years old took part in the study. Most of the participants had on average two children (with SD = 1.3). Their marital status shows that 29.2% were married and 13.9% had a cohabiting partner. The findings of the study showed that 99.3% lived in danger and the least common form of abuse was sexual assault, which accounted for 40.7%. Moreover, the severity of danger was higher among victims who still lived with their partners compared to those who lived with their partners. The Danger mean score was 8.2 (with SD = 3.1). The statistical results of their study confirm that the Danger Assessment Score were associated with PTSD symptoms. Also revealed that there was a moderate correlation between psychological ($r = 0.32$, $p < 0.001$) and physical assault ($r = 0.61$, $p < 0.001$) with a level of depression. According to these findings, abuse is associated with mental health consequences, as shown in the current study.

One further research demonstrated that the reported scores suggested by the Danger Assessment scale were quite high among victims of domestic violence and were connected with poor mental and physical health (Straus et al., 2009). This was not a major case in the current study.

The current data were in contrast with and challenged other research findings about the risk of homicide post-separation reported in several studies. Stöckl et al. (2013) conducted a systematic study that confirmed the link between IPV and murder, finding that an intimate partner was responsible for 13.5% of the total number of recorded killings. In addition, women were 6 times more likely to be victims of homicide than males. The prevalence of these killings was most prevalent in nations with high incomes. This was more specifically among those who had been in a violent relationship for an extended period of time. One of the key findings from the literature review indicates that the risk of homicide may increase after separation. Contrary to the current findings, the risk of danger was relatively low and did not indicate any serious homicide risk. This risk increases when partners separate; putting them at a greater risk of abuse or homicide, according to one study (Belfrage & Rying, 2004). However, it appears that this is not the case in the current research findings. Significant information was obtained from a study conducted in Italy to analyse the elements that may contribute to femicide or murder by an intimate partner (Zara & Gino, 2018). According to this study, 275 of the intimate partners of the deceased were responsible for their murders, while two victims were killed by strangers. More than half of the killings occurred during the day, and more than three-quarters of the victims were killed in the offender's or victim's house. Injury resulting from a physical confrontation was the leading cause of death in intimate partner femicide, accounting for 53.6% of all fatalities, whereas the average relationship lasted 13 years. According to the author, violent behaviour, persecutive reasoning, and contempt are the main causes of murder during heated arguments. Previous studies have revealed that those who have a history of being physically abused by their spouse have an increased probability of committing murder. In addition, the risk assessment score was high, and those who opted to leave an abusive spouse were nine times more likely to be murdered than those who stayed with the violent partner (Koziol-McLain et al., 2006).

Several similarities have been demonstrated in a study of a Western population. In 2018, a study was conducted to evaluate the impact of coercive control among women who experienced different forms of IPV. The participants were recruited from two different emergency departments who had abusive partners and were classified into two groups. The first group consisted of those who had experienced coercive control and the second group was a control group (Dichter et al., 2018). The participants' ages ranged from 18–62 years old, and there were 553 female victims of domestic abuse in total. More than half of the participants' annual income was less than $20,000 and almost half of the victims had a secondary school degree. The potential risk of femicide was assessed by the Danger Assessment Scale, and the scores for those who were under coercive control showed that 30% of them were under extreme danger and 25.9% were under variable danger. Meanwhile, for those who did not experience any form of coercive control, the danger assessment scores showed that they were in the lowest category level of other forms of danger, and only 2.7% fell under the highest and extreme danger level. The findings of the study also highlighted that regarding women who were in an economically detrimental position, most of them were in the coercive control group.

Any kind of aggression, whether mental or physical, may rapidly escalate into more serious forms of abuse, which in extreme situations can result in femicide. However, there are two likely causes for the differences between findings from the current study and other research findings. According to the participants, society is well protected by strong measures that prevent or reduce the risk of homicide.

Additionally, the cultural and religious domains are preventative factors that prevent the situation from getting out of hand. In contrast to the findings provided here, another study was conducted on female domestic violence victims who arrived at emergency departments with a range of different types of physical injuries. In this research, the likelihood of murder was assessed for 263 women aged 16 and older (Brignone & Gomez, 2017). The findings indicated varying degrees of susceptibility to femicide. Moreover, 25% of respondents scored highly on the DA scale, indicating a significant risk of femicide.

The results obtained from the first question in the study about the prevalence forms of domestic abuse challenge the prevailing belief that Qatari society does not suffer from domestic abuse. A lack of updated research and a lack of reporting undermines the existence and effects of domestic abuse against women.

6.2 Impact of Intimate Partner Violence on Women's Mental and Physical Health

A second set of analyses examines IPV's impact on women's mental health. IPV victims are at an increased risk of developing PTSD, anxiety, and depression according to the current findings. These findings confirm that IPV has adverse effects on women's mental health. In terms of mental health issues related to IPV, PTSD was the most rated, representing 48.5% of participants with PTSD symptoms. PTSD was significantly associated with minor and severe psychological aggression and minor physical assault. Anxiety was the second-rated mental health issue, and 49.7% of participants indicated severe anxiety. Participants' anxiety, depression and PTSD levels are significantly affected by psychological aggression, injury and minor physical assault in the current study. The least rated mental health issue was depression, almost half of the participants were classified as mildly depressed, and less than 7% as severely depressed.

In the current study, multiple regression analysis revealed that psychological aggression and economic abuse had significant effects on predicting PTSD. Economic abuse was also found to be a significant predictor of depression among study participants. Additionally, anxiety was significantly correlated with negotiation based on multiple regression analysis.

The findings from the qualitative data support the quantitative results, revealing recurring themes wherein a diverse array of distressing emotional states, including depression, anxiety, and PTSD, were recounted by the majority of respondents. These included decreases in self-confidence and diminished self-worth, as narrated by one participant: "He never requests anything from me. We live like two strangers. I am depressed and disappointed that he does not want to sort this situation out". Furthermore, some respondents reported complications related to pregnancy and reproductive health. The complex nature of IPV consequences confirm the findings of the study. Participants' narratives revealed overarching trends and configurations that yield significant illumination into domestic abuse's pervasive influence on women's mental well-being Some of the participants in the study shows that their symptomology differ based on how family of origin support system act as a preventive measure to reduce the overall psychological pain.

Participants' narratives have highlighted more plausible explanations of the current study, including the fact that parents continue to support them emotionally and financially after marriage, and physical assault is culturally stigmatized and punished severely. Psychology and economic forms of abuse accounted for the majority of painful experiences. In line with the current study findings, Sutherland et al. (2001) found that physical health was found significantly affecting women's health and increases among poor families.

As a result of the current research findings, an unequivocal conclusion has emerged. This indicates that the prevalence of posttraumatic stress disorder has been reported significantly by the participants. It may be explained by the fact that the abused wife cannot forget the abusive incident. Another explanation offered by victims is that they will not accept new changes imposed by the abuser as a coercive control measure to limit their autonomy. In some cases that helped to enrich the contextual understanding about IPV, participants narratives highlight family's concerns and tendency to normalize their feelings or to accept divorce, therefore the cycle of abuse continued and became traumatized. A study was carried out in 2001 to investigate the most common mental disorders associated with IPV, such as PTSD and MDD. The study was conducted on a group of 44 women who were selected from organisations in the United States that primarily deal with women who have been victims of domestic violence (Stein & Kennedy, 2001). This was used to examine different forms of physical abuse and psychological abuse. Researchers found that victims of intimate relationship abuse were significantly more likely to suffer from PTSD and major depression.

These stories and live experiences shared by the participants explains how IPV caused them to live in suffering and pain. They experienced a range of emotional and physical distress, some of which had received medical attention. The current findings are supported by a previous meta-analysis based on 207 studies, which found a significant correlation between anxiety, depression, and PTSD for those who have been exposed to partner violence (Spencer et al., 2019).

As evidenced in the current literature in Dubai and elsewhere, forms of abuse from intimate partners significantly increase the risk of mental disorders. For example, a study conducted near Qatar in the United Arab Emirates reached similar conclusions to the current study. Outpatients attending a mental health service in Dubai were screened for several mental health disorders, including PTSD, in 2012 (Lawton & Schulte, 2012). Fifty one percent of participants met the PTSD criteria, and high scores of PTSD were significantly associated with low self-esteem and high levels of stress. Furthermore, other studies have found similar results finding that participants reported having experienced sexual assault and being physically abused by their partner. PTSD and depression symptoms ranged from moderate to severe. Over half of the participants reported suffering from both conditions (Taft et al., 2009). Similar conclusions have been drawn from societies that are more tolerant of diversity and liberal. In 2015, Khadra et al. (2015) conducted an exploratory study in Lebanon to determine whether domestic violence victims have symptoms of PTSD. According to the study, the mean score of PTSD was 60.3 (SD = 14.2), which indicates a substantial association between physical assault and PTSD. The current findings are consistent with the pattern of adverse health outcomes mainly associated with IPV, such as elevated levels of depression, PTSD symptoms and unhappy marriage life (Varma et al., 2007).

In line with prior research findings, another study examined Arabic female victims of domestic abuse who have been abused within the past 12 months, revealing that they experience more signs of depression, lack of self-esteem and hopelessness (Cwikel et al., 2003). Moreover, the participants indicated that this uncomfortable feeling becomes persistent every day, resulting in them feeling more and more unwell. The current findings have been confirmed by other studies showing that anxiety and depression are another commonly reported mental health issues for women who have been in an abusive relationship, where the prevalence of depression was 15.5% and the anxiety score accounted for 5.6%, which was significantly associated with IPV (Mapayi et al., 2013).

Similarly, in a study conducted in Pakistan to examine the association between domestic violence against women and its adverse health impact, it was revealed that there was a positive correlation between psychological, physical, and sexual abuse, along with profound levels of anxiety, depression and poor quality of life among victims of domestic abuse (Malik et al., 2020). Their study findings reconfirmed the current findings that mental health disorders are common among female victims of domestic violence.

Several studies have found that the most common adverse health effects of being victims of intimate partner abuse are PTSD and depression (Sato-Dilorenzo & Sharps, 2007). One of the reasons behind this that were addressed by the participants was that the normalization of divorce is hard, especially a when divorced woman must justify herself to her family members. This was supported by a similar study (Hassouneh-Phillips, 2001) that was conducted on American female Muslims, suggesting that facing family disapproval and community stigma related to those women who seek to end their marriage are emotionally unbearable.

These findings are comparable to those that were found in research that was conducted by Thabet et al. (2015). These results reflect those of Bargai et al. (2007) who reported that 79% of the 102 female participants had experienced some kind of sexual or physical abuse in their relationships. Among all participants, 47% had a history of abuse in their families, whereas those with PTSD or depression were positively affected by a variety of types of violence. Husbands with domineering personalities and a history of abuse in their families were significantly more likely to be abusive. In line with other study conclusions regarding the association between IPV and elevated symptoms of depression, social ideation and PTSD. These conclusions were generated from 35 abused women from shelters, reporting that 34% of the participant women were emotionally and physically abused by their husbands (Karakurt et al., 2014).

Another interesting finding reported by literatures that helps to expand the understanding of how external factors such as war zones among victims do not alter their response toward developing mental health disorders when they exposed to IPV under war situations, similar psychological distributions toward IPV were observed. For example, in 2017, the Taylor Manifest Anxiety Scale was administered to domestic violence victims. Palestinian women living in Gaza participated in the study. A range of ages was represented in the study. ANOVA results showed that unmarried victims were significantly more anxious than married victims. Anxiety was extremely severe in 29.9% of victims. The current results are congruent with those of a previous study that evaluated the effects of IPV on 142 participants from a Primary HealthCare in Greece, the majority of whom were not victims (Dami et al., 2017). Eighty-seven point three percent of the total participants were female, while 12.7% were male. The Kruskal-Wallis test showed significant differences in income, residence, education, marital status, abuse, and depression between the groups. Similarly, depression and anxiety were reported among victims of IPV in a previous study (Messing et al., 2014).

A traumatic response to threatening situations is evident in these results, which is in agreement with other research that found anxiety levels higher among those who live in high-risk environments, such as war zones. There are remarkable similarities in results in a community that is always at risk and located in a conflict zone. This survey focused on families and children who were constantly threatened with murder or injury by military forces or bombings (Thabet et al., 2008). To assess the anxiety level of children and mothers who had experienced trauma, manifest anxiety scales were administered. The adolescents as well as the mothers showed clinically significant levels of anxiety. Another study that concluded similar findings was carried out on 214 refugee women within Syria, showing that victims who have been exposed to emotional abuse and sexual abuse were significantly associated with high levels of depression symptomology (Falb et al., 2019).

A study conducted in the US to measure the impact of IPV on young women of a mean age of 29 years old and $SD = 9.34$ (Wright et al., 2019) found that 15% had experienced different forms of domestic violence and reported a few depressive symptoms. Moreover, those who were abused within the past 12 months reported a statistically higher score on the depressive symptoms scale compared to those who were not abused.

However, psychological and economic abuse were found to be the most common forms of abuse in the current study, which attributed to most of the participants developing psychopathological symptoms., there was some consistency with prior studies in these results. For example one research has linked sexual abuse with mental illness. This contradicts the conclusions of the present study (Oram et al., 2017). Contrary to the findings of Choudhary et al. (2012), who investigated sexual assault against female victims of domestic abuse among a total of 61,187 representative samples of both genders, the current findings did not show any significant association between sexual coercion and the risk of developing anxiety among the participants. In contrast to Choudhary et al. (2012), this finding is contrary. Sexual abuse affects 5% of the population. Compared to men, women are at the highest risk. High levels of depression and anxiety were associated with those who were sexually assaulted. The current findings are consistent with other studies that confirm the negative effect of physical abuse on the risk of developing PTSD among participants. According to Cascardi et al. (1999), 17% of women who had been physically abused by their husbands also had PTSD and depression. However, the current findings are inconsistent with other studies indicating that economic abuse towards an intimate partner is associated with adverse mental health consequences, including depression, anxiety, and PTSD among female victims of domestic abuse (Davila et al., 2021). IPV-related adverse mental health issues were confirmed by other research looking at depression and abuse severity among married women (Esie et al., 2019). Seventy-seven point two percent of respondents reported experiencing psychological abuse, whereas 58.8% of respondents experienced sexual violence. Fewer than 45% of respondents experienced physical assault, and one-third of women had injuries as a consequence of physical violence. One in 16 IPV victims had severe depression. More often, older partners and spouses with lower education levels suffered from this condition.

Finally, this research has provided additional evidence with respect to the consequences of IPV, several works of the literature are in line with current research findings that IPV increases the risk of developing mental health issues among victims. The findings lead to a growing body of literature on this topic and emphasize the importance of screening IPV victims for PTSD, depression, and anxiety.

6.3 Risk Factor for Victimisation

Numerous studies in western cultures have examined the risk factors associated with risk of IPV victimization. This ground-breaking study stands out for its unprecedented exploration of risk factors associated with intimate partner violence (IPV) in Qatar. This study further elucidates the factors contributing to IPV within the Qatari context. Using the theoretical framework of the study, these factors included individuals, families, and society as independent variables, which were tested against different types of abuse.

6.3.1 Age at Marriage Time

The current study found that psychological aggression, physical assault, injuries, economic abuse was significantly affected by age at the time of marriage among the young age group who married at the age of 22 years or below, or and those who married at age of 33 years and above. As narrated by the participants in the current study the chance of pregnancy decreases among senior women. The second justification is that women who belong to a senior age group are more likely to know how to manage their lives. When they face a demanding husband who tends to exert power over the relationship, this might increase the risk of abuse among those who do not obey their husbands. Majority of the participants emphasise that marriage at such an early age might result in social pressure that forces couples to have children quickly. This is to prove that they are a healthy couple. The wife prefers to delay getting pregnant, while the husband faces social pressure and suggestions, he cannot make his wife pregnant. Different expectations create tension between couples during their first few years of marriage, especially when they are young.

It is important to understand how interrelated factors influence the risk of abuse from these findings. Similar, findings were observed in the present study. Approximately 20% of the participants in Speizer and Pearson's (2011) study said that when they were younger, their father physically abused their mother. Being married before the age of 18 and tolerating domestic violence are also important predictors of domestic abuse, although marriage for love is not a significant factor.

Following the results of this research, older couples with greater household earnings are less likely to engage in physical abuse towards the wife (Cheung & Choi, 2016). In addition, the present results are consistent with those of Cherlin (2017), who also discovered that the social dominance factor that rules society prevents women from terminating their marriage, even when it is legally authorised. In line with previous research, Physical violence was associated with those women who were married at a young age, with a lower financial status, poor education or unemployed, with two children or more, and those women whose marriage was arranged by their parents (Tokuç et al., 2010). Additionally, young age at the time of marriage and poor household income were both risk factors for domestic abuse against women (Bates et al., 2004). Many factors could explain increased IPV risk with age.

6.3.2 Age Difference Between Husband and Wife

The current findings support what has been hypothesized, that an increased age gap of 10 years and more between married partners may be associated with an increased chance of IPV, particularly increasing the risk of physical harm and causing injuries.

The qualitative data further confirm the trends observed in the quantitative analysis, showing that marriage time and age disparity between husband-and-wife influence the risk of IPV. Several participants concluded complex and varied reasons why age disparity in marriage matters, based mostly on different interpretations of family needs or having a shared interest in how they view the world. These findings broadly support the work of other research in this area linking age disparity between husband and wife with the risk of IPV. For example, findings of another study (Aizpurua et al., 2017) suggest older women are more likely to be psychologically abused than younger women. Psychological abuse is also more common among male partners with high incomes.

Another study found that the risk of IPV tends to increase among those aged between 5 years and more. Moreover, this covariate varies in nature depending on the cultural aspects that motivate this variance as a risk or protective factor (Otieno,

2017). However, in Qatar, the data shows a negative influence of age mismatch between married couples and the risk of spousal abuse. A study of individuals (Paris et al., 2004) contradicted the current findings, showing that the risk of physical violence was relatively lower among those whose age gap between couples was between 3 years, as opposed to those whose age difference was between 2 years and 2 years, as well as those from lower economic classes. In a marriage, a discrepancy in life objectives can cause tension. In addition, this variation might be culturally influenced. Women's occupational status and the age gap between intimate partners may influence abuse between couples, according to WHO reports. Cultural settings, however, can affect these factors (Abramsky et al., 2011) reflecting how everyone would like to prove that they are right. Meanwhile, some believe that financial trouble increases once there is an age mismatch, as the wife would prefer to enjoy her life in a similar way to which she was raised in her parents' house. One further explanation that was offered is that if there is any interference to support men financially this would be considered a direct threat to his manhood principle, and in such cases, the risk of abuse eventually tends to increase.

Contrary to the findings of the current research, in Nepal, women who marry at a young age are less likely to be able to protect themselves from spousal violence (Lamichhane et al., 2011). In line with the current study's findings, those who reported that they married at a younger age are at a greater risk of being exposed to some forms of domestic abuse which reveal that the association between spousal abuse and forced marriages was significant (Sheikhan et al., 2014).

A preliminary study conducted in Bangladesh confirms these findings. Participants with an average age difference of 8.5 years were identified as a risk factor for domestic violence (Das et al., 2016). Research indicates that the age difference between two spouses in the United States may be a predictor of the likelihood that one of them may murder the other. Over 10 years beginning in 1976 and ending in 1985, 16,595 verified homicides were collected from the Federal Bureau of Investigation. In 1976, this era ended (Mercy & Saltzman, 1989). The chance of being murdered by a male spouse is around 1,3 times higher than by a female partner, according to the study. When the woman's age was 2 or 3 years younger than the husband's age, there was a 3.6-fold increase in documented homicides, and women were at higher risk of sustaining major bodily injuries. There is an association between the age difference between the spouses in a relationship and the probability of murder.

In the United States, cross-sectional research was conducted on 155 female teenagers to examine the effect of the age difference between partners on the chance of suffering IPV. This research found, In line with the current study results, that the chance of suffering IPV rose with growing the age difference between spouses (Volpe et al., 2013). Forty seven percent of the participants reported being the victims of moderate kinds of psychological aggression, while 35% reported being the victims of severe forms of psychological aggression, 18% of the participants reported having suffered from severe forms of physical abuse. The average age difference between partners was 1.6 years, although this did not alter the types of domestic violence perpetrated against them or the low power dynamics within the relationships. On the other hand, this may be because the age gap between the spouses is less than it would be otherwise.

6.3.3 Marriage Types

This study revealed several key findings about IPV contributing factors that help explain why some marriage types are at greater risk of abuse. Approximately 50% of marriages in this study were arranged marriages, while 21% were love marriages. About 15.2% of all marriages were among relatives, while forced marriages accounted for about 4.5% of all marriages.

As pointed out by the participants, love marriages are quite uncommon in Arabic and conservative cultures. In the current study, love marriages and forced marriages were associated with a higher risk of IPV. Another important finding was that sexual coercion in this study was greater for those who married a polygamist partner than for victims who married a monogamist partner. Additionally, Physical harm such as minor injuries were associated with those who classified their marriage type either love or force marriages.

These types of marriages have a higher injury rate than those arranged marriages or consanguineous marriages, women's role, and marital type. The rationale behind forced marriages, as narrated by the participants, is that some of the parents or relatives might be unable to continue supporting women financially, therefore the force them to leave parents' house and to get married, so that the family expenses minimized.

There are several possible explanations for these results as narrated by the participants. Taking action against the tradition of the family's marriage structure leaves the abused wife to face their situation alone and protect their dignity from being blamed for their decisions. Alternatively, they may feel threatened by their parents' demands to end the marriage rather than resolve the conflict between the couple.

Consistent with the qualitative data, participants consistently expressed love marriages usually extend beyond the norms of society. This increases the social pressure on the married couple who step aside from tradition by forming a marriage that is culturally accepted and endorsed by all family members. These types of marriages might cause certain remarks, which could ruin the parent's social image and lead to their daughters losing control.

Several factors could explain this observation as narrated by the study participants, victims in this research are culturally influenced to fulfil their husband's sexual desires and wifely obligations. Current study results correlate with studies on why women rationalise violence. More women with more children have abusive husbands than those with fewer. Social or familial pressure and the expense of raising children are important reasons for moms to rethink staying in an abusive relationship, according to one research (Krause et al., 2016). In contrast to the present research, another found that women with more children are 60% less likely to be violent, and women's education level is linked to Intimate partner violence (Rahebi et al., 2019).

Contrary to the current findings, previous research in Zimbabwe found that when women belong to a senior age group (40 years and above), this was considered a protective factor against spousal abuse, as such women are more assertive and know how to deal with the complexity of abusive behaviour. Their results partially aligned with the current findings, that the younger the age group the increased their chances of victimization (Lasong et al., 2020).

Furthermore, physical abuse often happens during fights about money or family spending, according to studies for example, financially controlling husbands are three times more likely to assault their wives (Eldoseri & Sharps, 2017).

In Saudi Arabia, 18.5% of physical abuse included injuries, according to a survey (Eldoseri & Sharps, 2017). Young age, poverty, and planned marriage were major risk factors for Intimate partner violence, while love marriage was not (Ahinkorah, 2021).

Consistent with the current findings, previous research found that emotional, and physical abuse and economic hardship were associated with women whose marriage was classified as a forced marriage (Landau, 2016). Also, in line with the current results, one study found that forced marriages are still commonly practised in Islamic countries. This is because the wife-to-be does not have the free will to choose her life partner. Another argument related to arranged marriages in Arabic culture, namely arranged marriages in which pride plays a minor role in consent. According to Asli and Byouki (2016), this type of marriage is one of the most fundamental rights of a wife who is likely to be compromised or absent from the marriage. Still, Arab families practice and prefer arranged marriages that are permitted and authorized by both families' parents (Bromfield, 2014). In line with previous research relating to how family norms and traditions are persevered and protected above individuals and personal needs, arranged marriages are still preferred among Arab societies, and divorces are far more likely to be considered shameful, which causes parents to worry that they should encourage their daughters to continue and solve their disputes with their husbands (Hammad et al., 1999). These results support previous research into the area of intimate partner violence which links types of marriages, and educational attainment with a potential risk of intimate partner violence. A study was conducted in Sudan to measure the prevalence of domestic abuse against women via a cross-section survey (Ali et al., 2014). It was revealed that 33.5% of 1009 female respondents reported physical abuse, 17% reported being sexually abused, and 30.1% experienced psychological aggression. Moreover, the most common occurrences were shouting, divorce threats, or marrying another wife. The results showed that polygamous marriages and husbands' educational levels are significantly associated with IPV risk.

In line with the current findings, for women in love marriages, their risk of abuse increases twofold, and those couples are less likely to have family approval and full consent, which tends to cause tension among those spouses (Rocca et al., 2009). Clearly, among those who lean towards a more traditional attitude towards family structure and social image, being married at a young age and living in a low-income household increases their chances of IPV victimization (Daoud et al., 2020). Further research found that love marriage is usually packed with the emotion of guilt and shame, which can increase the chance of abuse, especially given women consider these abusive actions to be a challenge rather than a form of abuse (Bhandari, 2020).

Further interesting findings have been found in a study conducted on Pakistani and Bangladeshi populations in Northeast England (Gangoli et al., 2006). Abuse against women and men in the home was prevalent in all kinds of marriages within these groups. There was no direct link between forced marriage and domestic violence, however. Researchers discovered that males who were coerced into marrying a woman exhibited more emotionally abusive behaviour towards their spouses after the wedding. According to the findings of their research, it was typical for parents to engage in practices such as planned weddings and forced marriages. This was because they desire the finest for their children.

6.3.4 Polygamy and Marriage for the Second Time

The current study provided several key findings about marriage formation in Qatar. Around 79% of the analysed marriage categories in this study pertain to monogamous marriages, whereas polygamous marriages account for 20.5% of the total. Another important finding was that women who were married to polygamous partners experienced minor sexual coercion more often than women who were married to monogamous partners. Further confirmation of the trends observed in the quantitative analysis is provided by the qualitative data. Among those who married polygamous partners, many reported being subjected to sexual coercion and economic pressure. According to the senior wives of the participants, sexual abuse was recognized as a method of controlling marital life. It is meant to demonstrate the masculinity of husbands and to show that they are still in love with them.

Moreover, the findings of the study showed that the risk of physical and sexual violence increases among those in polygamous marriages. In previous research, it was found that the most common complaint among senior wives was economic hardship resulting from wealth distribution between co-wives, as well as emotional attention shifting to the new wife, especially when the senior wife was infertile (Dierickx et al., 2019). There were common complaints of feeling hopeless and psychologically abused, which manifested in husbands threatening to marry a second wife and avoiding and refusing to talk to their wives. As theorized in the present study, 68% of women in polygamous marriages are reported to be familiar with this marriage life arrangement, as their father has been married to more than one wife (Al-Krenawi & Graham, 2006).

Past research has suggested that a polygamous family setting is a risk factor for domestic violence against women (Tanimu et al., 2021). Another review study found that IPV victimisation is more likely in a family setting. The polygamous family structure, however, has been shown to have a dyadic effect as both a protective and a risk factor in communities that permit polygamy. Even so, inequalities in fulfilling the demands of family life in those marriages are a major factor contributing to IPV (Ruffin, 2021).

Another clarification made by participants was among those recently married wives who concurred that when marrying a polygamous husband, the sexual relationship must be maintained whenever it demands, and thus minor sexual coercion was frequently reported in the quantitative phases by the study participants. Another possible explanation for these results as reported by the study participants was the financial arrangements for co-wives or both families, unequal treatment, an imbalance in marital rights and being afraid of being abandoned by a husband and consequently living alone were among the most common concerns that made the participants feel depressed and anxious. Clearly, unequal treatment in polygamous marriages is one of the main challenges faced by women being the spouse of a polygamous partner (Den Otter, 2015).

The current study findings are in line with another cross-sectional study that explores the associated factors that increase the risk of IPV (Mapayi et al., 2013). The findings showed a significant difference in IPV scores between women in a polygamous marriage group by 48.9% more when compared to their counterparts from a monogamous group marriage, who scored 32.6%. In line with the current findings, previous research found that wives in polygamous marriages tend to feel lonely, endure economic hardship due to unequal financial support and distribution between co-wives and changes in the husband's priorities, resulting in them failing to maintain the health of their marital life (Naseer et al., 2021). Likewise, sudden divorce without any rational justification and the sudden news of remarried marriages were common complaints, justifying those traumatizing events. The study results obtained from Sudan confirm the present findings, with polygamous women having higher depression scores on average. In contrast, monogamous wives reported comparatively lower levels of depression. Furthermore, polygamous wives had higher anxiety levels than monogamous wives. This variance in scores was due to compromises in the wife's rights since she has co-wives who compete for financial resources and attention from their husband, along with negative social pressure that promotes the termination of the marriages (Al-Krenawi & Graham, 2006).

Another counterargument has been presented in a study from Saudi Arabia, in which 17% of polygamous marriages among Saudi women were not associated with spousal physical assault (Eldoseri & Sharps, 2017). Another line of thought was revealed by scholars who examined the impact of domestic abuse on Arabic Bedouin women's mental and physical health who lived in Israel. They pointed out there is no correlation between spousal abuse and polygamy. This finding might be inconsistent and requires some further investigation due to the inconvenient sample representing co-wives (Cwikel et al., 2003), given it is indicated that spousal violence most likely increases when a husband is unemployed compared to those who have a decent job (41.7% vs. 28.6%, x2 = 3.36, one-sided significance $p > 0.05$). Polygamy is quite a common practice among Arab Bedouin rather than non-Arab Bedouin families. Therefore, we should be cautious in concluding after controlling for the ethnicity of Arab families, to have a fair comparison between the groups.

Contrary to what has been previously theorized in the current study about the potential effect of polygamous families, according to Bird (2007) the study does not show any significant relationship between this covariate and the risk of IPV.

He argues that polygamy is considered a sign of having high-class social status in Uganda, and growing up in a polygamous family doesn't consistently negatively affect mental health. Similar findings were obtained via a household survey from a cross-sectional study carried out in Rwanda on 4338 couples, which measured the prevalence of domestic abuse against women (Thomson et al., 2015).

Regarding the second set of questions, the author investigates the risk of victimization among people who get married a second time. As a result of this investigation, vulnerable couples who remarry for a second time are better understood. Based on the current results, 11.5% of participants were married for the second time, while 88.5% got married for the first time. Furthermore, second marriages were significantly associated with economic abuse. Several participants reported feeling anxious and fearful if they were divorced a second time due to the pressure placed on them by family members. Participants also believed that they would have to compromise their financial rights, as compared to those getting married for the first time. As a result, the abuse escalated.

The qualitative findings offer several explanations for the risk of abuse in second marriages and confirm the findings of the quantitative phase. Participants reported that some second marriages were initiated by a husband's desire to improve his financial status by having control over his wife's financial resources. These findings are confirmed by another study that found that the rate of domestic abuse among remarried wives showed they were more likely to experience economic hardship, along with psychological and physical abuse compared to those who married for the first time (Eng et al., 2020). Like the current findings, experiencing an unsuccessful first marriage was found to increase tension and conflicts among couples in their second marriage (Qureshi, 2020).

These were plausible justifications provided by participants that aligned with quantitative data. Several significant findings from both the quantitative and qualitative results were consistent with those gathered by a separate study (Coleman et al., 2000). This study comprised a review and critique of theories and research focusing on both first marriage and remarriage instability conditions. Most divorced individuals remarry, and remarriages among older adult couples are more stable than first marriages. However, no concrete conclusion was reached regarding whether first or second marriages differed in terms of marital quality. Various factors influence couples' marriages or lead to divorce. In some cultures, stepfamilies are stigmatized and can have a bidirectional impact on family decision-making, quality of life, and certain behavioral problems. The current findings are consistent with a study conducted by Kalmuss and Seltzer (1986), which distinguishes between the risk of abuse among those who remarry after being divorced and those who marry for the first time. Their study findings revealed that the risk of intimate partner violence increases in marriages where one or both spouses remarried. This is compared with those who were married for the first time. Similar findings were observed in a study that took a cross-sectional approach; researchers looked at the experiences of 936 married Egyptian women who had been sexually abused by their husbands. They found that women who had been married more than once and had a lower level of education were significantly more likely to have been victims of spousal violence

(Elnashar et al., 2007). Consistent with the current findings (with few exceptions), a study (Bowlus & Seitz, 2000) found that the employment status of men and the decision to remain in wedlock or remarry is determined by a history of domestic abuse against women, where those who remarry are victims of IPV. The main protective factor was having a sufficient household income. Moreover, abuse tended to occur less among married couples, and victims with a history of parental abuse were more likely to remarry. The study concluded that the determinant factors of domestic abuse against women in second or first-time marriages are significantly correlated with younger-aged and less educated wives. The current findings are consistent with a study's findings in Bangladesh, which revealed that men in their second marriage tend to exhibit a violent attitude towards their wife if they cannot achieve their desired outcome of a second marriage, by having a son or being entitled to get a dowry for his new marriage (Das et al., 2016).

The current findings are consistent with a study conducted in the Philippines showing that among those women who participated in their study 66% had remarried and were young. Their marriage classification ranged between either married for the first, second or fourth time. Furthermore, nearly 33.3% of the participants met the criteria of depression, confirming that the likelihood of IPV victimisation increases among couples who remarried compared to other categories (Gultiano et al., 2009). Similar to the findings presented here, in a cross-sectional study conducted in Nepal examining the risk factors associated with spousal abuse, having two or more children, having low levels of education, and having love marriages were all significantly associated with physical and sexual abuse. Arranged marriages are less likely to experience spousal violence, however. Also, it is a common tradition in Nepal for parents to arrange weddings for their children (Dhungel et al., 2017). Compared to the present findings, the findings regarding arranged weddings are likely the most surprising. Arranged marriages have the potential to increase IPV risk among victims (Gebrewahd et al., 2020). Disparities in findings may be explained by cultural factors that affect the likelihood of abuse occurring throughout a marriage.

6.3.5 Employment and Educational Status

The current study reported several findings about the education disparity between husbands and wives contributing to the risk of IPV. Increased educational attainment was identified as a risk factor for abuse among women. In addition, working women were found to be substantially more likely to be subjected to harsh treatment. Moreover, the current findings showed a significant link between poor female education and victimization.

Furthermore, this study found that scores for severe psychological aggression, physical assault, and sexual coercion varied significantly among victims whose husbands had less than a high school diploma. Essentially, when women marry men with low educational attainment, they are more likely to experience abuse.

Meanwhile, the abuser's employment status, the victim's employment status, and the victim's education level have no influence on women's risk of abuse. The qualitative analysis reinforces the findings of the present study. Several factors related to victimization were identified. These factors suggest that husband concerns escalate into abusive actions whenever the wife pursues education, regains control over her property, or participates in major family decisions. These findings align with results from previous studies where the education variable increased the odds of domestic abuse against wives. Additionally, young and poorly educated individuals are far more likely to experience sexual abuse (Semahegn & Mengistie, 2015). According to another research, the likelihood of a woman becoming a victim of domestic violence increases by more than 23 times when she is younger than 30 years old at the time of marriage (Gebrewahd et al., 2020).

The findings of the current study corroborate previous research, which had indicated that a woman's level of education could influence her likelihood of experiencing IPV. However, the findings of this latest study contradict those prior findings. Data from household surveys were obtained for secondary research, investigating the connection between sociocultural factors and the risk of domestic violence against women. The study was conducted among a sample size of 400 people residing in Hong Kong (Wang et al., 2022). It was found that women with a higher education level were more likely to report being victims of IPV. This is compared to other groups of women with low educational attainment. This was in contrast to other groups of women with low educational attainment. It was observed that neither the working position nor the family income were significantly connected with IPV victimisation. A further study confirmed the current findings. It suggested that husbands who have low educational attainment or have not completed any formal education are more likely to abuse their wives. Additionally, the risk of domestic abuse increases among wives whose husbands witnessed their father abusing their mothers (Owusu Adjah & Agbemafle, 2016). The current finding is partially aligned with study findings revealing that the number of children, along with the education and employment status of the wife increases the likelihood of victimisation (Izugbara et al., 2020). However, in the present study, those variables were insignificant (except for the number of children). Similar to the current findings, other studies have found that husbands might strongly present a male identity in their marriage relationships, especially among those who have a lower social status and educational attainment (Jewkes, 2002).

According to the majority of participants in this study, education disparity between spouses was a significant risk factor that contributed to IPV. These findings are in line with those of previous studies showing a significant association between socioeconomic and demographic characteristics of the spouse and the risk of IPV conducted by Mojahed et al. (2020) on women living in Arabic countries. The present findings were confirmed by another study that demonstrates that an educational disparity between husband and wife increases the likelihood that a woman would become a victim of domestic violence, particularly when only the wife is illiterate or vice versa (Rahman et al., 2013). According to Almosaed (2015), research confirms that Saudi female victims of spousal abuse with less than a high school diploma or its equivalent are considerably more likely to accept domestic violence than Saudi female victims with a higher level of education When contrasted with findings of other studies, the association between a husband's degree of education and marital financial abuse is confirmed. Women are less likely to become victims of domestic abuse if their husbands have a high level of education and job (Alsawalqa, 2020).

Consistent with the present findings, a further study showed that women who have low-paid jobs are at a greater risk of experiencing spousal violence (Lamichhane et al., 2011). According to Rahman et al. (2013), study findings show that economic independence increases women's domestic violence risk, which was in line with the current study findings. Higher-income women are also more likely to experience relationship violence. In research on Indian female domestic abuse victims, those who earn more (Rs. 3000 and above per month) are more likely to encounter domestic violence (OR = 13.7, pb.05) than those who earn less (below Rs. 1000 per month) (Varma et al., 2007).

IPV victimisation was connected with low-educated women, whereas low-income males were more likely to be offenders because financial uncertainty increased men's feelings of vulnerability, leading them to be more aggressive against their spouses (Gass et al., 2011). There is a substantial correlation between domestic violence and factors such as poor family income, a low level of educational attainment for the husband, the presence of a postgraduate degree held by the wife, and the age of the woman at the time of marriage (Barnawi, 2017). In contrast to the results of the present study, data from prior research have shown that a woman's work position may be a possible risk factor for domestic violence against her. Two hundred participants were recruited from primary healthcare clinics to take part in exploratory research that was carried out in Jeddah to determine the extent to which violence is committed against women (Eldoseri et al., 2014). The results revealed that 44.5% of the total participants had been a victim of domestic violence, and it was also shown that the husband's unemployment status enhanced the probability of being a victim of domestic abuse. It was found that over 18.5% of the participants had been harmed, but only 6.5% were able to disclose their injuries to healthcare professionals.

These results further support the idea of the husband's education level, along with his social and employment status became a principal determining factor that increased the risk of abuse against women. For example, a national survey was conducted in Toronto to assess how sociodemographic factors can influence spouse abuse (Smith, 1990). The study findings showed that 27% of the low-income group were more likely to experience a form of abuse than their counterparts. The results indicated that 8% of respondents advised they had been abused by their partner. Unemployed and low status husbands were more likely to physically abuse their wives compared to those husbands with high social status and a decent job. Meanwhile, husbands with a low educational level and low income were essential predictors of wife abuse.

The given findings are supported by the findings of a nationwide survey of 4876 Kenyan women done in 2013. The goal of the research was to examine the risk factors that influence the occurrence of domestic violence against women and to identify the most common forms of abuse in these settings (Djamba & Kimuna, 2015). According to the survey, 36% of respondents reported being physically assaulted by their spouse, and 13% reported sexual coercion due to educational differences. There was also a high association between the wife's occupation and her likelihood of experiencing IPV. The likelihood of being a victim of physical abuse was also highly impacted by characteristics such as the number of children in the family, the age difference between the spouses, and household income. The risk of women being mistreated by their husbands was greater between 7 and 10 years of age difference than between less than 10 years. Many prior studies have been validated by this study. In Bahrain, a study found that 10.5% of pregnant women referred to primary healthcare centres had been physically abused. Furthermore, 29.1% of participants reported that their partner had grown up in a violent family (Al-Ekri et al., 1994).

6.3.6 Household Income

The household factor was set out as an indicator to explore when victims are more likely to be abused by their husbands. The current findings from Qualitative and Quantitative data provide evidence of the influence of household income factor on risk of victimization. This study shows that there was an increased risk of economic exploitation for women with household incomes below 25k per year compared to other income groups. It was also found that there was a significant increase in economic abuse among women from poor households.

Furthermore, women received meagre amounts of money and had limited financial resources. Consequently, their household income was minimal, putting them at an increased risk of abuse. Relying on their husbands as the primary source of income helped them meet their basic needs as wives and mothers. It is somewhat surprising that the financial status of women in this study was not a significant variable increasing their risk of abuse. This is because many parents in Qatar continue to provide financial support to their sons and daughters even after marriage. In the current study, neither the abuser's employment status nor the victim's employment status, nor even the victim's education level, had an effect on women's risk of abuse. Moreover, this study reveals that women play a minor role in decision-making and managing the family's finances. Clearly, the rationale behind this is to continue exerting power over women to keep them financially dependent. Another recurring finding from the qualitative data in this study offers several justifications. For example, false beliefs about traditional gender roles in the family structure, coupled with the husband's low educational attainment, result in poor financial management. This affects the entire household, making it unable to reprioritize household commitments over the husband's leisure or social activities, which consume the family's financial resources.

According to the findings of the current study, living in a household with a low income increases the likelihood of economic abuse. The current findings of the study are in line with the conclusions reached by Postmus et al. (2012) in their exploratory study of 120 female survivors of IPV. Seventy-eight percent of those polled admitted to having experienced employment sabotage at some point in their lives. Expenditures in the household were found to be a frequent demand from abusers. Eighty-eight percent of respondents reported economic control. Furthermore, psychological and physical aggressions were positively correlated with economic abuse. Despite the fact that a variety of risk factors have been investigated in published research, the precise time at which they become lethal across different populations remains unclear. Furthermore, there is little diversity in the samples that were examined (Messing et al., 2014).

Similar findings were suggested by Ali et al. (2014) in a study that found that women in male dominant societies are expected to put the family's interests first above their dreams and compromise her goals by focusing on nurturing her children. Another research has demonstrated a connection between having an unemployed male partner, substance abuse, violence in the family of origin, as well as physical and sexual abuse by their partner in a cross-sectional study of 1401 women in Columbia (Coker et al., 2000). This conclusion was inconsistent with current findings of the research that shows an internecine association between unemployment and risk of IPV.

It is imperative to acknowledge that there are some inconsistencies in the literature, with some studies reporting conflicting findings. In 2009, a study was conducted in Colombia with the objectives of determining the prevalence of domestic violence against women and finding the socioeconomic variables that predict such violence (Jones & Ferguson, 2009). The results of a national survey found that there was an increased likelihood of IPV when there was an age difference and an educational discrepancy between the husband and wife. Consistent with the current findings, significant indications were observed by Walton-Moss et al. (2005) in a study that aimed to identify risk factors associated with injuries among victims of domestic abuse. Women of a young age, male partners with less than a high school degree, coercive control imposed by a male partner, and a history of IPV arrest were associated with injuries. Another study that was done in the United States on 1155 women via a national survey confirmed that the likelihood of physical assault against a wife increases among those who live in an urban residence, as well as among relatively young women, and those who were mothers to four or more children. In addition, the likelihood of physical assault against a wife increases when the husband has a substance abuse problem (Lown & Vega, 2001).

The findings of this study are consistent with those of similar studies conducted in areas other than the West. Three hundred and ninety nine Chinese people responded to the economic abuse scale in 2019. Most of the participants in the study were housewives who were single, cohabiting, widowed, or divorced (Yau et al., 2019), and the results confirm economic abuse among women whose household income ranged between $10,000 and $14,000. Similar findings were found in another study (Abramsky et al., 2011) conducted between 2000 and 2003, which used a household survey. The current results are consistent with findings from previous research that suggest poor communication skills between couples that result in marital conflict increase the risk of domestic abuse (Alam & Islam, 2015). Similarly, previous research found that husbands tend to position themselves in charge of the financial resources, and the wife is assumed to have insufficient knowledge to manage the financial life of the family (Alsawalqa, 2020). Another research found that psychologically weary moms can't provide their children with the same social and economic lifestyle. This complicates leaving and hinders people from ending abusive relationships (Bruton & Tyson, 2018). Regarding financial maintenance or support for wives and children, the most prominent topic was that men often control the amount of monthly financial assistance provided. It was shown that 21% of divorced women pursue further legal proceedings to restore their financial rights (Siganporia, 1993a, b).

Similar results were confirmed by other studies, which found that the level of domestic abuse increased as the wife became powerless due to their lack of economic power in the relationship (Conroy, 2014). The current study confirms previous research findings in Jordan regarding the prevalence of economic abuse, which accounted for 38% of Arabic participants (Alsawalqa, 2020). Similar observations were found by Sharp-Jeffs (2015) in a study that found that when household income is below £50,000, then post-separation financial abuse occurs in the form of manipulating the child support system as a form of exerting power in retaliation against a wife. Poor household income tends to increase the risk of domestic abuse against women, as indicated by three Arabic countries (Egypt, Jordan and Lebanon). This is because men are considered the breadwinners in Arabic society and are held responsible for the family's expenses. This tends to have a negative influence on the tension between married couples (Djamba & Kimuna, 2015).

Other findings from previous research support the current study findings. When the abuser dominates the majority of household decisions, economic violence is also present. One percent of respondents said that their spouses did not respect or consult them with family financial problems (Btoush & Haj-Yahia, 2008). This was also shown by the study's findings, which suggested that 11 victims' narratives revealed economic abuse. Their remarks centred on the fact that they were financially exhausted, left with inadequate funds, took drastic means to avoid sharing money unless it was in their favour, or that their spouses were provided with little allowance to keep financial relations with them (Watson & Ancis, 2013).

Also, in contrast to the findings presented here, a study that was carried out in Ethiopia found that housewives and unemployed women have a risk of being abused by their partner that is more than 18 times higher than that of employed women, particularly in situations in which both the wife and the husband had a lower level of educational attainment. This finding stands in stark contrast to the findings presented here (Gebrewahd et al., 2020). Another interesting justification that emerged from Das et al. (2016) research suggests that women who worked outside the home were at greater risk of becoming a victim of IPV, as were those who were in love marriages. It was argued by the author that these variables could pose a threat to patriarchal culture, which is characterised by the fact that women often rely on their husbands. Additionally, the emotional stress brought on by the wife's need for financial support contributes to the increased incidence of violent behaviour. This is because people who are married to their romantic partners.

The current findings are strongly supported by gender resource theory. This theory claims that domestic violence increases when a husband is motivated by his ideological beliefs and traditional values of life. This in turn forms the basis of the relationship between both husband and wife. According to Atkinson et al. (2005), male breadwinners are viewed as privileged, giving them an advantage over their family members. The study demonstrates a significant correlation between the number of children mothers have and their risk of abuse.

In contrast to the findings of a cross-sectional study carried out in Albania with a random sample of 1039 women, the current findings suggest that the level of education of victims does not affect their probability of being victims of IPV. This is the conclusion that can be drawn from the data. The results of the poll showed that 37% of respondents had been victims of abuse in the past (Burazeri et al., 2005). Young women under the age of 35, husbands with the lowest education level, and women with tertiary education were all at substantial risk of IPV. When a husband thinks that he is unable to fulfil his role as the principal breadwinner in the family, the social status of the relationship suffers greatly. This is because of the societal notion of the husband's position and the expected contribution that they provide to the family. Previous research has revealed that a husband's level of education may be a risk factor for them becoming a violent spouse.

Another research has found some fascinating data on the economic mistreatment of women and the amount they contribute to the costs of raising a family. According to the results, women with increased incomes reported fewer instances of physical and sexual assault during the previous year at the time of the study's baseline (Abramsky et al., 2019). In addition to this, it has been shown that women who contribute more financially to their relationships than their spouses are at a much-increased risk of becoming the victim of sexual and physical violence. This was described in terms of women having scepticism about their husband's ability to provide enough financial resources for the family. In addition, they were required to meet the family's financial expenses. This in turn demonstrates that the probability of domestic violence against women was lower among those who were jobless, as the previous sentence said.

6.3.7 Pregnancy and Infertility

A growing amount of evidence points to a connection between intrauterine pregnancy loss and IPV. According to the findings of this study, various forms of physical and psychological abuse are associated with an increased risk of spontaneous abortion during pregnancy. This study found that 60.7% of participants did not encounter any abuse during their pregnancy, 39.3% did encounter abuse, and 7.1% did not complete their pregnancy owing to partner abuse. According to the results of the study, severe psychological abuse was grater for those who lose their pregnancy. Moreover, there was a significant association between economic abuse and pregnancy.

It is evident from the qualitative results that many participants were faced with similar challenges during their pregnancy, resulting in some participants losing their pregnancy due to repeated abusive behaviours. Most of the participants expressed the feeling of constantly being undervalued by their husbands as a psychological pattern, which consisted of threatening, screaming, or humiliating. Pregnant women in the quantitative analysis were found to have higher ratings of psychological aggression and economic abuse than their counterparts. Furthermore, severe psychological abuse is associated with higher pregnancy losses. These initial results from the current data suggest a link between psychological aggression and pregnancy as a risk factor for IPV victimisation. Two key observations have been used to confirm that pregnancy loss can be attributed to psychological and physical abuse. Several participants suggested that if such incidents were reported to an authority, divorce might result. As demonstrated in previous research conducted in Qatar, women are aware of the social pressure they may face if they escalate the abuse outside the family setting (Al Ghayathin, 2017).

In agreement with the current findings, a study conducted on 161 Omani females (like the Qatari cultural context) Women who suffered abuse during pregnancy and before pregnancy were relatively less likely to suffer abuse when they were not pregnant (Al Shidhani et al., 2020). Further research into this phenomenon reached a similar conclusion that psychologically abused pregnant women have an increased likelihood of pregnancy miscarriage or induced abortion as a result of a response to traumatic events, stress-related triggers, or even direct physical assault (Tiruneh et al., 2018). As confirmed by qualitative data, physical abuse is the second most common cause of pregnancy loss. Despite this, the quantitative results indicate that the association is insignificant. The results of this study are consistent with previous studies (Tanimu et al., 2021). According to previous research, the psychological and emotional experiences of multiple action victims ranged from a partner being unfaithful to their wife to being socially isolated from relatives and friends to excessive jealousy of a wife's social network, all of which were significant predictors of pregnancy loss for women (Tiruye et al., 2020).

The results of this study corroborate previous findings that suggest women who have experienced abuse from an intimate partner during pregnancy are more likely to have a miscarriage. Four hundred and one female victims of domestic violence participated in cross-sectional research conducted by Stöckl et al. (2013). The findings revealed that 29% of the total participants had their pregnancies terminated as a result of some form of physical abuse. In addition, it was discovered that women who had been the victims of physical abuse were much more likely (5.4 times) to lose their pregnancies compared to pregnant women who had not been abused. It is also consistent with the findings of Zakar et al. (2016) who found that 19.5% of participants who had been abused had experienced unintended pregnancies and 36.4% miscarried. Pakistani women of all ages were found to display similar findings. Physical abuse, emotional violence, and fatal losses all had a significant association $p < 0.001$. The current study confirms the results of previous research indicating the risk of pregnancy miscarriage and IPV victims (Tehreem et al., 2021).

An earlier study also found an association between IPV and pregnancy, supporting the current research. A total of 1200 pregnant women who reported to a postnatal clinic were randomly selected to take part in cross-sectional research to determine the frequency of experiencing domestic violence while they were pregnant (Ghazi & Isa, 2018). Approximately 33.3% of pregnant women suffered domestic abuse, according to the participants. The respondents reported emotional abuse at 29.8%, physical abuse at 29.8%, and sexual abuse at the least percentage. The results of previous studies that have come to similar conclusions are consistent with those of the present investigation. One of these studies included the screening of 2562 Cameroonian women to determine the possible risk of domestic violence and its consequences for the loss of pregnancy (Alio et al., 2009).

A second set of questions in the present study aimed to assess the association between IPV victimization and infertility. The analysis found that infertility conditions in women are not associated with abuse, as hypothesized. Consequently, childless women experience IPV less often than women with children. This finding was consistent with the qualitative data, where participants expressed feelings of guilt and isolation, and avoided heated arguments and topics that might cause their husbands to discuss infertility explicitly. However, this avoidance impacted the quality of their marital relationship and communication. Among the other valuable reasons given by participants to reduce marriage stress is the husband's approach to dealing with the wife's infertility with acceptance. Women are aware that marriage to a second wife is an alternative option, putting them under the pressure of unfaithfulness. In contrast to the current findings, a study conducted in Egypt revealed that infertile women were more likely to be abused by their husbands. Here, the form of abuse was manifested in verbal and psychological forms of abuse enacted by husbands, such as being verbally threatened with divorce or threats to marry another woman (Lotfy et al., 2019). The social background of families could determine the way they handle infertility conditions. However, there is variance among couples' reactions to the infertility condition, thus requiring multivariate analysis to understand this variation. In Bangladesh, Papreen et al. (2000) have found that social and community pressures are high among infertile women. Most commonly, threats of remarriage were used as a form of abuse, followed by labels such as incapable of providing happiness for the family, in which women are socially marginalized and disparaged for their inability to bear children. The result is that such women are fearful of rejection and insecure about their marriage life, which they fear may be terminated at any time because infertility forms the basis for remarrying or divorcing, which is accepted by the community. The current results were found to be contrary to a previous study conducted in western culture (Sheikhan et al., 2014). Furthermore, a cross-sectional study that was carried out on 400 infertile Iranian survivors of spousal abuse (Ahmadzad-Asl et al., 2016) revealed that 34.7% of the total participants suffered from domestic violence as a result of their infertility condition. When one partner in a married couple is unable to have children, increased levels of stress are correlated with a lack of educational understanding among couples on reproductive health. The current research findings confirmed that an inability to have children is not a sufficient excuse for spousal abuse. Another explanation was found in research justifying why infertility was not a contributing factor to IPV. This is because children don't need to work in agricultural jobs for their fathers to maintain the family's financial stability. In addition to this, it demonstrates that there was less rivalry amongst co-wives as a result of the decline of the polygamy notion in Nigeran culture (Solanke et al., 2018).

In contrast to the data shown here, research that was carried out on 142 women in Turkey revealed that psychological abuse was a prevalent kind of abuse. The prevalence of psychological abuse was evident. Economic status and low levels of education were also associated with IPV. IPV was reported by 47% of infertile spouses (Akpinar et al., 2019). In a study conducted by Aduloju et al. (2015), infertility for a longer period of time was associated with an increased risk of IPV.

6.3.8 Number of Children

As expected, the current study findings confirm previous research that has indicated that an increased number of children is associated with an increased likelihood of IPV. The most interesting findings was about moms with three or more children were more likely to experience IPV. In most cases, abuse was caused by a spouse's failure to provide sufficiently for the other partner. A further study supports the current findings that women who have a greater number of children are more likely to experience domestic abuse, such as emotional and physical abuse (Terrazas-Carrillo & McWhirter, 2015). This increase was attributed to the economic factor. This is contrary to the current findings where it is confirmed that the risk factor for the number of children increases with the odds of sexual coercion.

The risk of sexual abuse was particularly high in quantitative results. This study shows mothers who have more children than other groups show a positive correlation with severe sexual coercion. According to the findings from the Qualitative phase, these results are likely to be related to a wife's inability to maintain her wifely duties, including maintaining her husband's sexual needs, which were aggravated by a poor night's sleep, fatigue, and many other factors that interfered directly with the financial aspects of maintaining the needs of a newborn. Compared to women with one child, women with two or three children had a higher risk of experiencing domestic violence (Acevedo et al., 2013).

In line with previous research conducted in Jordan, the number of children was not shown to be associated with economic abuse (Alsawalqa, 2020). In line with previous literature, the age gap between married couples and the number of children is both risk factors for spousal abuse, showing that women with a greater number of children tend to be reluctant to engage in sexual relations with their partners. The number of children increases the chance of Intimate partner violence, according to another research (Cwikel et al., 2003).

The present results are consistent with those of previous research that investigated the sociodemographic characteristics that enhance the likelihood of IPV among a sample of 1402 Spanish women. According to the results of Ruiz-Pérez et al.'s (2006) research, moms who have three or more children and those whose home income is low are at greater risk of suffering an increased risk of experiencing all types of Intimate Partner Violence. Another research came to a similar conclusion, stating that the risk of young individuals having three or more children and having their husbands be between the ages of 24 and 35 was considerably increased when compared to the general population (Raj et al., 2006). Another substantial correlation was identified between women in Nepal who had two or more children and different types of physical and emotional abuse by their husbands or partners (Dhungel et al., 2017). In addition, another study reached several conclusions that contribute to IPV, in line with current research findings. Women who were separated or divorced or who had three or more children had a greater chance of experiencing sexual abuse or physical abuse by their life partner than women who didn't fall into any of these categories (Campbell et al., 2003).

6.3.9 Family of Origin Violence

In line with the hypothesis that witnessing a family of origin parental abuse influences women's adulthood victimisation, the current findings show that economic abuse is associated with husbands who had witnessed their fathers abusing their mothers during their childhood. Women who experience psychological abuse by their partner admit to having a history of family violence, having witnessed their father abuse their mother as children. Various reasons revolved around husbands emulating their fathers' actions to address conflicts as a common familial approach. Additionally, certain individuals held misconceptions about traditional masculinity, which diminished women's involvement in decision-making. Moreover, some were significantly impacted by their fathers' teachings about upholding family values, and when wives questioned these principles, the intensity of abuse escalated.

These results support social learning theory, which emphasizes the importance of modelling learned behaviour after observations (Bandura, 2019). Aggression is normalized as a tool to resolve conflict in abusive relationships. Therefore, victims are more tolerant of aggressive attitudes because of this (Laland & Rendell, 2010). The findings are reinforced by qualitative analysis. This revealed a common subtheme which was reported frequently by the participants about how the childhood history of husbands had a significant impact on their attitude. The emphasis was primarily on managing household expenses or resolving conflicts through screaming or throttling. Women who were mistreated as children or experienced parental violence build a stable relationship with their spouses, increasing their risk of IPV (Godbout et al., 2009). Young women exposed to violence are more inclined to accept it (Basar et al., 2019). In a similar vein, it was shown that among violent men, 55% of them either observed violence in their family of origin or were assaulted when they were children. This was found to be the case among violent spouses. The research identifies various risk factors that co-exist with a violent spouse, such as those who were mistreated as children, those whose husbands were from lower middle-class backgrounds, and those who had been married for more than 5 years (Fikree et al., 2005). In addition, the likelihood of adulthood victimisation of men increases by 60% for those who had witnessed parental violence (Kerley et al., 2010).

This discovery would imply, as the results of another research have shown, that those who have been abused as children might go on to abuse others as adults. Ahinkorah (2021) discovered that there was a statistically significant link between being exposed to violence as a kid and later being involved in an abusive relationship, and this was true for both sexes. In contrast to these results, it has been shown that women who have been victims of IPV are four times more likely to have seen violence in their families of origin or to have been the victims of physical abuse when they were children (Gass et al., 2011). The studies so far indicate that there is no substantial link between women's violent experiences in their families of origin and their adult victimisation.

This finding broadly supports the work of other studies in this area linking family of origin violence and adulthood victimisation. Hence, the results of our study support social learning theory's contention that the family environment plays an important role in shaping attitudes and behaviours towards domestic abuse. Correspondingly with another study (Kerley et al., 2010), 816 married Thai women were screened for the intergenerational impact of witnessing direct or indirect parental abuse on their adult victimization and offending. There was a significant association between witnessing parental violence during childhood and IPV victimisation. The physical assault odds increased by 66% among adult female IPV victims who had frequently witnessed their fathers abusing their mothers. This study is consistent with other studies showing that family of origin violence, such as witnessing parental abuse or tolerating partner violence, increases the likelihood of IPV victimisation (Tiruneh et al., 2018). Similarly, it has been found that exposure to family-of-origin violence or IPV increases the likelihood of developing depression, sleep deprivation, hypertension and abortion (Hawcroft et al., 2019).

Similar findings were supported by a study conducted in the United States with 14,564 male participants aged 20 and older yielded equivalent findings to the prior investigation. Four percent of all participants were found to have physically attacked their spouse at some time throughout their relationship (Roberts et al., 2010). According to the conclusions of a major study, there is a high correlation between having seen violence in one's own family of origin and being abused by one's spouse as an adult.

Emerging findings from current results are broadly consistent with earlier *the* intergenerational effects of witnessing parental abuse on victims' adulthood lives have been aligned with the Madruga et al.'s (2017) study which reported that participants who were abused by an intimate partner faced violence in their families of origin 16.6% of the time. Their chances of being victimized by IPV in adulthood were nearly four times higher. The risk was threefold higher than their counterparts who had not witnessed parental abuse. Furthermore, the risk of becoming a perpetrator was found to be heightened among those who had witnessed parental violence by 7.3%. The current findings are also consistent with other research showing that women who witnessed parental abuse are more likely to be victimized as adults. According to the findings, 33.7% of women who had witnessed violence in their families of origin had been psychologically abused, 39.6% had been physically abused, and 9.1% had been sexually abused. Furthermore, contrary to the findings of the present study, the same study found that younger women are less likely to experience domestic violence (Burgos-Muñoz et al., 2021). These results are in agreement with those obtained from cross-sectional research conducted in Turkey to identify the characteristics that raise a woman's risk of being a victim of IPV within 1 year of being exposed to it (Yüksel-Kaptanoğlu et al., 2012). Men who see their father physically beat their mother are more likely to physically and sexually abuse their future wives. There was no correlation between the husband's employment status and the likelihood of domestic violence.

Findings from a systematic review conducted in Ethiopia revealed that the risk of violence considerably increases when the husband turns out to have a history of family violence, when women are married before the age of 18, or when the wife's occupation status was a housewife (Semahegn & Mengistie, 2015). Moreover, the current findings highlight that when husbands have a history of witnessing parental violence this increases the likelihood of abusing their spouse economically in adulthood.

In line partly with the current findings, women who have partners with a secondary school degree or post-graduation degree are more likely to report a lower likelihood of IPV whereas females victims witnessing physical abuse against the mother in their family of origin are at a greater risk of being physically and sexually abused in their adulthood life (Thomson et al., 2015).

Domestic violence against women and family member maltreatment has both been proven to be influenced by a variety of significant variables, including a history of domestic abuse in the family of origin throughout childhood (Bracewell et al., 2021). It is probable that a perpetrator's financial obligations and unmet family expenses play a major part in their violent behaviour. Those who were convicted of criminal offences were more likely to engage in detrimental forms of abuse. This included the murder of a member of their own family or a love partner. According to the results of this research, exposure to domestic violence as a kid increases a person's likelihood of becoming a victim or perpetrator of violence as an adult. Two factors that may increase a person's risk of IPV are cultural preferences and the notion of masculine supremacy (Jewkes, 2002). The emphasis put on the notion that men are fundamentally superior to women tends to associate the masculinity principle with any strategies that may be used to establish control and authority over women.

6.4 Being Still Passive in an Abusive Relationship

Similar to the findings of other studies that shows child custody rights and post-divorce settlement can complicate and alter women decision to leave abusive relationship due to the complicated process that is often formed based on the child's best interests (Miller & Manzer, 2021). Similar concerns were noticed in this sample as well.

The current study offered several key findings contextualized understanding about why some women remain passive in abusive relationships, demonstrating their lack of action in response to violence. According to the Qualitative findings, the participants' major concerns were changes in child custody rights terms, family and social pressure, bureaucracy, preserving family dignity, and abuse after a divorce where patterns of concerns were centred around participants finding themselves in situations where they cannot afford a decent life after a divorce, which specifically affects divorced mothers. This shows that post-divorce economic hardship is created by the abuser who wishes to control the victim's life by limiting their financial resources. Husbands are more likely to threaten such a course of action when women seek to end an abusive relationship that keeps them thinking about their future life after marriage. Several participants expressed concerns that their ex-husbands are not fulfilling parental responsibilities as a form of emotional retaliation against them. Other concerns reported by quarters of the participants was about family pressure. For example, one participant stated "I prefer to continue with him until he changes instead of facing family pressure. I am so sad, no one cares anymore". A concern was raised that participants may be forced to normalize their emotions by their parents or relatives in some way. For example, one participant said "My mum told me that marriage life is quite a challenge. you go in a white dress, and you are allowed to come back only in a white shroud".

A plausible justification was also offered by the participants, who indicated that their children would benefit from remaining in bond with their husbands. Another emerging concern emerged from the findings concerning husbands' manhood ideology and social status. This is if a wife seeks professional help to end abuse or even to resolve a marital conflict. According to the participants, retaliation is exerted after divorce, especially when it comes to children's education and certificates, where the husband delays submitting or covering applications related to schools and travel. For example, one participant said "I cannot ask for professional help because I know it is a very sensitive subject that may worsen my post-marriage financial life by cutting Nafaqa or even cause problems by changing my children's school from private to public". Consequently, misperception of husband images could complicate marriages or even post-divorce settlements. Another participant raised concerns about attorneys' fees and the bureaucracy of the trails, which might deplete them financially or even disqualify their claim based on insufficient evidence. Due to these reasons, the leaving process is quite complex and requires multi-sectoral intervention to ensure that victims or abused mothers are left in a safe environment with their children during or after a divorce.

The current study findings reveal that women encounter a great deal of stress after ending their relationship. The ex-husband tries to stall the legal proceedings often by using children as a tool to retaliate against or cast their ex-wife as unfit parents to withdraw her child custody rights. This narrative agrees with a previous study that showed that child custody laws can deny women their rights and freedom. For example, a study that was carried out in Tunisia on the topic of violence against Arabic Muslim women found that the cohesion and unity of the family are significantly more important than any other personal rights and that they should be preserved at any cost (Douki et al., 2003).

The current findings show that some of the participants were concerned about post-divorce image and social status which is usually associated with shame and guilt of not being able to restore a married life. This concern was also confirmed by research conducted in Egypt found that 48% of people living in violent relationships were unwilling to be divorced owing to the shame associated with post-divorce life, which increases the probability of spousal abuse (Ibrahim et al., 2010). In order to safeguard the family's image, Arabic women who are victims of domestic violence often choose to resolve their marital conflicts inside the family, rather than seeking official or professional assistance, as seen by the fact that only 8% make formal requests (Cwikel et al., 2003). Arabic women who are victims of domestic violence prefer to seek professional assistance as a matter of custom.

These results are reinforced by another Saudi Arabian research that looked at why Saudi women accept abuse (Almosaed, 2015). Saudi women have fewer choices to cope with Intimate partner violence since their culture emphasises childcare as a wifely obligation, limiting their financial and civic independence. Another research found a link between kid number and maltreatment. In a study of Saudi female domestic violence victims, those with 3–5 children showed higher tolerance for abusive behaviour than those without children, who favoured divorce (Almosaed, 2015).

The present findings are supported by other literature showing reasons for common tactics used by ex-husbands when they get separated. The most common theme among the participants was their post-divorce concerns, which were related to their child support entitlement, which was usually manipulated or delayed by a former husband as a form of continuing exerting power over a spouse and to retaliate to being abandoned (Branigan & Grace, 2005). Usually, divorced mothers and their children alternatively live with their families of origin, especially when they are not economically sufficient or independent (Siganporia, 1993a, b).

Consistent with the current study's findings, in another qualitative study, 19 divorced women expressed their concerns about visitation in relation to child custody terms, where they have been frequently threatened by their ex-husbands that their child custody rights could change. This post-separation tactic imposes emotional distress on divorced mothers and leaves them with fear and insecurity about their children's welfare (Zeoli et al., 2013).

In Arabic, this kind of submission is known as "ta'a". These misunderstandings are commonly used to justify husband aggression, which is frequently misconstrued in a different context than intended (Yount, 2011). For example, in Arabic culture, women are trained to be submissive to their husbands, and as a result, they are culturally conditioned to suffer abuse more readily than women bred in other cultures (Barnawi, 2017). The findings of the current study are consistent with the beliefs of the male-dominated society and another study conducted in Tunisia on violence against Arabic Muslim women, which revealed that family cohesion and unity are significantly more important than any other personal rights and that unity must be maintained at any cost. The findings of the current study are also consistent with the findings of the other study (Douki et al., 2003). Another concern reported by the participants of the current study shows the personal vindictiveness of the abuser post-divorce in claiming child custody rights in their favour. In line with other research findings, many child custody procedure demands are motivated by the abuser's vindictiveness (Watson & Ancis, 2013).

A Jordanian study indicated that the number of children and a woman's monthly wages were insignificantly connected with economic violence (Alsawalqa, 2020). Most participants concerned in the current study were worried about post-divorce arrangements for children and that was one of the leading factors to deter their decision to terminate their marriage.

Several factors repeatedly expressed by the participants have associated costs of post-divorce arrangements, high attorney's fees, and change in child custody rights with key factors that contributed to women remaining passive in the abusive relationship linked to the bureaucracy of filing a divorce case and terminating their marriage. The views of the participants seem to corroborate with the ideas of Zeoli et al. (2013), who suggest that domestic abuse victims are desperate and unfamiliar with the court in terms of providing evidence to prove their claim. Thus, they fail to comply with the court's evidential mandate by providing less incriminating evidence, which has led to undermining victims' claims and prolonging the divorce procedure. The current findings outlined and confirmed the fear associated with women who wish to seek professional help to end or break the cycle of abuse which was confirmed by previous research. This data confirms the relationship between divorced women's shame in Arabic society and the likelihood of Intimate partner violence since it's unlikely to be reported to authorities (Abolfotouh & Almuneef, 2020). Indeed, professional advice in marital issues may be taken out of context, given that fear of penalties prevents individuals from seeking help. Research found that asking for professional aid or law enforcement to resolve a marital conflict might result in the woman being shunned by her community and blamed for any future complications that harm family unity (Douki et al., 2003).

The current findings supported by another research indicated that divorce lawyers tend to overlook the history of abuse and how a former partner's unexpected activities might extend the proceeding process to apply divorce terms in his favour (Hardesty & Ganong, 2006). There are also additional rights, such as the dowry, which is financial help offered to the woman if the marriage is dissolved (El Sheikh, 2019). As a consequence of this, it is very uncommon for an abuser to make threats about the child custody arrangement, and more serious and violent ex-husbands may on occasion try to kidnap the children (Hardesty & Ganong, 2006). Women who seek to end their relationship with the abuser by filing khulu cases—which are shown to be costly—drained them financially. This was in line with the Dray (1987) findings associated with khulu divorce, in which the dowry must be returned by the wife, and this process must be obtained by court order. Dray also outlined important aspects that are considered a widespread worry among divorced women who wish to remarry, or if she was found to be morally or physically unfit, then her default claim to child custody rights might be revoked.

This was also brought to light in a study that was conducted in 2013, in which respondents made similar comments regarding the complications associated with the current law article. This study sought to understand the reasons behind the high number of divorce cases that occur in countries along the Arab Gulf. According to the results of the research, the prevalence of divorce in Kuwait, Qatar, Bahrain, and the UAE varied between 34% and 46%, and the rate of spinsterhood indicators across these nations was between 15% and 20% of women who were unable to marry because of a lack of opportunity. In addition, the average age at which people get married has fallen, and the percentage of marriages that end in divorce is particularly high in the first 3 years. The prevalence of arranged weddings in many nations, where there is a noticeable lack of alternatives and access to information about whether a spouse is abusive before marriage, was one important element that significantly contributed to the deterioration of the marital situation (Anser, 2013).

In line with the present findings of the study that the option of getting remarried after divorce is quite challenging. Several findings have also been published regarding domestic abuse among married women. These findings indicate that a woman's decision to remain in an abusive relationship or become a second wife can be influenced by the frequency of abuse and the availability of alternative remarriages post-divorce. Thus, they may have to tolerate the stigma associated with a second marriage, which could negatively influence and consequently elevate the level of abuse between spouses (Adjei, 2017).

Financial factors contributed significantly to women's decisions to continue or leave abusive relationships in the present study. The current findings agree -in part- with a study conducted by Xu et al. (2005) in China showed that 1 in 5 women in the studied sample had been physically abused by their partners. The risk factors behind IPV increased when women had an unemployed partner, were forced to stay jobless, and when depended on their husbands to meet their financial needs. The results of the present research are congruent with those of a previous study that analysed the risk variables among 1004 women from various ethnic groups in order to determine the chance of victimisation. The data found that women with less than a high school diploma and a monthly income of less than $500 are more likely to experience partner violence (Bohn et al., 2004).

These are common tactics that are exerted to restrict women from leaving an abusive partner and encourage them to remain passive. These data build on existing evidence from previous research showing that the separation process is difficult due to the manipulative and non-compliance tactics that are used to drain the financial resources of the wife, by deliberately delaying court orders regarding post-divorce financial support and other incentives (Cameron, 2014). These relationships may partly be explained by Dhungel et al. (2017) of victims of spousal violence from Nepal, which attempted to quantify the risk variables of domestic abuse and found similar results. Who found that women who were financially reliant on their husbands were more susceptible to being subjected to physical abuse than women who were not economically dependent on their husbands. In addition, women who were financially dependent on their husbands were more likely to experience sexual assault. In addition, the number of women who experienced psychological abuse was three times more likely to occur in this population.

Another important finding related to women unable to end their relationship with their abusive husband was family pressure around being divorced which has an influence on a wife's decisions and can lead an abused wife to live with an abusive partner, suffer in silence and avoid seeking family support. The results of Rabaan et al.'s (2021) study conducted in Saudi Arabia are in agreement with current findings, where women were encouraged to tolerate unfavourable outcomes so that their marriages would be saved, and they would become more resilient to their husbands' actions. In accordance with the present results, previous studies have demonstrated that divorce is still a valid right, it is still in Arabic culture considered the least desirable solution and most of the criticism is associated with divorced mothers, given they are held accountable to protect the family unity and endure husbands' misbehaviour (Mendoza et al., 2020). There are several possible explanations for this result, social stigma and pressure from relatives are major concerns that push victims away from ending abuse. These are mostly driven by the social aspects of divorced daughters, who sometimes identify with their parent's failure to teach them how to be good wives, along with parenting manners to their daughters in order to be considered good wives. These results reflect those of Bromfield (2014) who also found that social stigma in patriarchal societies is still a public problem associated with social stigma relating to divorced women. In such contexts, the chances of remarrying are quite slim, especially for divorced mothers.

Another factor that may cause women to remain passive in abusive relationships is victims' rights following divorce. The majority of the participants in the current study highlighted their concerns regarding child custody status (which they were unfamiliar with) or suggested they might end up losing their custody rights if they wanted to seek a better opportunity with a new life partner. These results are consistent with previous research that was carried out in Egypt which found that women continue to have concerns relating to their post-divorce arrangements, specifically about their entitlement to child custody rights if they decide to remarry (Mendoza et al., 2020).

There are, however, other possible important explanations repeatedly reported by the participants about their post-divorce concerns. The option to remarry was a common concern among mothers who sought to separate since their child custody rights would be changed by default after remarrying. Moreover, post-divorce financial maintenance will differ drastically among mothers who have a high number of children of different age groups. These results are consistent with those obtained and explained by Campbell (2017), which show that abusers often threaten their wives with child custody to prevent them from ending their relationships.

It is critical to consider possible alternative explanations to understand these results. As revealed by several patterns in the participants' narratives, the current post-dissolution entitlement isn't enough for large family members. Mothers with a high number of children of different ages attending different school locations at the same time can find it challenging. The mother is unable to balance her role as mother and worker without additional assistance, resulting in a compromise between maintaining basic family needs and maintaining life balance. Often, an additional driver or housemaid is needed. The current findings are in line with previous research showing how difficult it is to manage changes in family arrangements after a divorce. This includes issues relating to leaving a home where they all once lived as a family. Furthermore, children's education is impacted due to these major life changes (Sheykhi, 2020).

After a divorce, the nature of the family's accommodation will change based on the court order, either via financial compensation paid on a monthly basis to the divorced mother and children, which will allow them to live in new the house, or otherwise to continue to live jointly in the same house with her ex-husband by splitting the floors, based on courts judgement. Regarding housing issues, sometimes the husband is asked by the court to pay for a new house so that the wife and children can live far away from their original house. This can result in difficulties for the mother in managing the commute to school and to work. This tactic is often used to retaliate against a wife for seeking divorce. This was supported by research findings from a previous study that identified an Egyptian study of 20 married Assiuiti Arab women of reproductive age. Men's revenge may worsen if family secrets are divulged to a stranger, as emphasised by responses that emphasised the guilt associated with seeking professional counselling or assistance. Society dictates that a respectable lady adheres to her husband's rules (Yount, 2011).

Consistent with the current findings, other research found that divorced mothers have limited financial resources and their housing allowance or accommodation options are at a disadvantage (Ferrari et al., 2019). These results match those observed in earlier studies, where it was found that the financial burdens on single parents, children's expenses and basic needs, an inability to live with the family of origin due to family disputes or being blamed for not being patient enough to save their marriage, along with getting proper accommodation are major concerns among divorced mothers (Rathi et al., 2018).

Another contributing factor to why some victims remain passive in the abusive relationship was the lack of familiarity with current family law which was observed among participants relating to their rights as a wife or as a divorced mother, which can leave them incapacitated and/or confused regarding how the violence can be ended. Some victims who couldn't pursue justice due to legal bills were financially dependent on their spouses (Campbell, 2017). When the abuse was committed equally by both parents and if the moms couldn't offer enough proof, the court may lessen the claim (Jaffe et al., 2008). The least common observation was that women with very limited financial resources are unable to maintain the court's requirement to file for a divorce case due to the high cost of attorneys, which leaves them to abandon their rights to obtain freedom by getting divorced. Previous studies indicated that losing a divorce lawsuit is expensive and might leave a woman in debt for attorney's expenses. There are also worries about the matter dragging on until the court call (King et al., 2017). Some participants said they couldn't report abuse to the authorities to save their marriage because men in Arabic culture are cautious and overprotect their social and personal image. Solving marriage conflicts outside the home could have negative consequences for the entire family, especially in a conservative and male-dominant society. In prior research in Qatar, it was determined that Qatari society is one of the world's most conservative, with conventional gender roles dictating that a good wife protects family interests and values (James-Hawkins et al., 2017).

6.5 Attitude Towards Women's Rights

These findings seem to be in line with the findings of prior studies, which discovered a connection between women's mindsets on gender roles and kinds of domestic violence that may be impacted by the women's beliefs (Harris et al., 2005). This study reported that 50.9% of participants indicated they were pro-feminist and egalitarian, while 49.1% were conservative. There were several significant findings regarding how women's mindset influences whether or not they are more traditional and conservative when it comes to abuse. Several salient patterns emerged from the analysis, each of which contributes to a more comprehensive understanding of the attitudes of victims of domestic abuse and their perceptions of women's role and rights in society, along with how their belief system can increase their likelihood of IPV victimisation. Findings from the quantitative analysis show that women who hold traditional and conservative views about women's rights were more likely to suffer severe sexual coercion and injury. Conversely, psychological aggression was associated with victims who were pro-feminist and held liberal views on women's rights. Furthermore, economic abuse was negatively correlated with attitudes towards women's rights. A possible explanation provided by the participants was that wives with traditional belief systems have been raised in a family where family values and traditions should be preserved, regardless of the cost, and are therefore more docile and tolerant of their abusive husbands. The more liberal women were more likely to report abuse and ask for more equal rights. There is a possibility that this argument resulted in her being psychologically abused. Another line of thought as that explains why liberal wives tend to be more likely psychologically abused because whenever they tries to preserve her rights or defend herself, they might be called stubborn women and might be punished for that said. Participants perceived that victims who endure traditional gender roles and docility find a cultural haven from abuse, as they are less likely to question their family's established approach to marital dynamics. However, once this established principle is disrupted, women often find themselves subjected to suppression within their own familial spheres as they breach the family traditional model.

As stated by one of the participants in this study "males in Arabic culture dislike being questioned about their financial choices". A recurring issue among participants pertains to meeting their husbands' expectations and requirements. Nevertheless, participants have astutely acknowledged the potential ambiguity in their husbands' perceptions of docility and submissiveness.

Hence, it could conceivably be hypothesised that different forms of abuse can be attributed to different mindset beliefs. Qualitative data complement quantitative findings since many participants shared narratives about their experiences holding a traditional mindset, which presumably reduced tension in their relationships. As a result of the passive attitude of women towards their husbands' prosperity, this occurs. During the qualitative phase, though more liberal in terms of response patterns, heated arguments can be rationalized since the wives are more aware of their rights which adds a plausible explanation for the quantitative results. Most participants of the current study constantly outline that husbands Domaine are culturally driven which is in line with the feminist theory principles in defining IPV.

Interestingly, these results are in keeping with the previous study that was carried out in 1996 that compared attitudes towards women's roles in Kuwaiti and Qatari societies (Abdalla, 1996). It was found that liberal opinions and a more equal approach towards women's roles were greater among Kuwaiti participants than Qatari participants (both genders). According to AWS, Qataris have more conservative and traditional views regarding women's rights. Participants' attitudes towards women were assessed based on their conformity to social gender norms and their belief that women play a role in society, as well as their belief that traditional gender roles are firmly segregated (Glick & Fiske, 1997). Patriarchal social belief systems tend to influence the traditional gender roles of the family. These results confirm the association between patriarchal societies and perceptions of women's roles in societies. In line with the current findings, a study conducted in the United Arab Emirates revealed that women score relatively higher on the attitude towards women scale. This is compared to male candidates. However, their scores still undermine women's role in the community, indicating that they shift more towards conservative and traditional roles in terms of women's participation in society. This influencing factor might account for the patriarchal family structure and conservative society, which defines and dictates women's contribution to society (Alibeli, 2015).

These results were consistent with DeGregoria's (1987) finding that liberal women were able to identify and address power imbalances in their marriages than women with traditional beliefs. Consistent with the current findings, previous research has also demonstrated the importance of understanding women's mindset in predicting forms of abuse. Suggesting that the more traditional the beliefs and attitudes women held the less likely they were to be abused by their partner. Justification is that they were unaware if the actions or tactics in question were considered forms of abuse (Harris et al., 2005). A number of findings have been made regarding domestic violence among married women, including the possibility of alternative remarriage opportunities after divorce and the frequency of abuse that women experience. These factors can influence a woman's decision to remain in a violent relationship or become a second wife after divorce. Due to this, they may be forced to tolerate the stigma associated with a second marriage, which could negatively affect and consequently escalate the level of abuse between husband and wife (Adjei, 2017).

The findings of this study were consistent with the conclusions reached out by a study conducted in 2014 in Jeddah. Among Saudi women who have been victims of domestic abuse in Jeddah, women who are more forceful and liberal in their ideas are more likely to have experienced intimate partner violence, while women who hold traditional values are less likely to have experienced spousal violence (Eldoseri et al., 2014). Another plausible explanation was provided which is in line with current study findings and reveals an important expansion of previous research studies that highlighted the association between spousal abuse and the power dynamic of the family, which is mainly driven by society's patriarchal belief system (Btoush & Haj-Yahia, 2008). A research of 291 Arabic married women from Israel found that the more traditional the woman and the more traditionally a husband regards their wife's gender position, the more likely they are to excuse their husband's aggressiveness, increasing their probability to be victims of Intimate partner violence (Haj-Yahia, 2002).

There are still some discrepancies in previous research findings on the influence of gender roles in families on the risk of IPV. Like the current findings, traditional gender roles were found to be a risk factor for IPV victimisation. This was in a sample of 157 male and female students who participated in a study to measure perceptions of wife abuse. It was revealed that men who indicated they were more traditional, and conservative were more likely to blame women and hold them accountable for provoking their husband's aggression (Kristiansen & Giulietti, 1990). Meanwhile, female students whose scores indicated a more liberal and egalitarian attitude were more likely to not attribute women's attitudes as a factor behind their partner's aggression.

Furthermore, it was found by another research that the ability of the current generation to protect the norms, values, and traditions of the previous generation by preventing further amendments in the marriage model that result in a decrease in the inherited value of the culture is a common concern in patriarchal societies. This concern is fundamentally centred around the ability of the current generation to protect the norms, values, and traditions of the previous generation (Sarkar & Rizzi, 2020).

In line with the current findings, Cavanaugh et al. (2011) also discovered that the psychological domain of the perpetrator includes women who refuse to fulfil their husband's sexual desires. Data showed this trend. In patriarchal cultures, spouses may respond forcefully when their masculinity is questioned, according to another research. Some researchers describe patriarchy as a male-dominated society in which males become the predominant breadwinner (Sultana, 2012). This idea arises when clerical gender roles impact how both genders behave. Gender inequality misinterprets religious provisions and oppresses women's rights. In male-dominated civilizations like Bangladesh, conventional gender roles persist (Sultana, 2012). The current findings are reinforced by similar results found in a study that was conducted on how gender and Islam shape egalitarianism among Egyptian and Saudi youth. Respondents who were religious and educated were more likely to highlight the significance of conventional gender roles in the house; nevertheless, young women were more likely to disagree with the declaration that they must always follow their husbands. When scores from Egypt and Saudi Arabia were compared, it was discovered that young Egyptians are more likely to embrace a more egalitarian social structure. The young Egyptians had a mean score of 6.12 ($SD = 2.56$), whereas their Saudi Arabian counterparts had a mean score of 4.75 ($SD = 3.05$). This finding was based on the fact that the mean score for Saudi Arabians was lower (Kucinskas, 2010).

In line with this point of view and the qualitative findings, one study that was conducted on 871 Chinese couples examined the association between husband and their spouse in relation to the risk of being physically assaulted due to differences in traditional gender attitudes. The findings revealed that the more liberal and non-traditional the wives' attitudes are, the more likely they are to be physically abused by their husbands. Such a mismatch in perceptions about gender roles thus resulted in poor communication style and negative outcomes (Cheung & Choi, 2016).

An additional school of thought concerning perspectives on gender roles was derived from a systematic study that was carried out on Ethiopian culture. This study was concerned with the idea that mistreated women prefer to keep quiet. This is partly because abuse is more likely to be regarded as a family secret, a phenomenon that also presents itself in a male-dominated society in which cultural conventions influence one's personal life. In addition, 18.2% of traditional ideas held by women about gender role models justify assault against women under specific circumstances, yet 39% of victims who have suffered physical abuse keep quiet about their experiences (Semahegn & Mengistie, 2015). One of the studies found that women's attitudes regarding domestic abuse are influenced by the patriarchal structure of society as well as gender inequality (Basar et al., 2019). It is less probable for men to behave aggressively against their wives if they have higher levels of education or if they have decent careers (Ibrahim et al., 2010).

Another study found that women who have a more egalitarian mindset are more likely to be victimized by IPV compared to those women who do not seek gender equality (Karakurt & Cumbie, 2012). Similarly, a study involving 466 intimate partners from Malawi confirmed the association between the risk of IPV and being in a male dominant relationship, where the gender role of men is empowered by suppressing gender equality and egalitarian attitudes among women (Conroy, 2014). Their study showed that the risk of sexual coercion increased by 216% among those who lived with a male dominant partner. This was in contrast to those couples living in an equal and unified relationship.

Other comparable results about shifting in women's mindset the results of one research were repeated in a second study. This study examined the attitudes of nursing students in Western Canadian universities between the years 1970 and 1990 using the complete Attitude Towards Women measure. This first study was conducted over a period of 20 years (Loo & Thorpe, 1998). The current research included a total of 152 undergraduate students, both male and female, as participants. In contrast, the previous study had 202 participants, both male and female, from the school of nursing and the faculty of management. AWS scores of the current sample of nursing students demonstrated more liberal and egalitarian attitudes in comparison to their historical counterparts. In addition, they showed that they held more liberal attitudes compared to the existing faculty of management. This was shown by the fact that they scored higher on the AWS. It is critical to note that the atmosphere and location of the healthcare setting are changing over time. Since women have gained equal status in society over the years, attitudes around the contributions that women are expected to make to the medical field have also undergone significant shifts.

As expected, family reputation was reported frequently by the current participants of this study which was in line with a previous literature. In 2010, a research conducted in Lebanon on 206 college students who identified as either Christian or Muslim. There were 97 females and 109 men, and their ages varied from 17 to 27 years (Obeid et al., 2010). To identify beliefs that are related to the role that women play in society in Lebanon, an Attitude Towards Women Scale consisting of 15 items was given. The results of the study indicated that female students are more likely to assist IPV victims. This suggests that sexually unfaithful spouses can cause tremendous damage to the family's reputation; many students justified wife beating under such circumstances.

Other research has shown that male-dominated civilizations whose cultural norms are the most significant factor in determining their attitudes about women are more likely to influence such attitudes. Enculturating attitudes about IPV were investigated in research that was carried out in Metro Detroit on 373 Gujarati men and women whose ages varied from 18 to 64. Participants in the study were from Gujarat (Yoshihama et al., 2014). The results of the Attitude Towards Women Scale indicated a significant connection between patriarchal gender role views and intimate partner enculturating attitudes. According to the results, when people followed cultural values, ideas, and clothing norms, this worked as a predictor for accepting domestic violence against women. This was shown to be true regardless of the culture the individuals followed. Additionally, the higher level of education among both men and women fosters a propensity to support an egalitarian society where non-traditional gender roles are prohibited.

Similar to the current findings, another study was carried out in the Philippines on 2050 married women who were recruited to understand when women are at increased risk of domestic violence (Hindin & Adair, 2002). The findings showed that when the gender role and decision-making process of the husband is challenged, this becomes a significant factor behind spouse abuse. Furthermore, the frequency of abuse against a spouse increases when financial resources are limited and where few assets are available, and especially when the husband is unemployed. The more household decisions are made by the wife the more likely abuse will occur. Moreover, 25% of domestic abuse against a spouse increases when there is no joint decision process between husband and wife.

A number of noteworthy results were found that shed light on the subject of how attitudes towards women's rights influence abuse risk among victims. Likewise, the current findings did not differ from other study findings that show that cultural roles and masculine ideologies influence husbands' aggression when their wives do not exhibit what is considered a "proper wife identity", as defined by culture (Dery, 2021). The current results provide evidence that husbands undermine women who favour gender equality. When it came to major family decisions, their opinions were suppressed and considered less reliable. The creation of IPV victimisation occurs when challenges are made against a husband's manhood as perceived by men or husbands. Another supported evidence from the current qualitative data suggests that women who seek higher education and decide to be in full control over their financial resources or their inheritance are more likely to be abused by their husbands because they do not want them to be financially independent. The current observations show that whenever the abuser feels that they are losing control they tend to act more aggressively.

In conclusion, this discussion chapter summarizes, interprets, and identifies the strengths, limitations, and policy implications of a research paper focused on Examining the impact of domestic abuse on Qatari women's mental health. Moreover, the paper highlights the importance of the research to advance knowledge, and it suggests the need for more comprehensive and coordinated multidisciplinary interventions that engage healthcare providers, lawyers, policymakers, and community service providers. A more family-friendly approach to domestic abuse against women is needed to address gender inequality.

References

Abdalla, I. A. (1996). Attitudes towards women in the Arabian gulf region. *Women in Management Review, 11*(1), 29–39. https://doi.org/10.1108/09649429610109271

Abolfotouh, M. A., & Almuneef, M. (2020). Prevalence, pattern and factors of intimate partner violence against Saudi women. *Journal of Public Health (United Kingdom), 42*(3), E206–E214. https://doi.org/10.1093/pubmed/fdz092

Abramsky, T., Lees, S., Stöckl, H., Harvey, S., Kapinga, I., Ranganathan, M., Mshana, G., & Kapiga, S. (2019). Women's income and risk of intimate partner violence: Secondary findings from the MAISHA cluster randomised trial in North-Western Tanzania. *BMC Public Health, 19*(1), 1108. https://doi.org/10.1186/s12889-019-7454-1

Abramsky, T., Watts, C. H., Garcia-Moreno, C., Devries, K., Kiss, L., Ellsberg, M., Jansen, H. A. F. M., & Heise, L. (2011). What factors are associated with recent intimate partner violence? Findings from the WHO multi-country study on women's health and domestic violence. *BMC Public Health, 11*. https://doi.org/10.1186/1471-2458-11-109

Acevedo, B. P., Lowe, S. R., Griffin, K. W., & Botvin, G. J. (2013). Predictors of intimate partner violence in a sample of multiethnic urban young adults. *Journal of Interpersonal Violence, 28*(15), 3004–3022. https://doi.org/10.1177/0886260513488684

Adjei, S. B. (2017). Sociocultural groundings of battered women's entrapment in abusive marital relationship in Ghana. *Journal of Aggression, Maltreatment and Trauma, 26*(8), 879–901. https://doi.org/10.1080/10926771.2017.1284171

Aduloju, P. O., Olagbuji, N. B., Olofinbiyi, A. B., & Awoleke, J. O. (2015). Prevalence and predictors of intimate partner violence among women attending infertility clinic in south-western Nigeria. *European Journal of Obstetrics and Gynecology and Reproductive Biology, 188*(February 2018), 66–69. https://doi.org/10.1016/j.ejogrb.2015.02.027

Ahinkorah, B. O. (2021). Polygyny and intimate partner violence in sub-Saharan Africa: Evidence from 16 cross-sectional demographic and health surveys. *SSM - Population Health, 13*(December 2020), 100729. https://doi.org/10.1016/j.ssmph.2021.100729

Ahmadzad-Asl, M., Davoudi, F., Zarei, N., Mohammad-Sadeghi, H., & Rasoulian, M. (2016). Domestic violence against women as a risk factor for depressive and anxiety disorders: Findings from domestic violence household survey in Tehran, Iran. *Archives of Women's Mental Health, 19*(5), 861–869. https://doi.org/10.1007/s00737-016-0626-4

Aizpurua, E., Copp, J., Ricarte, J. J., & Vázquez, D. (2017). Controlling behaviors and intimate partner violence among women in Spain: An examination of individual, partner, and relationship risk factors for physical and psychological abuse. *Journal of Interpersonal Violence, 36*(1–2), 231–254. https://doi.org/10.1177/0886260517723744

Akpinar, F., Yilmaz, S., Karahanoglu, E., Ozelci, R., Coskun, B., Dilbaz, B., & Tekin, Ö. M. (2019). Intimate partner violence in Turkey among women with female infertility. *Sexual and Relationship Therapy, 34*(1), 3–9. https://doi.org/10.1080/14681994.2017.1327711

Al Ghayathin, B. (2017). *Violence against women in Qatar: An exploratory study* [Master's thesis, Hamad Bin Khalifa University]. https://search.proquest.com/dissertations-theses/violence-against-women-qatar-exploratory-study/docview/1907499277/se-2?accountid=10673%0Ahttps://ed-primo.hosted.exlibrisgroup.com/openurl/44UOE/44UOE_VU2??url_ver=Z39.88-2004&rft_val_fmt=info:ofi/fmt:kev:m

Al Shidhani, N. A., Al Kendi, A. A., & Al Kiyumi, M. H. (2020). Prevalence, risk factors and effects of domestic violence before and during pregnancy on birth outcomes: An observational study of literate Omani women. *International Journal of Women's Health, 12*, 911–925. https://doi.org/10.2147/IJWH.S272419

Alam, M., & Islam, M. (2015). Factors affecting domestic violence against women in Bangladesh. *European Journal of Public Health, 25*(suppl_3). https://doi.org/10.1093/eurpub/ckv175.013

Al-Ekri, E., Al-Ubaidi, B. A., Husain, H., Bubshait, M., Al-Jamea, L., Al Ubaidi, B. A., Al-Dhubaib, D., Najem, W., & Husain, H. (1994). Prevalence of domestic violence & associated risk factors among adult females attending primary care in the Kingdom of Bahrain. *International Medical Journal, 28*(3), 4413–4425. https://www.researchgate.net/profile/Basem-Al-Ubaidi/publication/350515978_Prevalence_of_Domestic_Violence_Associated_Risk_Factors_among_Adult_Females_attending_Primary_Care_in_the_Kingdom_of_Bahrain/links/60646429a6fdcca78be013e2/Prevalence-of-Domestic-Violence-Associated-Risk-Factors-among-Adult-Females-attending-Primary-Care-in-the-Kingdom-of-Bahrain.pdf

Al-Ghanim, K. A. (2009). Violence against women in Qatari society. *Journal of Middle East Women's Studies, 5*(1), 80–93. https://doi.org/10.2979/mew.2009.5.1.80

Ali, A. A., Yassin, K., & Omer, R. (2014). Domestic violence against women in Eastern Sudan. *BMC Public Health, 14*, 1136. https://doi.org/10.1186/1471-2458-14-1136

Alibeli, M. A. (2015). Gender and attitudes toward women in the United Arab Emirates. *Perspectives on Global Development and Technology, 14*(1–2), 109–125. https://doi.org/10.1163/15691497-12341335

Alio, A. P., Nana, P. N., & Salihu, H. M. (2009). Spousal violence and potentially preventable single and recurrent spontaneous fetal loss in an African setting: Cross-sectional study. *The Lancet, 373*(9660), 318–324. https://doi.org/10.1016/S0140-6736(09)60096-9

Al-Krenawi, A., & Graham, J. R. (2006). A comparison of family functioning, life and marital satisfaction, and mental health of women in polygamous and monogamous marriages. *International Journal of Social Psychiatry, 52*(1), 5–17. https://doi.org/10.1177/0020764006061245

Almosaed, N. (2015). Why stay? Saudi Women's adaption's to violence. *International Journal of Humanities and Social Science, 5*(10(1)), 146–162. https://cawtarclearinghouse.org/storage/AttachementGender/Why%20Stay-%20Saudi%20Women%E2%80%99s%20Adaption%E2%80%99s%20to%20Violence.pdf

Alquaiz, A. M., Almuneef, M., Kazi, A., & Almeneessier, A. (2021). Social determinants of domestic violence among Saudi married women in Riyadh, Kingdom of Saudi Arabia. *Journal of Interpersonal Violence, 36*(3–4), NP1561–NP1585. https://doi.org/10.1177/0886260517746128

Alsawalqa, R. O. (2020). Economic abuse of women in Amman, Jordan: A quantitative study. *SAGE Open, 10*(4), 1–13. https://doi.org/10.1177/2158244020982616

Anser, L. (2013). Divorce in the Arab gulf countries: A major challenge to family and society. In A. Abela & J. Walker (Eds.), *Contemporary issues in family studies: Global perspectives on partnerships, parenting and support in a changing world* (pp. 59–73). Wiley-Blackwell. https://doi.org/10.1002/9781118320990.ch5

Asli, M. R., & Byouki, M. A. (2016). Forced marriage in Islamic countries: The role of violence in family relationships. In H. Kury, S. Redo, & E. Shea (Eds.), *Women and children as victims and offenders: Background, prevention, reintegration* (pp. 729–753). Springer. https://doi.org/10.1007/978-3-319-08398-8_26

Atkinson, M. P., Greenstein, T. N., & Lang, M. M. (2005). For women, breadwinning can be dangerous: Gendered resource theory and wife abuse. *Journal of Marriage and Family, 67*(5), 1137–1148. https://doi.org/10.1111/j.1741-3737.2005.00206.x

Bandura, A. (2019). Social learning: Theory. In K. N. Laland & L. Rendell (Eds.), *Encyclopedia of animal behavior* (pp. 380–386). Academic. https://doi.org/10.1016/B978-0-12-813251-7.00057-2

Bargai, N., Ben-Shakhar, G., & Shalev, A. Y. (2007). Posttraumatic stress disorder and depression in battered women: The mediating role of learned helplessness. *Journal of Family Violence, 22*(5), 267–275. https://doi.org/10.1007/s10896-007-9078-y

Barnawi, F. H. (2017). Prevalence and risk factors of domestic violence against women attending A primary care center in Riyadh, Saudi Arabia. *Journal of Interpersonal Violence, 32*(8), 1171–1186. https://doi.org/10.1177/0886260515587669

Basar, F., Demirci, N., Cicek, S., & Saglam, H. Y. (2019). Attitudes toward violence against women and the factors that affect them in Kutahya, Turkey. *African Journal of Reproductive Health, 23*(1), 16–26. https://doi.org/10.29063/AJRH2019/V23I1.2

Bates, L. M., Schuler, S. R., Islam, F., & Islam, K. (2004). Socioeconomic factors and processes associated with domestic violence in rural Bangladesh. *International Family Planning Perspectives, 30*(4), 190–199. https://doi.org/10.1363/3019004

Belfrage, H., & Rying, M. (2004). Characteristics of spousal homicide perpetrators: A study of all cases of spousal homicide in Sweden 1990–1999. *Criminal Behaviour and Mental Health, 14*(2), 121–133. https://doi.org/10.1002/cbm.577

Bhandari, P. (2020). Pre-marital relationships and violence: Experiences of working middle class women in Delhi. *Gender, Place and Culture, 27*(1), 13–33. https://doi.org/10.1080/0966369X.2019.1618795

Bird, K. (2007). *The intergenerational transmission of poverty: An overview* (CPRC Working Paper No. 99). SSRN Electronic Journal. https://doi.org/10.2139/ssrn.1629262.

Bohn, D. K., Tebben, J. G., & Campbell, J. C. (2004). Influences of income, education, age, and ethnicity on physical abuse before and during pregnancy. *Journal of Obstetric, Gynecologic & Neonatal Nursing, 33*(5), 561–571. https://doi.org/10.1177/0884217504269009

Bowlus, A., & Seitz, S. (2000). The economics of abuse. *International Economic Review*, 1–36. http://qed.econ.queensu.ca/pub/faculty/seitz/abuse.pdf

Bracewell, K., Jones, C., Haines-Delmont, A., Craig, E., Duxbury, J., & Chantler, K. (2021). Beyond intimate partner relationships: Utilising domestic homicide reviews to prevent adult family domestic homicide. *Journal of Gender-Based Violence, 6*(3), 535–550. https://doi.org/10.1332/239868021x16316184865237

Branigan, E., & Grace, M. (2005). *His money or our money: Financial abuse of women in intimate partner relationships.* 1–22. https://scholar.google.co.uk/scholar?q=his+money+or+our+money+financial+abuse+of+women+in+intimate+partner+relationships&btnG=&hl=en&as_sdt=0%2C5#0%5Cnhttp://csmc.org.au/wp-content/uploads/2014/05/Financial_Abuse.pdf

Brignone, L., & Gomez, A. M. (2017). Double jeopardy: Predictors of elevated lethality risk among intimate partner violence victims seen in emergency departments. *Preventive Medicine, 103*, 20–25. https://doi.org/10.1016/j.ypmed.2017.06.035

Bromfield, N. (2014). Interviews with divorced women from the United Arab Emirates: A rare glimpse into lived experiences. *Families, Relationships and Societies, 3*(3), 339–354. https://doi.org/10.1332/204674313X13842674567773

Bruton, C., & Tyson, D. (2018). Leaving violent men: A study of women's experiences of separation in Victoria, Australia. *Australian & New Zealand Journal of Criminology, 51*(3), 339–354. https://doi.org/10.1177/0004865817746711

Btoush, R., & Haj-Yahia, M. M. (2008). Attitudes of Jordanian society toward wife abuse. *Journal of Interpersonal Violence, 23*(11), 1531–1554. https://doi.org/10.1177/0886260508314313

Burazeri, G., Roshi, E., Jewkes, R., Jordan, S., Bjegovic, V., & Laaser, U. (2005). Factors associated with spousal physical violence in Albania: Cross sectional study. *British Medical Journal, 331*(7510), 197–201. https://doi.org/10.1136/bmj.331.7510.197

Burgos-Muñoz, R. M., Soriano-Moreno, A. N., Bendezu-Quispe, G., Urrunaga-Pastor, D., Toro-Huamanchumo, C. J., & Benites-Zapata, V. A. (2021). Intimate partner violence against reproductive-age women and associated factors in Peru: Evidence from national surveys, 2015–2017. *Heliyon, 7*(7), E07478. https://doi.org/10.1016/j.heliyon.2021.e07478

Cameron, P. (2014). *Relationship problems and money: Women talk about financial abuse.* Research Report. WIRE Women's Information. https://apo.org.au/sites/default/files/resource-files/2014-08/apo-nid41025.pdf

Campbell, E. (2017). How domestic violence batterers use custody proceedings in family courts to abuse victims, and how courts can put a stop to it. *UCLA Women's Law Journal, 24*(1) https://escholarship.org/uc/item/31z272j1

Campbell, J. C., Webster, D. W., & Glass, N. (2008). The danger assessment. *Journal of Interpersonal Violence, 24*(4), 653–674. https://doi.org/10.1177/0886260508317180

Campbell, J. C., Webster, D., Koziol-McLain, J., Block, C., Campbell, D., Curry, M. A., Gary, F., Glass, N., McFarlane, J., Sachs, C., Sharps, P., Ulrich, Y., Wilt, S. A., Manganello, J., Xu, X., Schollenberger, J., Frye, V., & Laughon, K. (2003). Risk factors for femicide in abusive relationships: Results from a multisite case control study. *American Journal of Public Health, 93*(7), 1089–1097. https://doi.org/10.2105/ajph.93.7.1089

Cascardi, M., O'Leary, K. D., & Schlee, K. A. (1999). Co-occurrence and correlates of posttraumatic stress disorder and major depression in physically abused women. *Journal of Family Violence, 14*(3), 227–249. https://doi.org/10.1023/A:1022827915757

Cavanaugh, C. E., Messing, J. T., Del-Colle, M., O'sullivan, C., & Campbell, J. C. (2011). Prevalence and correlates of suicidal behavior among adult female victims of intimate partner violence. *Suicide and Life-threatening Behavior, 41*(4), 373–383. https://doi.org/10.1111/j.1943-278x.2011.00035.x

Cherlin, A. J. (2017). Introduction to the special collection on separation, divorce, repartnering, and remarriage around the world. *Demographic Research, 37*(1), 1275–1296. https://doi.org/10.4054/DemRes.2017.37.38

Cheung, A. K. L., & Choi, S. Y. P. (2016). Non-traditional wives with traditional husbands: Gender ideology and husband-to-wife physical violence in Chinese society. *Violence Against Women, 22*(14), 1704–1724. https://doi.org/10.1177/1077801216632615

Choudhary, E., Smith, M., & Bossarte, R. M. (2012). Depression, anxiety, and symptom profiles among female and male victims of sexual violence. *American Journal of Men's Health, 6*(1), 28–36. https://doi.org/10.1177/1557988311414045

Coker, A. L., Smith, P. H., McKeown, R. E., & King, M. J. (2000). Frequency and correlates of intimate partner violence by type: Physical, sexual, and psychological battering. *American Journal of Public Health, 90*(4), 553–559. https://doi.org/10.2105/AJPH.90.4.553

Coleman, M., Ganong, L., & Fine, M. (2000). Reinvestigating remarriage: Another decade of progress. *Journal of Marriage and Family, 62*(4), 1288–1307. https://doi.org/10.1111/j.1741-3737.2000.01288.x

Collins, T. W., Grineski, S. E., & Morales, D. X. (2017). Environmental injustice and sexual minority health disparities: A national study of inequitable health risks from air pollution among same-sex partners. *Social Science & Medicine, 191*, 38–47. https://doi.org/10.1016/j.socscimed.2017.08.040

Conroy, A. A. (2014). Gender, power, and intimate partner violence. *Journal of Interpersonal Violence, 29*(5), 866–888. https://doi.org/10.1177/0886260513505907

Cwikel, J., Lev-Wiesel, R., & Al-Krenawi, A. (2003). The physical and psychosocial health of Bedouin Arab women of the Negev Area of Israel. *Violence Against Women, 9*(2), 240–257. https://doi.org/10.1177/1077801202239008

Dami, C., Karathanos, V., Dimitakopoulou, V. I., Damigos, D., & Gouva, M. (2017). Intimate Partner violence in primary settings and consequences in mental health. *International Journal of Caring Sciences, 10*(1), 17–29. http://www.internationaljournalofcaringsciences.org/docs/3_gouva_original_10_1.pdf

Daoud, N., Sergienko, R., & Shoham-Vardi, I. (2020). Intimate partner violence prevalence, recurrence, types, and risk factors among Arab, and Jewish immigrant and nonimmigrant women of childbearing age in Israel. *Journal of Interpersonal Violence, 35*(15–16), 2869–2896. https://doi.org/10.1177/0886260517705665

Das, T. K., Bhattacharyya, R., Alam, M. F., & Pervin, A. (2016). Domestic violence in Sylhet, Bangladesh: Analysing the experiences of abused women. *Social Change, 46*(1), 106–123. https://doi.org/10.1177/0049085715618561

Davila, A. L., Johnson, L., & Postmus, J. L. (2021). Examining the relationship between economic abuse and mental health among Latina intimate partner violence survivors in the United States. *Journal of Interpersonal Violence, 36*(1–2), NP287–NP310. https://doi.org/10.1177/0886260517731311

Decima Research Inc. (2002). *National profile of family caregivers in Canada 2002.* Health Canada https://www.canada.ca/content/dam/hc-sc/migration/hc-sc/hcs-sss/alt_formats/hpb-dgps/pdf/pubs/2002-caregiv-interven/2002-caregiv-interven-eng.pdf

DeGregoria, B. (1987). Sex role attitude and perception of psychological abuse. *Sex Roles, 16*(5–6), 227–235. https://doi.org/10.1007/BF00289951

Den Otter, R. C. (2015). Three may not be a crowd: The case for a constitutional right to plural marriage. *Emory Law Journal, 64*(6), 1977–2046. https://scholarlycommons.law.emory.edu/elj/vol64/iss6/8

Dery, I. (2021). "Give her a slap or two.. She might change": Negotiating masculinities through intimate partner violence among rural Ghanaian men. *Journal of Interpersonal Violence, 36*(19–20), 9670–9690. https://doi.org/10.1177/0886260519869066

Dhungel, S., Dhungel, P., Dhital, S. R., & Stock, C. (2017). Is economic dependence on the husband a risk factor for intimate partner violence against female factory workers in Nepal? *BMC Women's Health, 17*(1), 1–9. https://doi.org/10.1186/s12905-017-0441-8

Dichter, M. E., Thomas, K. A., Crits-Christoph, P., Ogden, S. N., & Rhodes, K. V. (2018). Coercive control in intimate partner violence: Relationship with women's experience of violence, use of violence, and danger. *Psychology of Violence, 8*(5), 596–604. https://doi.org/10.1037/vio0000158

Dierickx, S., Coene, G., Jarju, B., & Longman, C. (2019). Women with infertility complying with and resisting polygyny: An explorative qualitative study in urban Gambia. *Reproductive Health, 16*(1), 1–11. https://doi.org/10.1186/s12978-019-0762-1

Djamba, Y. K., & Kimuna, S. R. (Eds.). (2015). *Gender-based violence: Perspective from Africa, the Middle East, and India.* Springer. https://doi.org/10.1007/978-3-319-16670-4

Douki, S., Nacef, F., Belhadj, A., Bouasker, A., & Ghachem, R. (2003). Violence against women in Arab and Islamic countries. *Archives of Women's Mental Health, 6*(3), 165–171. https://doi.org/10.1007/s00737-003-0170-x

Dray, J. A. W. (1987). International conflicts in child custody: United States v. Saudi Arabia. *Loyola of Los Angeles International and Comparative Law Review, 9*(2), 413–443. https://digitalcommons.lmu.edu/ilr/vol9/iss2/5

El Sheikh, M. A. (2019). Post-divorce financial support from the Islamic perspective (Mutʿat al-Ṭalāq). In M. Ayoub (Ed.), *Contemporary approaches to the Quran and Sunnah* (pp. 172–196). International Institute of Islamic Thought. https://doi.org/10.2307/j.ctvk8w26p.14

Eldoseri, H. M., & Sharps, P. (2017). Risk factors for spousal physical violence against women in Saudi Arabia. *Journal of Interpersonal Violence, 35*(5–6), 1269–1293. https://doi.org/10.1177/0886260517696861

Eldoseri, H. M., Tufts, K. A., Zhang, Q., & Fish, J. N. (2014). Adverse health effects of spousal violence among women attending Saudi Arabian primary health-care clinics. *Eastern Mediterranean Health Journal, 20*(11), 717–725. https://applications.emro.who.int/emhj/v20/11/EMHJ_2014_20_11_717_725.pdf

Elnashar, A. M., El-Dien Ibrahim, M., Eldesoky, M. M., Aly, O. M., & El-Sayd Mohamed Hassan, M. (2007). Sexual abuse experienced by married Egyptian women. *International Journal of Gynecology & Obstetrics, 99*(3), 216–220. https://doi.org/10.1016/j.ijgo.2007.05.049

Eng, S., Szmodis, W., & Grace, K. (2020). Cambodian remarried women are at risk for domestic violence. *Journal of Interpersonal Violence, 35*(3–4), 828–853. https://doi.org/10.1177/0886260517691520

Esie, P., Osypuk, T. L., Schuler, S. R., & Bates, L. M. (2019). SSM - population health intimate partner violence and depression in rural Bangladesh: Accounting for violence severity in a high prevalence setting. *SSM – Population Health, 7*(August 2018), 100368. https://doi.org/10.1016/j.ssmph.2019.100368

Falb, K. L., Blackwell, A., Stennes, J., Hussein, M., & Annan, J. (2019). Depressive symptoms among women in Raqqa Governorate, Syria: associations with intimate partner violence, food insecurity, and perceived needs. *Global Mental Health (Cambridge, England), 6*, e22. https://doi.org/10.1017/gmh.2019.20

Ferrari, G., Bonnet, C., & Solaz, A. (2019). "Will the one who keeps the children keep the house?" Residential mobility after divorce by parenthood status and custody arrangements in France. *Demographic Research, 40*(February), 359–394. https://doi.org/10.4054/DEMRES.2019.40.14

Fikree, F. F., Razzak, J. A., & Durocher, J. (2005). Attitudes of Pakistani men to domestic violence: A study from Karachi, Pakistan. *Journal of Men's Health and Gender, 2*(1), 49–58. https://doi.org/10.1016/j.jmhg.2005.01.004

Gangoli, G., Razak, A., & McCarry, M. (2006, June). *Forced marriage and domestic violence among South Asian communities in North East England*. School for Policy Studies, University of Bristol. https://research-information.bris.ac.uk/files/188679401/Final_report.pdf

Gass, J. D., Stein, D. J., Williams, D. R., & Seedat, S. (2011). Gender differences in risk for intimate partner violence among South African adults. *Journal of Interpersonal Violence, 26*(14), 2764–2789. https://doi.org/10.1177/0886260510390960

Gebrewahd, G. T., Gebremeskel, G. G., & Tadesse, D. B. (2020). Intimate partner violence against reproductive age women during COVID-19 pandemic in Northern Ethiopia 2020: A community-based cross-sectional study. *Reproductive Health, 17*(1), 152. https://doi.org/10.1186/s12978-020-01002-w

Ghazi, H. F., & Isa, Z. (2018). Women's attitude and its influence on violence during pregnancy in northern state of peninsular Malaysia: Cross-sectional study. *Journal of Interpersonal Violence, 36*(5–6), 1–25. https://doi.org/10.1177/0886260518759059

Glick, P., & Fiske, S. T. (1997). Hostile and benevolent sexism: Measuring ambivalent sexist attitudes toward women. *Psychology of Women Quarterly, 21*(1), 119–135. https://doi.org/10.1111/j.1471-6402.1997.tb00104.x

Godbout, N., Dutton, D. G., Lussier, Y., & Sabourin, S. (2009). Early exposure to violence, domestic violence, attachment representations, and marital adjustment. *Personal Relationships, 16*(3), 365–384. https://doi.org/10.1111/j.1475-6811.2009.01228.x

Gultiano, S., Hindin, M., & Upadhyay, U. (2009). Marital status and psychological Well-being of Filipino women. *Philippine Population Review, 8*(1), 16–33. https://www.pssc.org.ph/wp-content/pssc-archives/Philippine%20Population%20Review/2009/05_Martal%20Status%20And%20Psychological%20Well_Being%20Of%20Filipino%20Women.pdf

Haj-Yahia, M. M. (2002). Attitudes of Arab women toward different patterns of coping with wife abuse. *Journal of Interpersonal Violence, 17*(7), 721–745. https://doi.org/10.1177/08862605020170070

Hammad, A., Kysia, R., Rabah, R., Hassoun, R., & Connelly, M. (1999). *Arab community center for economic and social services guide to Arab culture: Health care delivery to the Arab American community*. ACCESS Community Health Center. https://my.vanderbilt.edu/globalhealth/files/2013/04/Guide-to-Arab-Culture-Health-care-delivery-to-the-Arab-American-Community.pdf

Hardesty, J. L., & Ganong, L. H. (2006). How women make custody decisions and manage co-parenting with abusive former husbands. *Journal of Social and Personal Relationships, 23*(4), 543–563. https://doi.org/10.1177/0265407506065983

Harris, R. J., Firestone, J. M., & Vega, W. A. (2005). The interaction of country of origin, acculturation, and gender role ideology on wife abuse. *Social Science Quarterly, 86*(2), 463–483. https://doi.org/10.1111/j.0038-4941.2005.00313.x

Hassouneh-Phillips, D. (2001). American Muslim women's experiences of leaving abusive relationships. *Health Care for Women International, 22*(4), 415–432. https://doi.org/10.1080/07399330119163

Hawcroft, C., Hughes, R., Shaheen, A., Usta, J., Elkadi, H., Dalton, T., Ginwalla, K., & Feder, G. (2019). Prevalence and health outcomes of domestic violence amongst clinical populations in Arab countries: A systematic review and meta-analysis. *BMC Public Health, 19*(1), 315. https://doi.org/10.1186/s12889-019-6619-2

Hindin, M. J., & Adair, L. S. (2002). Who's at risk? Factors associated with intimate partner violence in The Philippines. *Social Science and Medicine, 55*(8), 1385–1399. https://doi.org/10.1016/S0277-9536(01)00273-8

Ibrahim, K., Fahimi, F., Ismail, H., Mamdouh, H., Muhammad, Y., Tawfik, M., El-Sharkawy, O., Sallam, H., (2010, September). *Spousal violence in Egypt*. Population Reference Bureau. https://www.prb.org/wp-content/uploads/2010/09/09282010-spousalviolence-egypt.pdf

Izugbara, C. O., Obiyan, M. O., Degfie, T. T., & Bhatti, A. (2020). Correlates of intimate partner violence among urban women in sub-Saharan Africa. *PLoS One, 15*(3), 1–21. https://doi.org/10.1371/journal.pone.0230508

Jaffe, P. G., Johnston, J. R., Crooks, C. V., & Bala, N. (2008). Custody disputes involving allegations of domestic violence: Toward a differentiated approach to parenting plans. *Family Court Review, 46*(3), 500–522. https://doi.org/10.1111/j.1744-1617.2008.00216.x

James-Hawkins, L., Qutteina, Y., & Yount, K. M. (2017). The patriarchal bargain in a context of rapid changes to normative gender roles: Young Arab women's role conflict in Qatar. *Sex Roles, 77*(3–4), 155–168. https://doi.org/10.1007/s11199-016-0708-9

Jewkes, R. (2002). Intimate partner violence: Causes and prevention. *The Lancet, 359*(9315), 1423–1429. https://doi.org/10.1016/S0140-6736(02)08357-5

Jones, J. H., & Ferguson, B. (2009). Demographic and social predictors of intimate partner violence in Colombia: A dyadic power perspective. *Human Nature, 20*(2), 184–203. https://doi.org/10.1007/s12110-009-9064-6

Kalmuss, D., & Seltzer, J. A. (1986). Continuity of marital behavior in remarriage: The case of spouse abuse. *Journal of Marriage and the Family, 48*(1), 113–120. https://doi.org/10.2307/352234

Karakurt, G., & Cumbie, T. (2012). The relationship between egalitarianism, dominance, and violence in intimate relationships. *Journal of Family Violence, 27*(2), 115–122. https://doi.org/10.1007/s10896-011-9408-y

Karakurt, G., Smith, D., & Whiting, J. (2014). Impact of intimate partner violence on women's mental health. *NIH Public Access Author Manuscript, 29*(7), 693–702. https://doi.org/10.1038/jid.2014.371

Kerley, K. R., Xu, X., Sirisunyaluck, B., & Alley, J. M. (2010). Exposure to family violence in childhood and intimate partner perpetration or victimization in adulthood: Exploring intergenerational transmission in urban Thailand. *Journal of Family Violence, 25*(3), 337–347. https://doi.org/10.1007/s10896-009-9295-7

Khadra, C., Wehbe, N., Lachance Fiola, J., Skaff, W., & Nehmé, M. (2015). Symptoms of post-traumatic stress disorder among battered women in Lebanon: An exploratory study. *Journal of Interpersonal Violence, 30*(2), 295–313. https://doi.org/10.1177/0886260514534774

King, K., Murray, C. E., Crowe, A., Hunnicutt, G., Lundgren, K., & Olson, L. (2017). The costs of recovery: Intimate partner violence survivors' experiences of financial recovery from abuse. *Family Journal, 25*(3), 230–238. https://doi.org/10.1177/1066480717710656

Koziol-McLain, J., Webster, D., McFarlane, J., Block, C. R., Ulrich, Y., Glass, N., & Campbell, J. C. (2006). Risk factors for femicide-suicide in abusive relationships: Results from a multisite case control study. *Violence and Victims, 21*(1), 3–21. https://doi.org/10.1891/0886-6708.21.1.3

Krause, K. H., Gordon-Roberts, R., VanderEnde, K., Schuler, S. R., & Yount, K. M. (2016). Why do women justify violence against wives more often than do men in Vietnam? *Journal of Interpersonal Violence, 31*(19), 3150–3173. https://doi.org/10.1177/0886260515584343

Kristiansen, C. M., & Giulietti, R. (1990). Perceptions of wife abuse. *Psychology of Women Quarterly, 14*(2), 177–189. https://doi.org/10.1111/J.1471-6402.1990.TB00013.X

Kucinskas, J. (2010). A research note on Islam and gender egalitarianism: An examination of Egyptian and Saudi Arabian youth attitudes. *Journal for the Scientific Study of Religion, 49*(4), 761–770. https://doi.org/10.1111/j.1468-5906.2010.01545.x

Kutin, J., Russell, R., & Reid, M. (2017). Economic abuse between intimate partners in Australia: Prevalence, health status, disability and financial stress. *Australian and New Zealand Journal of Public Health, 41*(3), 269–274. https://doi.org/10.1111/1753-6405.12651

Laland, K. N., & Rendell, L. (2010). Social learning: Theory. In *Encyclopedia of animal behavior* (2nd ed., pp. 380–386). Elsevier Ltd.. https://doi.org/10.1016/B978-0-12-813251-7.00057-2

Lamichhane, P., Puri, M., Tamang, J., & Dulal, B. (2011). Women's status and violence against young married women in rural Nepal. *BMC Women's Health, 11*, 19. https://doi.org/10.1186/1472-6874-11-19

Landau, E. M. (2016). Custom or Crime?: Part II of IV: Legal remedies. *American Journal of Family Law, 30*(1), 46–57. https://preventforcedmarriage.org/wp-content/uploads/2016/05/Elizabeth-Landau_Custom-or-Crime-II.pdf

Lasong, J., Zhang, Y., Muyayalo, K. P., Njiri, O. A., Gebremedhin, S. A., Abaidoo, C. S., Liu, C. Y., Zhang, H., & Zhao, K. (2020). Domestic violence among married women of reproductive age in Zimbabwe: A cross sectional study. *BMC Public Health, 20*(1), 354. https://doi.org/10.1186/s12889-020-8447-9

Lawton, J., & Schulte, S. J. (2012). The prevalence of mental health symptoms among outpatients in the United Arab Emirates. *Arab Journal of Psychiatry, 23*(2), 138–147. https://platform.almanhal.com/Files/2/17304

Loo, R., & Thorpe, K. (1998). Attitudes toward women's roles in society: A replication after 20 years. *Sex Roles, 39*(11–12), 903–912. https://doi.org/10.1023/a:1018832823010

Lotfy, M., Hamdy, M. A., Mansour, A. F. I., Gharib, W. F., Ghoneim, H. M., Abbas, A. M., Ahmed, W. A. S., & Ibrahim, Z. M. (2019). Prevalence and risk factors for domestic violence among infertile Egyptian women: A cross-sectional study. *European Journal of Contraception and Reproductive Health Care, 24*(5), 362–367. https://doi.org/10.1080/13625187.2019.1642467

Lown, E. A., & Vega, W. A. (2001). Prevalence and predictors of physical partner abuse among Mexican American women. *American Journal of Public Health, 91*(3), 441–445. https://doi.org/10.2105/AJPH.91.3.441

Madruga, C. S., Viana, M. C., Abdalla, R. R., Caetano, R., & Laranjeira, R. (2017). Pathways from witnessing parental violence during childhood to involvement in intimate partner violence in adult life: The roles of depression and substance use. *Drug and Alcohol Review, 36*(1), 107–114. https://doi.org/10.1111/dar.12514

Malik, M., Munir, N., Usman Ghani, M., & Ahmad, N. (2020). Domestic violence and its relationship with depression, anxiety and quality of life: A hidden dilemma of Pakistani women. *Pakistan Journal of Medical Sciences, 37*(1), 1–4. https://doi.org/10.12669/pjms.37.1.2893

Mapayi, B., Makanjuola, R. O. A., Mosaku, S. K., Adewuya, O. A., Afolabi, O., Aloba, O. O., & Akinsulore, A. (2013). Impact of intimate partner violence on anxiety and depression amongst women in Ile-Ife, Nigeria. *Archives of Women's Mental Health, 16*(1), 11–18. https://doi.org/10.1007/s00737-012-0307-x

Mendoza, J. E., Tolba, M., & Saleh, Y. (2020). Strengthening marriages in Egypt: Impact of divorce on women. *Behavioral Sciences, 10*(1), 1–8. https://doi.org/10.3390/bs10010014

Mercy, J. A., & Saltzman, L. E. (1989). Fatal violence among spouses in the United States, 1976–85. *American Journal of Public Health, 79*(5), 595–599. https://doi.org/10.2105/ajph.79.5.595

Messing, J. T., Campbell, J. C., Brown, S., Patchell, B., Androff, D. K., & Wilson, J. S. (2014). The Association between protective actions and homicide risk: Findings from the Oklahoma lethality assessment study. *Violence and Victims, 29*(4), 543–563. https://doi.org/10.1891/0886-6708.VV-D-13-00013

Miller, S. L., & Manzer, J. L. (2021). Safeguarding children's well-being: Voices from abused mothers navigating their relationships and the civil courts. *Journal of Interpersonal Violence, 36*(9–10), 4545–4569. https://doi.org/10.1177/0886260518791599

Mojahed, A., Alaidarous, N., Shabta, H., Hegewald, J., & Garthus-Niegel, S. (2020). Intimate partner violence against women in the Arab countries: A systematic review of risk factors. *Trauma, Violence & Abuse, 23*(2), 1–18. https://doi.org/10.1177/1524838020953099

Moshtagh, M., Amiri, R., Sharafi, S., & Arab-Zozani, M. (2021). Intimate partner violence in the Middle East region: A systematic review and meta-analysis. *Trauma, Violence, and Abuse, 24*(2), 613–631. https://doi.org/10.1177/15248380211036060

Mshweshwe, L. (2020). Understanding domestic violence: Masculinity, culture, traditions. *Heliyon, 6*(10), e05334. https://doi.org/10.1016/j.heliyon.2020.e05334

Naseer, S., Farooq, S., & Malik, F. (2021). Causes and consequences of polygamy: An understanding of coping strategies by co-wives in polygamous marriage. *ASEAN Journal of Psychiatry, 22*(9), 1–10. https://doi.org/10.54615/2231-7805.47221

Obeid, N., Chang, D. F., & Ginges, J. (2010). Beliefs about wife beating: An exploratory study with Lebanese students. *Violence Against Women, 16*(6), 691–712. https://doi.org/10.1177/107780 1210370465

Oram, S., Khalifeh, H., & Howard, L. M. (2017). Violence against women and mental health. *The Lancet Psychiatry, 4*(2), 159–170. https://doi.org/10.1016/S2215-0366(16)30261-9

Otieno, F. O. (2017). *A Meta-analysis of the association between intimate partner violence and age disparity in sub-Saharan Africa* [Master's thesis, University of Stellenbosch]. SUNScholar. https://scholar.sun.ac.za/server/api/core/bitstreams/6651d00b-23bc-482f-bdb5-c649c649010a/content

Owusu Adjah, E. S., & Agbemafle, I. (2016). Determinants of domestic violence against women in Ghana. *BMC Public Health, 16*, 368. https://doi.org/10.1186/s12889-016-3041-x

Usta, J., Makarem, N. N., & Habib, R. R. (2013). Economic Abuse in Lebanon: Experiences and Perceptions. *Violence Against Women, 19*(3), 356–375. https://doi.org/10.1177/107780121348 6313

Papreen, N., Sharma, A., Sabin, K., Begum, L., Ahsan, S. K., & Baqui, A. H. (2000). Living with infertility: Experiences among urban slum populations in Bangladesh. *Reproductive Health Matters, 8*(15), 33–44. https://doi.org/10.1016/S0968-8080(00)90004-1

Paris, W. L., Wang, T., Laumann, E. O., Pan, S., & Luo, Y. (2004). Intimate partner violence in China: National prevalence, risk factors and associated health problems. *International Family Planning Perspectives, 30*(4), 174–181. https://doi.org/10.1363/3017404

Peltzer, K., Pengpid, S., McFarlane, J., & Banyini, M. (2013). Mental health consequences of intimate partner violence in Vhembe district, South Africa. *General Hospital Psychiatry, 35*(5), 545–550. https://doi.org/10.1016/j.genhosppsych.2013.04.001

Postmus, J. L., Plummer, S. B., McMahon, S., Murshid, N. S., & Kim, M. S. (2012). Understanding economic abuse in the lives of survivors. *Journal of Interpersonal Violence, 27*(3), 411–430. https://doi.org/10.1177/0886260511421669

Qureshi, K. (2020). Transnational divorce and remarriage between Pakistan and Britain: Intersectionality, harmful immigration rules and internal racism. *Population, Space and Place,* (September), e2396. 1–11. https://doi.org/10.1002/psp.2396

Rabaan, H., Young, A. L., & Dombrowski, L. (2021). Daughters of men: Saudi women's sociotechnical agency practices in addressing domestic abuse. *Proceedings of the ACM on Human-Computer Interaction, 4*(CSCW3), 1–31. https://doi.org/10.1145/3432923

Rahebi, S. M., Rahnavardi, M., Rezaie-Chamani, S., Nazari, M., & Sabetghadam, S. (2019). Relationship between domestic violence and infertility. *Eastern Mediterranean Health Journal, 25*(8), 537–542. https://doi.org/10.26719/emhj.19.001

Rahman, M., Nakamura, K., Seino, K., & Kizuki, M. (2013). Does gender inequity increase the risk of intimate partner violence among women? Evidence from a national Bangladeshi sample. *PLoS One, 8*(12), e82423. https://doi.org/10.1371/journal.pone.0082423

Raj, A., Santana, M. C., La Marche, A., Amaro, H., Cranston, K., & Silverman, J. G. (2006). Perpetration of intimate partner violence associated with sexual risk behaviors among young adult men. *American Journal of Public Health, 96*(10), 1873–1878. https://doi.org/10.2105/ AJPH.2005.081554

Rathi, P., Pachauri, J., & Pooja Rathi, C. (2018). Problems faced by divorced women in their pre and post-divorce period: A sociological study with reference to District Meerut. *Journal of Pharmacognosy and Phytochemistry, 7*(1), 207–212. https://www.phytojournal.com/archives/2018/vol7issue1/PartC/6-6-234-823.pdf

Roberts, A. L., Gilman, S. E., Fitzmaurice, G., Decker, M. R., & Koenen, K. C. (2010). Witness of intimate partner violence in childhood and perpetration of intimate partner violence in adulthood. *Epidemiology, 21*(6), 809–818. https://doi.org/10.1097/EDE.0b013e3181f39f03

Rocca, C. H., Rathod, S., Falle, T., Pande, R. P., & Krishnan, S. (2009). Challenging assumptions about women's empowerment: Social and economic resources and domestic violence among young married women in urban South India. *International Journal of Epidemiology, 38*(2), 577–585. https://doi.org/10.1093/ije/dyn226

Ruffin, A. K. (2021). *Family structure and women's experiences of intimate partner violence* [Unpublished doctoral dissertation]. University of Pennsylvania.

Ruiz-Pérez, I., Plazaola-Castaño, J., Álvarez-Kindelán, M., Palomo-Pinto, M., Arnalte-Barrera, M., Bonet-Pla, Á., et al. (2006). Sociodemographic associations of physical, emotional, and sexual intimate partner violence in Spanish women. *Annals of Epidemiology, 16*(5), 357–363. https://doi.org/10.1016/j.annepidem.2005.03.007

Sarkar, K., & Rizzi, E. (2020). Love marriage in India. Document de Travail 14, Centre de recherche en démographie. *Louvain-la-Neuve*, 1–42. https://doi.org/10.13140/RG.2.2.14596.55687

Sato-Dilorenzo, A., & Sharps, P. W. (2007). Dangerous intimate partner relationships and women's mental health and health behaviors. *Issues in Mental Health Nursing, 28*(8), 837–848. https://doi.org/10.1080/01612840701493535

Semahegn, A., & Mengistie, B. (2015). Domestic violence against women and associated factors in Ethiopia: Systematic review. *Reproductive Health, 12*(1), 78. https://doi.org/10.1186/s12978-015-0072-1

Sharp-Jeffs, N. (2015). *Money matters: Research into the extent and nature of financial abuse within intimate relationships in the UK*. London Metropolitan University. http://repository.londonmet.ac.uk/1481/1/Money-Matters.pdf

Sheikhan, Z., Ozgoli, G., Azar, M., & Alavimajd, H. (2014). Domestic violence in Iranian infertile women. *Medical Journal of the Islamic Republic of Iran, 28*(1), 152. https://pubmed.ncbi.nlm.nih.gov/25695010/

Sheykhi, M. T. (2020). World perspective of divorce in selected countries: A sociological appraisal. *World Family Medicine, 18*(6), 66–70.

Siganporia, M. (1993a). Indian Muslim women: Post divorce problems and social support. *Indian Journal of Social Work, 54*(3), 355–355. TISS – The Indian Journal of Social Work Achieve. https://journals.tiss.edu/archive/index.php/ijswarchive/article/view/3274

Siganporia, M. (1993b). Indian Muslim women: Post divorce problems and social support. *Indian Journal of Social Work, 54*(3), 355–355. https://journals.tiss.edu/archive/index.php/ijswarchive/article/view/3274

Smith, M. D. (1990). Sociodemographic risk factors in wife abuse: Results from a survey of Toronto women. *Canadian Journal of Sociology, 15*(1), 39. https://doi.org/10.2307/3341172

Solanke, B. L., Bisiriyu, A. L., & Oyedokun, A. (2018). Is the likelihood of spousal violence lower or higher among childless women? Evidence from Nigeria demographic and health surveys. *BMC Women's Health, 18*(1), 1–12. https://doi.org/10.1186/s12905-018-0514-3

Speizer, I. S., & Pearson, E. (2011). Association between early marriage and intimate partner violence in India: A focus on youth from Bihar and Rajasthan. *Journal of Interpersonal Violence, 26*(10), 1963–1981. https://doi.org/10.1177/0886260510372947

Spencer, C., Mallory, A. B., Cafferky, B. M., Kimmes, J. G., Beck, A. R., & Stith, S. M. (2019). Mental health factors and intimate partner violence perpetration and victimization: A meta-analysis. *Psychology of Violence, 9*(1), 1–17. https://doi.org/10.1037/vio0000156

Stein, M. B., & Kennedy, C. (2001). Major depressive and post-traumatic stress disorder comorbidity in female victims of intimate partner violence. *Journal of Affective Disorders, 66*(2–3), 133–138. https://doi.org/10.1016/S0165-0327(00)00301-3

Stöckl, H., Devries, K., Rotstein, A., Abrahams, N., Campbell, J., Watts, C., & Moreno, C. G. (2013). The global prevalence of intimate partner homicide: A systematic review. *The Lancet, 382*(9895), 859–865. https://doi.org/10.1016/S0140-6736(13)61030-2

Straus, H., Cerulli, C., McNutt, L. A., Rhodes, K. V., Conner, K. R., Kemball, R. S., Kaslow, N. J., & Houry, D. (2009). Intimate partner violence and functional health status: Associations with severity, danger, and self-advocacy behaviors. *Journal of Women's Health, 18*(5), 625–631. https://doi.org/10.1089/jwh.2007.0521

Sultana, A. (2012). Patriarchy and women's subordination: A theoretical analysis. *Arts Faculty Journal, 4*(2010–2011), 1–18. https://doi.org/10.3329/afj.v4i0.12929

Sutherland, C. A., Sullivan, C. M., & Bybee, D. I. (2001). Effects of intimate partner violence versus poverty on women's health. *Violence Against Woman, 7*(10), 1122–1143. https://doi.org/10.1177/10778010122183775

Taft, C. T., Resick, P. A., Watkins, L. E., & Panuzio, J. (2009). An investigation of posttraumatic stress disorder and depressive symptomatology among female victims of interpersonal trauma. *Journal of Family Violence, 24*(6), 407–415. https://doi.org/10.1007/s10896-009-9243-6

Tanimu, T. S., Yohanna, S., & Omeiza, S. Y. (2021). The pattern and correlates of intimate partner violence among women in Kano, Nigeria. *African Journal of Primary Health Care and Family Medicine, 8*(1), 1–7. https://doi.org/10.4102/phcfm.v8i1.1209

Tashkandi, A., & Rasheed, F. P. (2009). Wife abuse: a hidden problem. A study among Saudi women attending PHC centres. *Eastern Mediterranean health journal = La revue de sante de la Mediterranee orientale = al-Majallah al-sihhiyah li-sharq al-mutawassit, 15*(5), 1242–1253. http://apps.who.int/iris/bitstream/handle/10665/117755/15_5_2009_1242_1253.pdf?sequence=1&isAllowed=y

Tehreem, A., Zakar, R., Khan, B. S., Hussain, M. F., & Afza, R. (2021). Factors associated with termination of pregnancy among married adolescent girls in Pakistan: Secondary analysis of data from Pakistan demographic and health survey. *JAMDC, 3*(3), 95–102. https://doi.org/10.51127/JAMDCV3I3OA01

Terrazas-Carrillo, E. C., & McWhirter, P. T. (2015). Employment status and intimate partner violence among Mexican women. *Journal of Interpersonal Violence, 30*(7), 1128–1152. https://doi.org/10.1177/0886260514539848

Thabet, A. A., Tawahina, A. A., El Sarraj, E., & Vostanis, P. (2008). Exposure to war trauma and PTSD among parents and children in the Gaza strip. *European Child and Adolescent Psychiatry, 17*(4), 191–199. https://doi.org/10.1007/s00787-007-0653-9

Thabet, A., Tawahina, A., Victoria, T., & Vostanis, P. (2015). PTSD, depression, and anxiety among Palestinian women victims of domestic violence in the Gaza strip. *British Journal of Education, Society & Behavioural Science, 11*(2), 1–13. https://doi.org/10.9734/bjesbs/2015/18960

Thomson, D. R., Bah, A. B., Rubanzana, W. G., & Mutesa, L. (2015). Correlates of intimate partner violence against women during a time of rapid social transition in Rwanda: Analysis of the 2005 and 2010 demographic and health surveys. *BMC Women's Health, 15*(1), 1–13. https://doi.org/10.1186/s12905-015-0257-3

Tiruneh, F. N., Chuang, K. Y., Ntenda, P. A. M., & Chuang, Y. C. (2018). Unwanted pregnancy, pregnancy loss, and other risk factors for intimate partner violence in the Democratic Republic of the Congo. *Women and Health, 58*(9), 983–1000. https://doi.org/10.1080/03630242.2017.1377800

Tiruye, T. Y., Harris, M. L., Chojenta, C., Holliday, E., & Loxton, D. (2020). Intimate partner violence against women in Ethiopia and its association with unintended pregnancy: A national cross-sectional survey. *International Journal of Public Health, 65*(9), 1657–1667. https://doi.org/10.1007/s00038-020-01510-3

Tokuç, B., Ekuklu, G., & Avcioğlu, S. (2010). Domestic violence against married women in Edirne. *Journal of Interpersonal Violence, 25*(5), 832–847. https://doi.org/10.1177/0886260509336960

Varma, D., Chandra, P. S., Thomas, T., & Carey, M. P. (2007). Intimate partner violence and sexual coercion among pregnant women in India: Relationship with depression and post-traumatic stress disorder. *Journal of Affective Disorders, 102*(1–3), 227–235. https://doi.org/10.1016/j.jad.2006.09.026

Volpe, E. M., Hardie, T. L., Cerulli, C., Sommers, M. S., & Morrison-Beedy, D. (2013). What's age got to do with it? Partner age difference, power, intimate partner violence, and sexual risk in urban adolescents. *Journal of Interpersonal Violence, 28*(10), 2068–2087. https://doi.org/10.1177/0886260512471082

Walton-Moss, B. J., Manganello, J., Frye, V., & Campbell, J. C. (2005). Risk factors for intimate partner violence and associated injury among urban women. *Journal of Community Health, 30*(5), 377–389. https://doi.org/10.1007/s10900-005-5518-x

Wang, T., Wong, J. Y. H., & Fong, D. Y. T. (2022). Subjective socioeconomic status: An indicator of intimate partner violence in middle-aged adults in Hong Kong. *Health and Social Care in the Community, 30*(5), 1–8. https://doi.org/10.1111/hsc.13760

Watson, L. B., & Ancis, J. R. (2013). Power and control in the legal system: From marriage/relationship to divorce and custody. *Violence Against Women, 19*(2), 166–186. https://doi.org/10.1177/1077801213478027

Wright, E. N., Hanlon, A., Lozano, A., & Teitelman, A. M. (2019). The impact of intimate partner violence, depressive symptoms, alcohol dependence, and perceived stress on 30-year cardiovascular disease risk among young adult women: A multiple mediation analysis. *Preventive Medicine, 121*(August 2018), 47–54. https://doi.org/10.1016/j.ypmed.2019.01.016

Xu, X., Zhu, F., O'Campo, P., Koenig, M. A., Mock, V., & Campbell, J. (2005). Prevalence of and risk factors for intimate partner violence in China. *American Journal of Public Health, 95*(1), 78–85. https://doi.org/10.2105/AJPH.2003.023978

Yau, J. H. Y., Wong, J. Y. H., Choi, E. P. H., & Fong, D. Y. T. (2019). Transcultural validation of the 12-item scale of economic abuse in Chinese population. *Violence and Victims, 34*(5), 804–817. https://doi.org/10.1891/0886-6708.VV-D-17-00164

Yoshihama, M., Blazevski, J., & Bybee, D. (2014). Enculturation and attitudes toward intimate partner violence and gender roles in an Asian Indian population: Implications for community-based prevention. *American Journal of Community Psychology, 53*(3–4), 249–260. https://doi.org/10.1007/s10464-014-9627-5

Yount, K. M. (2011). Women's conformity as resistance to intimate partner violence in Assiut, Egypt. *Sex Roles, 64*(1–2), 43–58. https://doi.org/10.1007/s11199-010-9884-1

Yüksel-Kaptanoğlu, I., Türkyilmaz, A. S., & Heise, L. (2012). What puts women at risk of violence from their husbands? Findings from a large, nationally representative survey in Turkey. *Journal of Interpersonal Violence, 27*(14), 2743–2769. https://doi.org/10.1177/0886260512438283

Zakar, R., Nasrullah, M., Zakar, M. Z., & Ali, H. (2016). The association of intimate partner violence with unintended pregnancy and pregnancy loss in Pakistan. *International Journal of Gynecology & Obstetrics, 133*(1), 26–31. https://doi.org/10.1016/j.ijgo.2015.09.009

Zara, G., & Gino, S. (2018). Intimate partner violence and its escalation into femicide. Frailty thy name is "violence against women". *Frontiers in Psychology, 9*, 1–11. https://doi.org/10.3389/fpsyg.2018.01777

Zeoli, A. M., Rivera, E. A., Sullivan, C. M., & Kubiak, S. (2013). Post-separation abuse of women and their children: Boundary-setting and family court utilization among victimized mothers. *Journal of Family Violence, 28*(6), 547–560. https://doi.org/10.1007/s10896-013-9528-7

Chapter 7
Conclusions and Policy Implications

The purpose of this study was to examine how domestic abuse affects the mental health of Qatari women. Several questions were sought to be addressed in this study concerning the prevalence and forms of IPV exerted on Qatari women and the potential risk of homicide they may encounter. PTSD, Depression, and Anxiety were considered adverse outcomes of IPV on mental health in this study. This study investigated factors associated with IPV victimisation, attitudes towards women, and the reasons behind women's passive attitudes towards ending the cycle of abuse.

Intimate partner violence and its adverse effects on mental health are discussed in the introduction chapter. This chapter provides an overview of the research problem, research questions, and study objectives. Several scholars' arguments presented in this chapter discuss how oil discovery has led to increased consumerism and dependency on the government, while the 'core institutions' remain less impacted. A detailed discussion of family social structure is conducted, demonstrating that many arguments suggest that the government follows Islamic principles, and that the family is primarily responsible for socialization. Furthermore, this chapter offers an overview of Qatar, where the research was conducted, and explains the Arabic family structure. It also discusses the significance of the study and the rationale for conducting it.

Following the introduction, the review of literature was carried to support the assertion that there was lack of research not just in Qatar but also Arab world in general related to domestic violence. The findings of this current study provided valuable insights into the phenomenon under investigation through an explanatory sequential mixed method approach that draws on theoretical frameworks influenced by social learning theory, gendered resource theory, feminist theory, and ecological model of domestic abuse. Both quantitative and qualitative findings were integrated with the support of an existing body of knowledge that examined similar covariates. Both phases of the study contributed explanations and theoretical insights to the interpretation of the findings.

K. Al-Naama, *Domestic Abuse and Mental Health in Qatar*, Gulf Studies 23,
https://doi.org/10.1007/978-981-96-7392-6_7

This design facilitated the investigation and provided valuable insights into IPV prevalence and the various forms of violence present in Qatar. By using this methodology, a gap in previous research was addressed, and a greater understanding of domestic abuse against women was gained. The information and rationale presented in this chapter support the use of a mixed method approach and statistical measures. Previous research has predominantly employed qualitative or quantitative approaches, which indicates a need for an integrative approach. This creates an urgent need for an integrative approach to understanding IPV in Qatar. By combining findings from both approaches, a comprehensive understanding can be achieved by offsetting the limitations of each approach due to Qatari society's tendency to avoid discussing family issues in public or in formal settings, which results in a lack of reliable information about domestic abuse current status, and access to data and gatekeepers is quite challenging in order to gain a comprehensive understanding of IPV.

To address the research questions, several scales were implemented, including the CTS-2 and SEA-2 to measure the forms and severity of abuse to which victims were exposed. Additionally, the PCL-C, PHQ-9, and TMAS scales were used to measure and examine the effects of domestic abuse on PTSD, depression, and anxiety. The DA scale was used to assess the risk of homicide, and the AWS-25 scale was used to measure women's rights in society from the victims' perspectives. Semi-structured interviews were employed in the qualitative phases to gain deeper insights and expand upon the findings from the quantitative results.

Based on the results of the current study, PCLC was an effective measure to assess symptoms of PTSD among victims of domestic abuse. These results are not substantially different from those obtained from a student population that was investigated in the year 2012. Undergraduate students at a major institution located in the eastern region of the United States were given a PCL-C checklist to complete.

Furthermore, this chapter reflects on findings from previous studies conducted in Qatar and discusses several key limitations adopted for this study. The Introduction chapter continues to provide a framework for understanding domestic violence in Qatar, drawing from anecdotes, the voices of victims, and concealed stories. Conducting research in Qatar has become a necessity for several reasons, given the potential grave danger faced by those involved. This research has added another layer to seeking justice by presenting victims' claims that have prompted global responses from international human rights organizations and activists, leading to scrutiny of current human rights laws, family policies, the effectiveness of social welfare and protection systems, and local organizations that assist victims of domestic violence.

It underscores the fact that not enough attention has been paid to understanding the nature, prevalence, negative consequences, and reasons why victims remain passive in abusive relationships. Only a few descriptive studies have been conducted, resulting in a lack of comprehensive knowledge. Domestic violence in Qatar has suffered from a scarcity of information due to limited resources and a gendered perspective on women's rights. The absence of empirical research methodologies in previous studies conducted in Qatar necessitates a scientific approach to understanding domestic abuse in the country. Consequently, it becomes challenging to compare the types of abuse reported in Qatar with those occurring in other places.

An extensive review of the existing literature pertaining to domestic abuse against women and its impact on mental health is presented in the literature review chapter. This chapter also delves into the prevalence of domestic abuse, the various forms it can take, and the risk of homicide. Multiple studies have indicated that the risk of domestic abuse is prevalent, encompassing physical, sexual, psychological, and economic forms of intimate partner violence. According to the literature review, psychological abuse is the most prevalent form of abuse experienced by women in Arabic culture, among a few other forms. The severity and frequency of abuse have been associated with cumulative adverse mental and physical health outcomes, including pregnancy complications or miscarriage.

Additionally, this chapter discusses the adverse mental health outcomes associated with domestic abuse, including depression, anxiety, and post-traumatic stress disorder (PTSD). A growing body of literature has shown that various forms of intimate partner violence (IPV) can significantly influence the development of PTSD, depression, anxiety, and other mental health issues. In the literature, inconsistencies have been found regarding when abuse may be considered a risk factor for homicide, with more concerns raised about the risk of homicide during the separation process. Few studies have been conducted to measure the potential risk of murder in GCC countries, particularly Qatar, where such research has been lacking. In light of the current findings, it can be cautiously concluded that the risk of homicide is relatively low, but this conclusion should be interpreted with caution due to the small sample size.

A literature review discussed several theoretical frameworks for determining and explaining domestic abuse in some situations. It highlighted several risk factors that have been examined in western societies and cross-sectional studies that have proven their significance with variance. The majority of studies regarding IPV in Qatar are descriptive in nature, so there is not enough scientific evidence to assess the risk of IPV in Qatar. It was also identified in the chapter that women face barriers in seeking assistance when seeking to end their relationship with an abuser. Ending an abusive relationship with an intimate partner presents a great deal of difficulties, including financial obstacles, homicide risk, social pressure, and concerns about post-marriage arrangements.

In addition, attitudes towards women's rights as well as societal norms and family structure have been discussed as potential influences on IPV risk. Researchers have reported that a key element in understanding IPV risk is women's mindset and traditional gender roles within the family. Clearly, there is a lack of research on the impact of family and social structure on influencing the risk of abuse among the less fortunate in Qatar. There are several sources of ambiguity regarding the impact of women's rights in society on their risk of abuse, which was discussed extensively in literature reviews to provide an overview of the risk factors that should be considered when investigating IPV risk. In prior studies conducted in Qatar, such findings have not been replicated.

Moreover, the sample representation was biased and did not accurately reflect the full spectrum of abuse in society. There is a tendency for domestic abuse cases in Qatar to go unreported, as it is in many other Arab countries in the region. The reason for this is that many victims suffer in silence while their abusers go free. Being a victim of IPV is most likely to lead to social shame, which cannot be proven without scientific evidence. Understanding Qatari culture and social values is essential when it comes to domestic abuse.

Western nations have paid considerable attention to the issue of domestic violence against women. In the discussion, there was a lot of discussion about how living in a multicultural society has influenced Qatari culture and preferences. Among the major issues associated with IPV is the social shame associated with being a victim. Without evidence-based research, this cannot be proven. In this chapter, the importance of understanding Qatari culture and social values is emphasized. The author argues that domestic violence against women is a growing epidemic in the Middle East, where victims suffer in silence while their abusers remain at large, it also discusses outdated social systems that could negatively impact victims' lives. There were several points raised about the impact of inadequate social protection systems and laws on women's decision to leave abusive marriages. It reveals how societal stigma and reputation concepts prioritise family and group cohesion over individual interests.

An overview of the historical, political, and cultural context of the evolving transition of Arab families was provided. Families' traditional gender roles were revealed. During the discussion, the context was analysed in relation to how current debates about Arab populations in the Middle East have been shaped by dealing with victims of domestic abuse claims. There has been a narrowing of perspectives and attitudes about the traditional female role as a result of these debates.

In a family, one's status is determined by age and sex. Numerous arguments revolve around patrilineal, patrilocal, patriarchal, and endogamous relationships, which shape the dynamics among family members, with age and sex playing pivotal roles in determining one's position. Additionally, traditional views regarding women's roles in public life were examined. The discussion also delves into the reasons why elders continue to influence their sons' and daughters' decisions after marriage. This highlights the significance of preserving the dignity of the tribe and maintaining family stability.

Another significant aspect discussed was the cultural taboo against discussing domestic abuse in Arab nations, which contributes to the public perception that domestic violence does not exist. Qatar lacks studies on domestic violence and its consequences on health, despite a few studies on the topic.

The findings of this study confirm that IPV significantly contributes to the development of women's mental health conditions, including PTSD, depression, and anxiety. These findings indicate that patriarchal norms, family structure, and attitudes towards women's rights significantly influence the risk of IPV among women. Several findings were discussed in detail in the discussion chapter. They showed that there is a significant association between mothers with a high number of children, intermarriage, and second marriage associated with sexual coercion. Poor educational attainment, low household income, and forced or love marriages, as well as age disparity between husband and wife of 10-year period or more, are all associated with the occurrence of IPV, including economic abuse. While infertility and employment were insignificantly associated with the risk of IPV.

This study has made a valuable contribution to understanding why women often remain passive in abusive relationships. It has also revealed that many victims face substantial barriers when attempting to leave an abusive relationship. These barriers encompass post-divorce abuse, societal pressures stemming from divorce, and the complexities associated with child custody.

The study highlighted the need for a multifaceted approach that involves raising community awareness levels about the devastating risk of domestic abuse on women's mental and reproductive health, outlining the importance of reducing gender discrimination by challenging an outdated social and cultural norm. Practitioners may be able to benefit from this insight in order to better understand the problem and develop appropriate interventions. This will assist in protecting the family member during and after divorce in situations where there are abusive relationships.

The study has also provided evidence supporting the importance of implementing a screening tool to identify and protect IPV victims. By training medical, health, and legal professionals to use this tool, it will enable them to respond appropriately and potentially save the lives of victims. The study underscores the pressing need for more comprehensive support services for women who have experienced abuse at home.

The current research fills a significant knowledge gap in Qatar regarding IPV. Despite some limitations in our approach, it provides novel insights into the complexities of domestic violence against women. This dissertation has made a substantial contribution to the field of domestic abuse and mental health, with findings that have far-reaching implications for policy and practice.

These findings serve as a foundation for further research in this area, utilizing advanced statistical methods to predict forms of abuse and their impacts. It is hoped that the results of this study will contribute to ongoing efforts to address domestic abuse at the national level. This could involve a review of outdated family policies, which can play a significant role in the lives of victims. Such policies can serve as a means of protecting families and breaking the cycle of abuse, enabling victims to make more informed decisions. Moreover, future studies should delve into the causes and effects of domestic abuse, while also examining various cultural and societal norms. Investigating socio-economic status in relation to financial abuse and post-divorce arrangements can provide valuable insights into preventing women from enduring abusive relationships.

The outcomes of this research provide a comprehensive and nuanced insight into IPV in Qatar. Nevertheless, the results of this study should be interpreted with caution due to the small sample size and other limitations. A reflection on the key findings of this research is provided in this chapter. Participants regarded psychological aggressiveness and economic abuse as primary types of violence, and symptomology of depression, anxiety, and PTSD was often connected with victims of domestic abuse in Qatar.

The new research serves to fill an important need in the existing body of research about the dynamics of abusive relationships in the home in Qatar. In addition to this, it expands upon the research that has been done earlier in Qatar by Al Ghayathin (2017) and Al-Ghanim (2009). In addition, the findings of this study will assist policymakers in rethinking the current family policy in order to improve it and cut the abuse rate among vulnerable groups. The goal of this is to create a secure environment for families in order to improve their health and strengthen their bonds with one another. This study will also improve our understanding of how important it is to provide additional assistance to abused single parents during the pre- and post-divorce phases in order to preserve the previous family's financial and emotional status. This will be accomplished through the preservation of the previous family. The individual, societal, and familial factors that most likely evolved and changed over time should be taken into consideration when analysing the risk factors that were investigated in this study because they will help future research to extend knowledge about the complex nature of domestic abuse in Qatar. It is also suggested that future research should concentrate more on patriarchal standards and family structure, both of which may contribute adversely to the fact that women endure domestic violence. I provide a summary of the strengths and contributions to existing knowledge in the next section.

7.1 Contributions to the Field

The findings of this study have contributed to the existing literature on intimate partner violence (IPV) in several ways. Notably, it was the first study in Qatar to investigate IPV and economic abuse, as well as the risk of homicide –topics that had never been examined before.

The greatest strength of the current study lay in the diversity of its participants. Although the sample size was relatively small, it was highly representative as participants were recruited from various sources. This inclusiveness extended to victims who had experienced threats of homicidal violence and severe forms of abuse, who were sourced from the Protection Social Rehabilitation Center (AMAN), as well as individuals who visited family counseling centers to discuss post-dissolution rights and disputes related to child custody and visitation rights. Furthermore, this research actively engaged non-governmental organizations (NGOs) like WAYAK, mental health associations, the CCQ, and the wider public domain to identify unreported and hidden cases of IPV, thus ensuring a comprehensive understanding of this domain.

Second, the quantitative phase of this study revealed substantial evidence that participants reported psychological and economic abuse as the most common forms of abuse. A number of findings emerged from the qualitative phase regarding economic hardship post-divorce and child custody rights for breaking the cycle of abuse and preventing them from remarrying. The study findings contribute to filling a gap in knowledge in the literature among women who experienced IPV who were found to display significantly higher levels of depression, anxiety, and (PTSD) symptoms in Qatar, which have previously not been studied. This finding underlines the importance of addressing the mental health needs of IPV survivors. The study also sheds light on the possibility of integrating IPV interventions that address physical and mental health consequences.

Third, the methodology empirical approach adopted in this study enabled the enrichment of data collection with a sequential explanatory method and provided a nuanced understanding of pretested questionnaires that have been addressed in Western cultures and peer-reviewed articles that have been tested for the first time in Qatar. In this study, the theoretical framework ecological model guided the development of the research questions which enabled the testing of the broader impact of individual, community, and family factors on the increasing risk of victimisation. Previous research conducted in Qatar raised concerns about the prevalence and types of domestic abuse among university students. To expand on previous research findings, this study provides further insights into when IPV victims are at greater risk of being murdered by their husbands.

Fourth, the current findings confirm the assumption that IPV significantly affects women's mental and physical health, challenging the notion that it's a minor and private issue. These findings underscore the importance of advanced intervention programs aimed at educating society about the risks of abuse. Additionally, they emphasize the need to equip healthcare providers with screening toolkits to identify a broad range of abuse as a protective measure, which is essential for preserving the public health of individuals.

Fifth, understanding family structure was enhanced through a number of useful insights such as marriage type, age at marriage time, age disparity between husband and wife, polygamous marriages, second marriages, husband and wife mindset and terms and conditions involved with divorce cases filed. These factors were found to be significantly associated with vulnerability to victimisation or with concerns about leaving an abusive relationship where surprisingly, husband and wife unemployment and women's infertility were not associated with risk of victimisation which provides another line of thought to consider future research if these conditions were examined with reference to societal factor. In this preliminary exploration-related study across the Gulf region, significant synergies and novelty have been introduced. This contribution to knowledge has the potential to inform policy development not only in Qatar but also in the wider Gulf states within the Arab world. Given the existing gap in research on domestic abuse, further studies are needed. This study aims to contribute to the development of future research by providing valuable grassroots knowledge.

This is the first study of its kind to capture unique psychological data. It's the first study within Qatar of this scale to examine the issue of domestic violence, where both recorded figures and psychometric data were guided by victims of domestic violence. Additionally, study results highlight the importance of understanding adverse mental health outcomes associated with various forms of domestic violence among the Arab population. This is the first mixed-method study to have been conducted in Qatar, measuring various forms of domestic abuse against women using a pre-established questionnaire that has been employed in both cross-cultural and Western studies. This process has enabled the author to build upon existing literature and shed light on domestic abuse patterns and consequences in Qatar for future studies.

7.2 Policy Implications

The research results represent a further step towards developing a better understanding of domestic abuse and its psychopathological effects. In order to provide long-term care for victims and their families, an integrative modelling approach is a key measure of combating IPV. There is a need for a common synergy between healthcare providers, policy advocates, and legal institutes to work more proactively to raise awareness about equal rights to deconstruct traditional gender roles that suppress women's rights and promote power imbalance between life partners (Di Napoli et al., 2019).

Another practical implication suggests several courses of action helps to mitigate risks that extend beyond victims' mental health and social well-being. Various indicators, such as the gender pay gap, gender inequality, and low economic participation in the labour force, should be continuously monitored. This will enable governments and civil society organisations to gain a comprehensive understanding of how policy options may contribute to the lives of fragmented families (Vujadinovi et al., 2023).

The implications of this include the possibility of revisiting current socio-legal policy, professional training for healthcare providers, and the development of mental health and social welfare services. Furthermore, women suffering from IPV are more likely to seek help from healthcare providers (HCPs), but they often do not report the violence. Thus, it is important to train HCPs how to identify victims of IPV, take care of them, preserve their privacy, and refer them to specialists as needed leading to more positive health results for these women and their children (Kalra et al., 2021). For instance, WHO (2021) launched a revised edition of a training programme for healthcare providers about how to enhance identification, communication, and support skills for better care of victims of IPV. One policy reasonable approach is to modify a validated screening tool that can be used in clinical settings. This will facilitate the identification of domestic abuse victims in the emergency department (Houry et al., 2007). It is possible that these victims may have unreported suicidal thoughts or mental health problems.

According to the findings of this study, violence in the family of origin is associated with future victimisation or perpetration in adulthood. Consequently, the screening process should emphasize the defects of family members who have been affected by domestic violence, in particular children. Furthermore, children who get abused are in danger of suffering from extended physical and psychological health issues. Even those who just observe violence against their mother may suffer from mental problems due to living in a tense and unfriendly habitat (Basile et al., 2021). Trained paediatrics and healthcare providers are required to identify an abused child, ask about his/her safety during screening, and decide whether it is necessary to report the violence encountered by this child. Some programs in hospitals, in the paediatric departments, in the USA, take care of both children and their mothers such as "Advocacy for Women and Kids in Emergencies, "AWAKE, which is found at Children's Hospital in Boston. This program provides referrals for medical, legal, social, and psychological help (Culross, 1999). In addition, as shown by the current findings that pregnant women were at greater risk of abuse. For this reason, antenatal clinics should adopt comprehensive screening protocols to detect concealed cases of abuse.

As another critical aspect, legal, health, and child protection services must embrace a multidisciplinary approach to understanding and addressing domestic abuse. Domestic abuse cases demand unique handling and reliance on diverse resources to minimize the serious harm inflicted on victims (Newman, 2010). Healthcare providers and criminal justice officers should undergo professional training to recognize less obvious forms of abuse, such as emotional abuse (Walklate et al., 2018). There is a recognized need for protocols that guide practitioners in responding to traumatized victims and their family members, based on scientific evidence that elucidates the power dynamics within abusive relationships. The quality of intervention and inter-organizational collaboration are essential in extricating the victim from the abusive relationship. This may involve providing victims with accommodation options, such as staying in a shelter or with a trusted relative or friend, with the ultimate goal of breaking the cycle of abuse. Moreover, these professionals bear the responsibility of helping the victim make informed decisions regarding her future and safety, as well as the safety of any children involved (Enache et al., 2019).

Furthermore, the economic situation also plays a crucial role in the reintegration of women victims into society. To leave a violent relationship, women need good financial standing. Cultural perspectives may, however, contribute to domestic violence against women and children, as some societies tolerate such abuse. Similarly, Fahmy et al. (2016) demonstrates that recognizing domestic violence against a spouse as a crime and improving the law enforcement response is a key policy implication that has to be considered. The researcher further elaborate that women's financial abuse may continue after divorce due to inadequate child support orders and inadequate childcare options. It is, therefore, necessary to reconsider and evaluate post-divorce financial maintenance policy, especially among divorced mothers, as narrated by the participants in the current study. To manage the mental health effects of traumatized women and their families, ongoing efforts are required to make social support programs and psychotherapy options available to survivors of domestic abuse, either remotely or in person (Ogbe et al., 2020).

The environment and the social and cultural background of victims of domestic violence must be considered in order to help them build their capacities to become more active socially so that they can attain the essential conditions for a good life (Enache et al., 2019). Awareness programs also require continual evaluation of their effectiveness. It has recently been found that the New York City Department of Education has implemented a variety of preventive and education programs, and the survey's results indicate that inspection of such programs may be beneficial to enhance awareness and observers' involvement throughout society (Lambson & Reich, 2017).

The development of social and legal policies is essential to support victims of domestic violence. For example, Romania utilizes Law 227/2003, with some adjustments made in 2015, and Law 211/2005 with specific adjustments concerning victim protection. These two laws grant significant rights to victims, including access to special protection measures such as restraining orders that prevent the abuser from approaching the victim, free legal consultation, free social consultation to identify various sources of economic assistance programs for victims, and free emergency healthcare (Enache et al., 2019). Moreover, marriage instability and divorce were reported among the study participants. It is therefore important to invest in premarital education programs, encourage early disclosures of abuse, and provide early intervention programs for low-income households as a means to maintain family stability through reliable protective measures (Lawrence, 2002).

While some women may not disclose the nature of their violent relationships, the current findings underscore the crucial role of healthcare providers in protecting them from further and more severe forms of aggressive behaviour. Implementing proactive screening policies for females visiting antenatal clinics, emergency rooms, and primary care centres, particularly those who may not be adequately screened for abuse, can help prevent more serious assaults. This, in turn, can facilitate the management of treatment programs in mental health hospitals and facilities. Additionally, campaigns can be developed to educate the public about the often-underrecognized effects of domestic violence on mental health.

WIFAQ and AMAN demonstrate their commitment to understanding the adverse effects of abuse on mental health and educating the public. The Community Police Department is determined to combat violent behaviour against women, and danger assessment scales can play a pivotal role in protecting victims of domestic abuse by detecting and diagnosing potential lethal crimes earlier. The findings of this study have the potential to guide policymakers and advocates in revising socially equitable policies that safeguard people's rights. This could involve the development of rehabilitation programs employing a holistic approach to ensure social justice for both husbands and wives. Additionally, a more systematic approach to improving data accuracy can be implemented by adapting validated scales to current reporting protocols. One approach that may encourage the disclosure of traumatic experiences is the adaptation of self-rated scales in clinical settings. Given the sensitive nature of abuse, self-rated scales may be more suitable than traditional diagnostic tools such as face-to-face interviews (MacMillan et al., 2006). These scales can be introduced to healthcare providers as a practical screening measure for domestic abuse. Furthermore, the use of restraining orders may be one of the most effective measures in protecting the rights of victims during and after divorce, despite its current underutilization.

References

Al Ghayathin, B. (2017). *Violence against women in Qatar: An exploratory study* [Master's thesis, Hamad Bin Khalifa University]. https://search.proquest.com/dissertations-theses/violence-against-women-qatar-exploratory-study/docview/1907499277/se-2?accountid=10673%0Ahttps://ed-primo.hosted.exlibrisgroup.com/openurl/44UOE/44UOE_VU2??url_ver=Z39.88-2004&rft_val_fmt=info:ofi/fmt:kev:m

Al-Ghanim, K. A. (2009). Violence against women in Qatari society. *Journal of Middle East Women's Studies, 5*(1), 80–93. https://doi.org/10.2979/mew.2009.5.1.80

Basile, K. C., Jones, K., Smith, S. G., & RAINN Staff. (2021, February 15). *Effects of domestic violence on children.* The Office on Women's Health, National Center for Injury Prevention and Control, Centers for Disease Control and Prevention (CDC). https://www.womenshealth.gov/relationships-and-safety/domestic-violence/effects-domestic-violence-children

Culross, P. L. (1999). Health care system responses to children exposed to domestic violence. *The Future of Children, 9*(3), 111–121. https://doi.org/10.2307/1602785

Di Napoli, I., Procentese, F., Carnevale, S., Esposito, C., & Arcidiacono, C. (2019). Ending intimate partner violence (IPV) and locating men at stake: An ecological approach. *International Journal of Environmental Research and Public Health, 16*(9), 1652. https://doi.org/10.3390/ijerph16091652

Enache, R. G., Matei, R. S., & Tuşa, E. (2019). Specialized intervention for protecting victims of domestic violence. *Revista De Asistenta Sociala, 1*, 127–137. https://www.proquest.com/scholarly-journals/specialized-intervention-protecting-victims/docview/2440936908/se-2

Fahmy, E., Williamson, E., & Pantazis, C. (2016). *Evidence and policy review: Domestic violence and poverty* (pp. 1–42). Joseph Rowntree Foundation. https://research-information.bristol.ac.uk/files/80376377/JRF_DV_POVERTY_REPORT_FINAL_COPY_.pdf

Houry, D., Kemball, R. S., Click, L. A., & Kaslow, N. J. (2007). Development of a brief mental health screen for intimate partner violence victims in the emergency department. *Academic Emergency Medicine, 14*(3), 202–209. https://doi.org/10.1197/j.aem.2006.09.056

Kalra, N., Hooker, L., Reisenhofer, S., Di Tanna, G. L., & García-Moreno, C. (2021). Training healthcare providers to respond to intimate partner violence against women. *Cochrane Database of Systematic Reviews, 5*(5), CD012423–CD012423. https://doi.org/10.1002/14651858.CD012423.pub2

Lambson, S. H., & Reich, W. A. (2017). *Intimate partner violence as a community problem community perspectives from Bedford-Stuyvesant, Brooklyn.* Center for Court Innovation. http://www.courtinnovation.org/sites/default/files/documents/BedStuy_IPV_Research_Report.pdf

Lawrence, S. (2002). *Domestic violence and welfare policy research findings that can inform policies on marriage and child well-being*. National Center for Children in Poverty, Columbia University. https://doi.org/10.7916/D87D33S1

MacMillan, H. L., Wathen, C. N., Jamieson, E., Boyle, M., McNutt, L. A., Worster, A., Lent, B., Webb, M., & McMaster Violence Against Women Research Group. (2006). Approaches to screening for intimate partner violence in health care settings: A randomized trial. *JAMA, 296*(5), 530–536. https://doi.org/10.1001/jama.296.5.530

Newman, C. (2010). Expert domestic violence risk assessments in the family courts. *Respect*, 1–19. http://www.fsa.me.uk/uploads/7/6/5/6/7656227/respect_dv_risk_assessment_review_-_c_newman_c_bell.pdf

Ogbe, E., Harmon, S., van den Bergh, R., & Degomme, O. (2020). A systematic review of intimate partner violence interventions focused on improving social support and/ mental health outcomes of survivors. *PLoS One, 15*(6), 1–27. https://doi.org/10.1371/journal.pone.0235177

Vujadinovi, D., Fröhlich, M., & Giegerich, T. (Eds.). (2023). *Gender-competent legal education.* Springer. https://doi.org/10.1007/978-3-031-14360-1

Walklate, S., Fitz-Gibbon, K., & McCulloch, J. (2018). Is more law the answer? Seeking justice for victims of intimate partner violence through the reform of legal categories. *Criminology and Criminal Justice, 18*(1), 115–131. https://doi.org/10.1177/1748895817728561

World Health Organization (WHO). (2021). *Caring for women subjected to violence: a WHO training curriculum for health care providers (Revised edition)*. https://apps.who.int/iris/handle/10665/349539

Appendices

Appendix 1—CTS-2 Short Version of Conflict Tactics Scale

Relationship Behaviours

	How often this happens in the past year	Once	Twice	3–5 times	6–10 times	11–20 times	More than 20 times	Never
1	My partner showed care for me even though we disagreed	1	2	3	4	5	6	0
2	My partner explained his or her side of a disagreement to me	1	2	3	4	5	6	0
3	My partner showed respect for my feelings about an issue	1	2	3	4	5	6	0
4	My partner said he or she was sure we could work out a problem	1	2	3	4	5	6	0

(continued)

K. Al-Naama, *Domestic Abuse and Mental Health in Qatar*, Gulf Studies 23,
https://doi.org/10.1007/978-981-96-7392-6

(continued)

	How often this happens in the past year	Once	Twice	3–5 times	6–10 times	11–20 times	More than 20 times	Never
5	My partner suggested a compromise to a disagreement	1	2	3	4	5	6	0
6	My partner agreed to try a solution to a disagreement I suggested	1	2	3	4	5	6	0
7	My partner insulted or swore at me	1	2	3	4	5	6	0
8	My partner shouted or yelled at me	1	2	3	4	5	6	0
9	My partner stomped out of the room or house or yard during a disagreement	1	2	3	4	5	6	0
10	My partner did something to spite me	1	2	3	4	5	6	0
11	My partner accused me of being a lousy lover	1	2	3	4	5	6	0
12	My partner called me fat or ugly	1	2	3	4	5	6	0
13	My partner destroyed something that belonged to me	1	2	3	4	5	6	0
14	My partner threatened to hit or throw something at me	1	2	3	4	5	6	0

(continued)

(continued)

	How often this happens in the past year	Once	Twice	3–5 times	6–10 times	11–20 times	More than 20 times	Never
15	My partner threw something at me that could hurt	1	2	3	4	5	6	0
16	My partner twisted my arm or hair	1	2	3	4	5	6	0
17	My partner pushed or shoved me	1	2	3	4	5	6	0
18	My partner grabbed me	1	2	3	4	5	6	0
19	My partner slapped me	1	2	3	4	5	6	0
20	My partner used a knife or gun on me	1	2	3	4	5	6	0
21	My partner punched or hit me with something that could hurt	1	2	3	4	5	6	0
22	My partner choked me	1	2	3	4	5	6	0
23	My partner slammed me against a wall	1	2	3	4	5	6	0
24	My partner beat me up	1	2	3	4	5	6	0
25	My partner burned or scalded me on purpose	1	2	3	4	5	6	0
26	My partner kicked me	1	2	3	4	5	6	0
27	I had a sprain, bruise, or small cut because of a fight with my partner	1	2	3	4	5	6	0

(continued)

(continued)

	How often this happens in the past year	Once	Twice	3–5 times	6–10 times	11–20 times	More than 20 times	Never
28	I felt physical pain that still hurt the next day because of a fight with my partner	1	2	3	4	5	6	0
29	I passed out from being hit on the head by my partner in a fight	1	2	3	4	5	6	0
30	I went to a doctor because of a fight with my partner	1	2	3	4	5	6	0
31	I needed to see a doctor because of a fight with my partner but I did not	1	2	3	4	5	6	0
32	I had a broken bone from a fight with my partner	1	2	3	4	5	6	0
33	My partner made me have sex without a condom	1	2	3	4	5	6	0
34	My partner insisted that I have sex when I did not want to (but did not use physical force)	1	2	3	4	5	6	0

(continued)

(continued)

	How often this happens in the past year	Once	Twice	3–5 times	6–10 times	11–20 times	More than 20 times	Never
35	My partner insisted I have oral or anal sex (but did not use physical force)	1	2	3	4	5	6	0
36	My partner used force to make me have oral or anal sex	1	2	3	4	5	6	0
37	My partner used force to make me have sex	1	2	3	4	5	6	0
38	My partner used threats to make me have oral or anal sex	1	2	3	4	5	6	0
39	My partner used threats to make me have sex	1	2	3	4	5	6	0

Appendix 2—The Scale of Economic Abuse – 12 (SEA-12)

Scale of Economic Abuse—12 (SEA-12)

Postmus, J.L., Plummer, S.B., & Stylianou, A.M. (2016). Measuring Economic Abuse in the Lives of Survivors: Revising the Scale of Economic Abuse. *Violence Against Women, 22*(6), 692–703.

I'm going to go through a list of things some individuals do to hurt their partner or ex-partner financially. Could you tell me, to the best of your recollection, how frequently your partner or ex-partner has done any of the following things in the last 12 months. Your answer can range from 1 to 5. 1 = Never, 2 = Hardly ever, 3 = Sometimes, 4 = Often, 5 = Quite Often.

Economic Exploitation (3 items)	
1.	Pay bills late or not pay bills that were in your name or in both of your names.
2.	Spend the money you needed for rent or other bills.
3.	Build up debt under your name by doing things like use your credit card or run up the phone bill.
Economic Control (5 items)	
4.	Demand to know how money was spent.
5.	Make important financial decisions without talking with you about it first.
6.	Keep financial information from you.
7.	Demand that you give him receipts and/or change when you spent money.
8.	Make you ask him for money.
Employment Sabotage (4 items)	
9.	Do things to keep you from going to your job
10.	Demand that you quit your job.
11.	Threaten you to make you leave work.
12.	Beat you up if you said you needed to go to work.

Appendix 3—Danger Assessment Scale (DA)

Danger Assessment

Jacquelyn C. Campbell, PhD, R.N. Copyright, 2003; update 2019; www.dangerassessment.com

Several risk factors have been associated with an increased risk of homicides (murders) of women and men in violent relationships. We cannot predict what will happen in your case, but we would like you to be aware of the danger of homicide in situations of abuse and for you to see how many of the risk factors apply to your situation.

Using the calendar, please mark the approximate dates during the past year when you were abused by your partner or ex-partner. Write on that date how bad the incident was according to the following scale:

1. Slapping, pushing; no injuries and/or lasting pain
2. Punching, kicking; bruises, cuts, and/or continuing pain
3. "Beating up"; severe contusions, burns, broken bones
4. Threat to use a weapon; head injury, internal injury, permanent injury, miscarriage or choking* (use a © in the date to indicate choking/strangulation/cut off your breathing- example 4©)
5. Use of weapon; wounds from weapon

(If **any** of the descriptions for the higher number apply, use the higher number.)

Mark **Yes** or **No** for each of the following. ("He" refers to your husband, partner, ex-husband, ex-partner, or whoever is currently physically hurting you.)

_____ 1. Has the physical violence increased in severity or frequency over the past year?
_____ 2. Does he own a gun?
_____ 3. Have you left him after living together during the past year?

3a. (If you have *never* lived with him, check here:)

_____ 4. Is he unemployed?
_____ 5. Has he ever used a weapon against you or threatened you with a lethal weapon? (If yes, was the weapon a gun? check here:)
_____ 6. Does he threaten to kill you?
_____ 7. Has he avoided being arrested for domestic violence?
_____ 8. Do you have a child that is not his?
_____ 9. Has he ever forced you to have sex when you did not wish to do so?
_____ 10. Does he ever try to choke/strangle you or cut off your breathing?

10a. (If yes, has he done it more than once, or did it make you pass out or black out or make you dizzy? check here: __)

_____ 11. Does he use illegal drugs? By drugs, I mean "uppers" or amphetamines, "meth", speed, angel dust, cocaine, "crack", street drugs or mixtures.
_____ 12. Is he an alcoholic or problem drinker?
_____ 13. Does he control most or all of your daily activities? For instance, does he tell you who you can be friends with, when you can see your family, how much money you can use, or when you can take the car? (If he tries, but you do not let him, check here: __)
_____ 14. Is he violently and constantly jealous of you? (For instance, does he say: "If I can't have you, no one can.")
_____ 15. Have you ever been beaten by him while you were pregnant? (If you have never been pregnant by him, check here: __)
_____ 16. Has he ever threatened or tried to commit suicide?
_____ 17. Does he threaten to harm your children?
_____ 18. Do you believe he is capable of killing you?
_____ 19. Does he follow or spy on you, leave threatening notes or messages, destroy your property, or call you when you don't want him to?
_____ 20. Have you ever threatened or tried to commit suicide?
_____ Total "Yes" Answers

Thank you. Please talk to your nurse, advocate, or counsellor about what the Danger Assessment means in your situation.

Appendix 4—Attitudes Towards Women Scale (Spence et al., 1978)—Short version

Instructions The statements listed below describe attitudes towards the roles of women in society which different people have. There are no right or wrong answers, only opinions. You are asked to express your feeling about each statement by indicating whether you (A) agree strongly, (B) agree mildly, (C) disagree mildly, or (D) disagree strongly.

1. Swearing and obscenity are more repulsive in the speech of a woman than of a man.

A	B	C	D
Agree strongly	Agree mildly	Disagree mildly	Disagree strongly

2* Women should take increasing responsibility for leadership in solving the intellectual and social problems of the day.

A	B	C	D
Agree strongly	Agree mildly	Disagree mildly	Disagree strongly

3.* Both husband and wife should be allowed the same grounds for divorce.

A	B	C	D
Agree strongly	Agree mildly	Disagree mildly	Disagree strongly

4. Telling dirty jokes should be mostly a masculine prerogative.

A	B	C	D
Agree strongly	Agree mildly	Disagree mildly	Disagree strongly

5. Intoxication among women is worse than intoxication among men.

A	B	C	D
Agree strongly	Agree mildly	Disagree mildly	Disagree strongly

6.* Under modern economic conditions with women being active outside the home, men should share in household tasks such as washing dishes and doing the laundry.

A	B	C	D
Agree strongly	Agree mildly	Disagree mildly	Disagree strongly

7.* It is insulting to women to have the "obey" clause remain in the marriage service.

A	B	C	D
Agree strongly	Agree mildly	Disagree mildly	Disagree strongly

8.* There should be a strict merit system in job appointment and promotion without regard to sex.

A	B	C	D
Agree strongly	Agree mildly	Disagree mildly	Disagree strongly

9.* A woman should be free as a man to propose marriage.

A	B	C	D
Agree strongly	Agree mildly	Disagree mildly	Disagree strongly

10. Women should worry less about their rights and more about becoming good wives and mothers.

A	B	C	D
Agree strongly	Agree mildly	Disagree mildly	Disagree strongly

11.* Women earning as much as their dates should bear equally the expense when they go out together.

A	B	C	D
Agree strongly	Agree mildly	Disagree mildly	Disagree strongly

12.* Women should assume their rightful place in business and all the professions along with men.

A	B	C	D
Agree strongly	Agree mildly	Disagree mildly	Disagree strongly

13. A woman should not expect to go to exactly the same places or to have quite the same freedom of action as a man.

A	B	C	D
Agree strongly	Agree mildly	Disagree mildly	Disagree strongly

14. Sons in a family should be given more encouragement to go to college than daughters.

A	B	C	D
Agree strongly	Agree mildly	Disagree mildly	Disagree strongly

15. It is ridiculous for a woman to run a locomotive and for a man to darn socks.

A	B	C	D
Agree strongly	Agree mildly	Disagree mildly	Disagree strongly

16. In general, the father should have greater authority than the mother in the bringing up of children.

A	B	C	D
Agree strongly	Agree mildly	Disagree mildly	Disagree strongly

17. Women should be encouraged not to become sexually intimate with anyone before marriage, even their fiancés.

A	B	C	D
Agree strongly	Agree mildly	Disagree mildly	Disagree strongly

18.* The husband should not be favored by law over the wife in the disposal of family property or income.

A	B	C	D
Agree strongly	Agree mildly	Disagree mildly	Disagree strongly

19. Women should be concerned with their duties of childbearing and house tending rather than with desires for professional or business careers.

A	B	C	D
Agree strongly	Agree mildly	Disagree mildly	Disagree strongly

20. The intellectual leadership of a community should be largely in the hands of men.

A	B	C	D
Agree strongly	Agree mildly	Disagree mildly	Disagree strongly

21.* Economic and social freedom is worth far more to women than acceptance of the ideal of femininity which has been set up by men.

A	B	C	D
Agree strongly	Agree mildly	Disagree mildly	Disagree strongly

22. On average, women should be regarded as less capable of contributing to economic production than men.

A	B	C	D
Agree strongly	Agree mildly	Disagree mildly	Disagree strongly

23. There are many jobs in which men should be given preference over women in being hired or promoted.

A	B	C	D
Agree strongly	Agree mildly	Disagree mildly	Disagree strongly

24.* Women should be given equal opportunity with men for apprenticeship in the various trades.

A	B	C	D
Agree strongly	Agree mildly	Disagree mildly	Disagree strongly

25.* The modern girl is entitled to the same freedom from regulation and control that is given to the modern boy.

A	B	C	D
Agree strongly	Agree mildly	Disagree mildly	Disagree strongly

In scoring the items, A=0, B=1, C=2, and D=3 except for the items with an asterisk where the scale is reversed. A high score indicates a profeminist, egalitarian attitude while a low score indicates a traditional, conservative attitude.

References

Spence, J. T., Helmreich, R., & Stapp, J. (1973). A short version of the Attitudes toward Women Scale (AWS). *Bulletin of the Psychonomic Society*, 2, 219-220. https://doi.org/10.3758/BF03329252

Spence, J. T. & Helmreich, R. L. (1978). *Masculinity and femininity: Their psychological dimensions, correlates, and antecedents*. University of Texas Press.

Appendix 5—PTSD Checklist—Civilian Version (PCL-C)

Below is a list of problems and complaints that people sometimes have in response to stressful life experiences. Please read each one carefully, and pick the answer that indicates how much you have been bothered by that problem *in the last month.*

No.	Response	Not at all (1)	A little bit (2)	Moderately (3)	Quite a bit (4)	Extremely (5)
1.	Repeated, disturbing *memories, thoughts, or images* of a stressful experience from the past?					
2.	Repeated, disturbing *dreams* of a stressful experience from the past?					
3.	Suddenly *acting* or *feeling* as if a stressful experience *were happening* again (as if you were reliving it)?					
4.	Feeling *very upset* when *something reminded* you of a stressful experience from the past?					
5.	Having *physical reactions* (e.g., heart pounding, trouble breathing, or sweating) when *something reminded* you of a stressful experience from the past?					
6.	Avoid *thinking about* or *talking about* a stressful experience from the past or avoid *having feelings* related to it					
7.	Avoid *activities* or *situations* because they *remind you* of a stressful experience from the past					
8.	Trouble *remembering important parts* of a stressful experience from the past?					
9.	Loss of *interest in things that you used to enjoy*?					
10.	Feeling *distant* or *cut* off from other people?					
11.	Feeling *emotionally numb* or being unable to have loving feelings for those close to you?					
12.	Feeling as if your *future* will somehow be *cut short*?					
13.	Trouble *falling* or *staying asleep*?					
14.	Feeling *irritable* or having *angry outbursts*?					

(continued)

(continued)

No.	Response	Not at all (1)	A little bit (2)	Moderately (3)	Quite a bit (4)	Extremely (5)
15.	Having *difficulty concentrating*?					
16.	Being "*super alert*" or watchful on guard?					
17.	Feeling *jumpy* or easily startled?					

PCL-M for DSM –IV (11/1/94) Weathers, Litz, Huska, & Keane National Center for PTSD-Behavioral Science Div.

How is the PCL Scored?

1) Add up all items from each of the 17 items for a total severity score (range = 17–85)

17–29 This cutoff shows little to no severity.
28–29 Some PTSD symptoms—If you are seeing or will be seeing a therapist, print the results of this Quiz and take them to your therapist for further evaluation.
30–44 Moderate to Moderately High severity of PTSD symptoms—If you are seeing or will be seeing a therapist, print the results of this Quiz and take to your therapist for further evaluation.
45–85 High Severity of PTSD symptoms—If you are seeing or will be seeing a therapist, print the results of this Quiz and take to your therapist for further evaluation.

Appendix 6—Taylor Manifest Anxiety Scale

Circle the items that are true of you.

1. I do not tire quickly.
2. I am troubled by attacks of nausea.
3. I believe I am no more nervous than most others.
4. I have very few headaches.
5. I work under a great deal of tension.
6. I cannot keep my mind on one thing.
7. I worry about money and business.
8. I frequently notice my hand shakes when I try to do something.
9. I blush no more often than others.
10. I have diarrhoea once a month or more.
11. I worry quite a bit over possible misfortune.
12. I practically never blush.
13. I am often afraid that I am going to blush.
14. I have nightmares every few nights.

15. My hands and feet are usually warm.
16. I sweat very easily even on cool days.
17. Sometimes when embarrassed, I break out in a sweat.
18. I hardly ever notice my heart pounding and I am seldom short of breath.
19. I feel hungry almost all the time.
20. I am very seldom troubled by constipation.
21. I have a great deal of stomach trouble.
22. I have had periods in which I lost sleep over worry.
23. My sleep is fitful and disturbed.
24. I dream frequently about things that are best kept to myself.
25. I am easily embarrassed.
26. I am more sensitive than most other people.
27. I frequently find myself worrying about something.
28. I wish I could be as happy as others seem to be.
29. I am usually calm and not easily upset.
30. I cry easily.
31. I feel anxiety about something or someone almost all the time.
32. I am happy most of the time.
33. It makes me nervous to have to wait.
34. I have periods of such great restlessness that I cannot sit long in a chair.
35. Sometimes I become so excited that I find it hard to get to sleep.
36. I have sometimes felt that difficulties were piling up so high that I could not overcome them.
37. I must admit that I have at times been worried beyond reason over something that did not matter.
38. I have very few fears compared to my friends.
39. I have been afraid of things or people that I know could not hurt me.
40. I certainly feel useless at times.
41. I find it hard to keep my mind on a task or job.
42. I am usually self-conscious.
43. I am inclined to take things hard.
44. I am a high-strung person.
45. Life is a trial for me much of the time.
46. At times I think I am no good at all.
47. I am certainly lacking in self-confidence.
48. I sometimes feel that I am about to go to pieces.
49. I shrink from facing a crisis of difficulty.
50. I am entirely self-confident.

Source: Spence, J. T. (1953). Taylor Manifest Anxiety Scale is A personality scale of manifest anxiety. *Journal of Abnormal and Social Psychology.* Copyright © 1953.

Appendix 7—Patient Health Questionnaire-9

Over the <u>last 2 weeks</u>, how often have you been bothered by any of the following problems? *(Use "✔" to indicate your answer)*	Not at all	Several days	More than half the days	Nearly every day
1. Little interest or pleasure in doing things	0	1	2	3
2. Feeling down, depressed, or hopeless	0	1	2	3
3. Trouble falling or staying asleep, or sleeping too much	0	1	2	3
4. Feeling tired or having little energy	0	1	2	3
5. Poor appetite or overeating	0	1	2	3
6. Feeling bad about yourself — or that you are a failure or	0	1	2	3
7. Trouble concentrating on things, such as reading the	0	1	2	3
8. Moving or speaking so slowly that other people could have noticed? Or the opposite — being so fidgety or restless that you have been moving around a lot more than usual	0	1	2	3
9. Thoughts that you would be better off dead or hurting yourself in some way	0	1	2	3

For Office Coding: 0 + + + = Total Score:

If you checked off <u>any</u> problems, how <u>difficult</u> have these problems made it for you to do your work, take care of things at home, or get along with other people?

Not difficult at all	Somewhat difficult	Very difficult	Extremely difficult
D	**D**	**D**	**D**

Appendix 8 (Interview Protocol)—Qualitative Phase

I will be carrying out structured in-depth interviews (19 open-ended questions and probes, as needed). Open-ended questions and topics will be used to obtain in-depth information about the proposed topic.

1. Opening: I will extend a warm welcome and express gratitude to the interviewee for dedicating their time and participating in the study. This is aimed at fostering an environment conducive to open and uninhibited idea exchange. I will ensure the participants are relaxed and comfortable.
2. I will remind the interviewee about the objective and length of the interview.
3. I will prepare the participants for the topics which will be addressed during the interview.
4. I will brief the interviewee with her rights in general.

5. I will ask the interviewee if she has any questions or concerns which need to be addressed during the interview process. I will remind the interviewee that she can ask questions or request breaks during the interview process.
6. I will ask if there are any questions regarding what I have just explained.
7. I will inquire whether they are inclined to engage in the interview.
8. Singe consent form.
9. Closing Remarks.

I'd like to express my appreciation for your time in meeting with me today. My name is Khalid AL-Naama and I would like to talk to you about your domestic abuse experiences. We greatly value your participation, which will make a valuable contribution to our study on the impact of domestic abuse on the mental health of Qatari women. The insights gained will be instrumental in shaping future interventions. The interview should take less than an hour. I'd like to request your permission to record our meeting as it's essential for ensuring that no perspective in your comments is overlooked, and I want to preserve the session accurately. Throughout our interview, I plan to make important notes, yet I understand they may not encompass your entire perspective. To ensure a comprehensive understanding, I believe it's crucial to record our conversation and thoroughly review it. Therefore, may I request your consent for audio recording? Because we're on tape, please be sure to speak up so that we don't miss your comments.

All responses will be kept confidential. This means that your interview responses will only be shared with the supervisor of the study. I will ensure that any information we include in our report does not identify you as the respondent. Keep in mind that you are not obligated to discuss any topic you are uncomfortable with, and you have the freedom to conclude the interview whenever you choose.

1. Are there any questions about what I have just explained?
2. Would you be open to taking part in this interview

Name of participant: ______________________________
Signature: ______________________________
Date: ______________________________

Appendix 9—Consent Proforma

Consent for the participant (adult) to be recorded + recordings archived and used for future research and teaching.
CONSENT TO BE AUDIO-RECORDED, AND FOR STORAGE AND FUTURE USE OF DATA

Please initial box
I agree to be audiotaped for this study. ☐
Initial ***one box only*** *to show how long you want recordings to be kept for*

EITHER

2a) For as long as the Library exists, for future research. I know that future researchers will sign a CAVA Repository End User License Agreement to respect my confidentiality, rights and dignity, and use my data in a responsible way. ☐

OR

2b) until the project team has finished their work in [date]. Then they will be destroyed ☐
3. I know that when the project team labels my recordings, writes articles and talks about the project they will use a false name, not my real name. ☐
4. I agree that my data can be used for presenting research findings (e.g., at conferences); for further analysis in research to be conducted in the future [and/or for teaching purposes]. ☐
5. I know that the information collected about me may be audited by the research sponsor, [name], to ensure the research is being conducted appropriately. ☐

Name of participant: ______________________________
Signature: ______________________________
Date: ______________________________

Appendix 10—Interview Questions

No	In-depth Interview questions	Probes
1	What is your understanding of domestic abuse?	-Could you provide me with an example? Can you elaborate on that idea? Would you explain that further? Anything else you want to add? I'm not sure I understand what you're saying. I see you are exhausted do you want to have...? Give me an example that…
2	Is there anything you can tell me about the types of abuse you have suffered?	
3	Can you tell me some of the things that you remember about this experience? Please explain.	
4	Did you feel your life was in danger or that it might escalate to murder?	
5	Why do you think you have experienced this form of abuse? Please elaborate.	
6	Why do these factors make victims more likely to be victimized, and how do they contribute? Could you share your thoughts on…?	
7	Is there a possibility that women's mindset can affect their risk of IPV? Would you be able to elaborate on that?	
8	What impact has abuse had on your physical and mental health?	
9	What physical or emotional symptoms have you experienced since the violent incident?	

(continued)

(continued)

No	In-depth Interview questions	Probes
10	Are there any specific reasons why you have not acted to stop or leave the abuser?	
11	Are there any obstacles you have encountered when trying to end or break the cycle of abuse, if any?	
12	What is like to experience the process of leaving intimate partner violence?	
13	How did you think others experience domestic abuse?	
14	Can you talk me through what would happen if you were to stand up for yourself?	
15	To return to the previous question, can I ask you a little bit more about the role of your family and relatives?	
16	How did the abuser react to what you said?	
17	Do you mean that your decision changed when he said …….?	
18	Finally, are there any other reasons that could lead women to continue their relationship with their abuser?	
19	Is there anything more you would like to add?	
Closing Remarks	I'll be analysing the information you and others have given me. I'll be happy to send you a copy to review at that time, if you are interested. Thank you for your time.	

Appendix 11—Participant Information Sheet

University of
HUDDERSFIELD
Inspiring global professionals

Version 001
UNIVERSITY OF HUDDERSFIELD
PARTICIPANT INFORMATION SHEET

An examination of the impact of domestic abuse on Qatari women's mental health
Khalid Jamal AL-Naama

You are invited to take part in this study. Before you decide to take part, it is important that you understand why the research is being done, what it will involve and what will happen to the data you provide.

Please take the time to read the following information carefully and discuss it with us if you wish. Please do not hesitate to ask if there is anything that is not clear, or if you would like more information.

Thank you for reading this information. If you decide to take a part, you will be given a copy of this information sheet and your signed consent form.

WHAT IS THE STUDY ABOUT?

This study seeks to examine the impact of domestic abuse on Qatari women's mental health. The research and the interviews are designed to address the impact of domestic abuse on women's mental health and will study the potential of anxiety, depression and post-traumatic stress disorder among Qatari women facing domestic abuse. In addition to that, it will aid to understand factors associated with women's likelihood of experiencing intimate partner violence and women's inaction.

WHO IS THE TARGET AUDIENCE?

Adult Qatari women who have been exposed to or experienced domestic abuse from their life partner or family members.

WHAT WILL I NEED TO DO?

Should you decide to take part in the study, you will be asked to provide your consent by signing your name or ticking a box. Then, you will receive a survey questionnaire which will take 30 min to complete. You will also be asked whether you would like to participate in a follow-up interview conducted at a later date. This is entirely optional - you will be asked to provide your email address only if you would like to take part.

The face-to-face interview will last for no longer than 45 min, with as many breaks as you require. The interview will consist of open-ended questions regarding your experiences of domestic abuse. The exact questions cannot be predicted, and you have the right to decline to answer questions. The interview is recorded in order to accurately record the information that you provide. It will also be used for transcription purposes (optional). After the interview, you will receive a copy of the transcripts before their analysis in the event that you want to add or remove anything you have said from the final report.

The location and time of the interview will be arranged in one of the following places: Hamad Hospital, WEYAK the Media Centre for Youth meeting room. The location will be agreed upon prior to the interview between us. You are free to have a chaperone during the interview and there will be no other requirements involved.

DO I HAVE TO TAKE PART?

This study is completely voluntary. It is up to you to decide if you want to take part. I will describe the study and go through this information sheet, which I will then give to you. I will then ask you to sign a consent form to show that you have agreed to take part. The decision not to take part will not affect you in any way and will not affect your treatment or legal rights. You are free to withdraw from the research at any time without giving a reason and you have the right to decline to answer certain questions. The final date of data withdrawal is one month after the interview. A decision to withdraw will not affect you in any way.

WHO IS CONDUCTING THE RESEARCH?

The research is conducted for academic purposes by PhD student Khalid AL-Naama in the school of human and health science, at the University of Huddersfield. The project is self-funded by the researcher. You can contact the researcher through email: khalid.al-naama@hud.ac.uk. Should you have any questions, you can also contact Dr. John Synott the supervisor of the study j.p.synnott@hud.ac.uk.

WHO WILL HAVE ACCESS TO THE DATA?

The data will be collected from Qatar and restricted access to data is being granted throughout the research. The access will be granted only to the researcher and supervisors of the research.

WHAT WILL HAPPEN TO THE DATA COLLECTED?

Personal data shared by participants in an examination of the impact of domestic abuse on Qatari women's mental health.

Collected data will be held confidentially by the University of Huddersfield in accordance with the requirements of the General Data Protection Regulation (GDPR) and Data Protection Act 2018. The University is the Data Controller and is responsible for its security management. The research team and transcribers are the data processors. No information provided will be shared in a way that would allow the participants to be personally identified *except where legal obligations would necessitate disclosure by the researchers to appropriate personnel.*

Below are the following criteria which may affect your right to privacy:

1. Personal information will remain confidential unless the participant states that they or anyone else is at risk of serious harm, or unless they reveal a criminal offence for which they have not been convicted.
2. If any permitted access is granted to any organisation or individuals other than the researcher or examiners, the participants shall be informed prior to taking part in the study.

The data will be securely stored for 10 years, It will then be safely destroyed in line with UoH and GDPR guidelines. Quotes used in any resulting book/article/report or other publication will be anonymised or pseudonymised. The collected data will be presented in my dissertation by the end of the study.

Audio recording during the interview can help with the accuracy of the data and with transcriptions after the interview. The University's standard retention period is 10 years. However, this research considers audio recording as an optional part of the research. The data will be transferred to the United Kingdom.

The University of Huddersfield is the Data Controller. Complaints should be addressed to the University Solicitor (the Data Protection Officer) at enquiriesvco@hud.ac.uk

Appeals can be made to the Information Commissioner's Office if a participant is not satisfied with the response from the University.

Ethical Approval
The project has obtained ethical approval from the **Human and Health Science** School of Research Ethics Committee at the University of Huddersfield or another external organisation].

Appendix 12—Participant Consent Form

University of
HUDDERSFIELD
Inspiring global professionals

Version 001
UNIVERSITY OF HUDDERSFIELD
PARTICIPANT CONSENT FORM

An examination of the impact of domestic abuse on Qatari women's mental health
Khalid Jamal Al-Naama

Thank you for your interest in this project. Before agreeing to participate, please read the information sheet. If you have any questions, please ask a researcher. You will be given a copy of this consent form, and one will be retained by the researcher.

I understand that if I decide to no longer take part in this research I can leave and withdraw my data from the study within the time limits outlined in the Information Sheet (during or after one month of the interview/questionnaire), without giving a reason for my withdrawal or to decline to answer any particular questions in the study without any consequences to my future treatment by the

I understand that should I wish to withdraw my contribution I can contact the researcher through his email address—khalid.Al-Naama@hud.ac.uk and let him know that I no longer wish to participate in the research without giving a reason. A follow-up email will be received to confirm that my data has been marked for deletion.

I understand that my personal information will be processed only for the purposes of this research. I understand that such information will be treated as confidential, except where legal obligations require information to be shared with relevant personnel and handled in accordance with the provisions of the General Data Protection Regulation (GDPR) and the UK Data Protection Act 2018.

I understand that the information I share, including anonymised direct quotes, may be included in any resulting report or future publications.

[RECOMMENDED] I consent to the research team having access to any results derived from this study for any subsequent analyses or publications in the future. I understand that any identifying information would be kept confidential (except where legal obligations require information to be shared with relevant personnel), and access is limited strictly to the original study team and database team.

I understand that the information collected about me will be used to support other research in the future and may be shared anonymously with other researchers.

I understand that this research considers audio recording optional throughout the study and that it is only used for the purposes of data accuracy and transcription.

I understand that the information I provide will be retained for 10 YEARS UNLESS OTHERWISE REQUIRED and destroyed after this time in line with UoH and GDPR guidelines. Once the questioner completed and submitted, still you will be able to access and modify your answers within 48 h after the submission.

I agree that the project named above has been explained to me to my satisfaction and I agree to take part in this research. I have read and understood the institution's Privacy Statement https://www.hud.ac.uk/informationgovernance/dataprotection/ and consent to the researchers processing my data accordingly.

I have read the information sheet and understand the purpose of the research.

I agree that (please tick)

☐ Agree to Participate
☐ Disagree to Participate

PRINT NAME: ______________________________
SIGNATURE: ______________________________
DATE: ______________________________

References

Abdul Hak, N., Mansor, A. M., & Che Soh, R. (2019). Resolution of child custody dispute: Legislative foundation and contemporary application of Sulh in the Shariah court of Malaysia. *Journal of Islam in Asia, 53*(9), 1689–1699. https://journals.iium.edu.my/jiasia/index.php/jia/article/view/990/451

Abolfotouh, M. A., & Almuneef, M. (2020). Prevalence, pattern and factors of intimate partner violence against Saudi women. *Journal of Public Health (United Kingdom), 42*(3), E206–E214. https://doi.org/10.1093/pubmed/fdz092

Abraham, M. (2005). Domestic violence and the Indian diaspora in the United States. *Indian Journal of Gender Studies, 12*(3), 427–451. https://doi.org/10.1177/097152150501200212

Abramsky, T., Lees, S., Stöckl, H., Harvey, S., Kapinga, I., Ranganathan, M., Mshana, G., & Kapiga, S. (2019). Women's income and risk of intimate partner violence: Secondary findings from the MAISHA cluster randomised trial in North-Western Tanzania. *BMC Public Health, 19*(1), 1108. https://doi.org/10.1186/s12889-019-7454-1

Abramsky, T., Watts, C. H., Garcia-Moreno, C., Devries, K., Kiss, L., Ellsberg, M., Jansen, H. A. F. M., & Heise, L. (2011). What factors are associated with recent intimate partner violence? Findings from the WHO multi-country study on women's health and domestic violence. *BMC Public Health, 11*. https://doi.org/10.1186/1471-2458-11-109

Abu-Lughod, L. (2018). Do Muslim women really need saving? Anthropological reflections on cultural relativism and its others. *American Anthropologist, 104*(3), 783–790. https://doi.org/10.1525/AA.2002.104.3.783

Abu-Ras, W. (2007). Cultural beliefs and service utilization by battered Arab immigrant women. *Violence Against Women, 13*(10), 1002–1028. https://doi.org/10.1177/1077801207306019

Acevedo, B. P., Lowe, S. R., Griffin, K. W., & Botvin, G. J. (2013). Predictors of intimate partner violence in a sample of multiethnic urban young adults. *Journal of Interpersonal Violence, 28*(15), 3004–3022. https://doi.org/10.1177/0886260513488684

Adams, A. E., Sullivan, C. M., Bybee, D., & Greeson, M. R. (2008). Development of the scale of economic abuse. *Violence Against Women, 14*(5), 563–588. https://doi.org/10.1177/1077801208315529

Adelman, M. (2000). No way out: Divorce-related domestic violence in Israel. *Violence Against Woman, 6*(11), 1223–1254. https://doi.org/10.1177/10778010022183613

Adjei, S. B. (2017). Sociocultural groundings of battered women's entrapment in abusive marital relationship in Ghana. *Journal of Aggression, Maltreatment and Trauma, 26*(8), 879–901. https://doi.org/10.1080/10926771.2017.1284171

Aduloju, P. O., Olagbuji, N. B., Olofinbiyi, A. B., & Awoleke, J. O. (2015). Prevalence and predictors of intimate partner violence among women attending infertility clinic in south-western Nigeria.

K. Al-Naama, *Domestic Abuse and Mental Health in Qatar*, Gulf Studies 23,
https://doi.org/10.1007/978-981-96-7392-6

European Journal of Obstetrics and Gynecology and Reproductive Biology, 188(February 2018), 66–69. https://doi.org/10.1016/j.ejogrb.2015.02.027

Afifi, Z. E., Al-Muhaideb, N. S., Hadish, N. F., Ismail, F. I., & Al-Qeamy, F. M. (2011). Domestic violence and its impact on married women's health in Eastern Saudi Arabia. *Saudi Medical Journal, 32*(6), 612–620. http://www.emro.who.int/imemrf/Saudi_Med_J/Saudi_Med_J_2011_32_6_612_620.pdf

Ahinkorah, B. O. (2021). Polygyny and intimate partner violence in sub-Saharan Africa: Evidence from 16 cross-sectional demographic and health surveys. *SSM - Population Health, 13*(December 2020), 100729. https://doi.org/10.1016/j.ssmph.2021.100729

Ahmadzad-Asl, M., Davoudi, F., Zarei, N., Mohammad-Sadeghi, H., & Rasoulian, M. (2016). Domestic violence against women as a risk factor for depressive and anxiety disorders: Findings from domestic violence household survey in Tehran, Iran. *Archives of Women's Mental Health, 19*(5), 861–869. https://doi.org/10.1007/s00737-016-0626-4

Ahmed, A. M., & Elmardi, A. E. (2005). A study of domestic violence among women attending a medical centre in Sudan. *Eastern Mediterranean Health Journal, 11*(1–2), 164–174. https://pubmed.ncbi.nlm.nih.gov/16532685/

Aizpurua, E., Copp, J., Ricarte, J. J., & Vázquez, D. (2017). Controlling behaviors and intimate partner violence among women in Spain: An examination of individual, partner, and relationship risk factors for physical and psychological abuse. *Journal of Interpersonal Violence, 36*(1–2), 231–254. https://doi.org/10.1177/0886260517723744

Akpinar, F., Yilmaz, S., Karahanoglu, E., Ozelci, R., Coskun, B., Dilbaz, B., & Tekin, Ö. M. (2019). Intimate partner violence in Turkey among women with female infertility. *Sexual and Relationship Therapy, 34*(1), 3–9. https://doi.org/10.1080/14681994.2017.1327711

Al Ghayathin, B. (2017). *Violence against women in Qatar: An exploratory study* [Master's thesis, Hamad Bin Khalifa University]. https://search.proquest.com/dissertations-theses/violence-against-women-qatar-exploratory-study/docview/1907499277/se-2?accountid=10673%0Ahttps://ed-primo.hosted.exlibrisgroup.com/openurl/44UOE/44UOE_VU2??url_ver=Z39.88-2004&rft_val_fmt=info:ofi/fmt:kev:m

Al Meezan. (2022a). Articles 61–73. Law No. 22 of 2006 Promulgating 'The Family Law'. Date:29/06/2006, Official Gazette: Issue:8. Starting Date: 28/08/2006. https://www.almeezan.qa/LawArticles.aspx?LawTreeSectionID=8748&lawId=2558&language=en

Al Meezan. (2022d). *Article 170. Law No. 22 of 2006 Promulgating 'The Family Law'*. Date:29/06/2006, Official Gazette: Issue:8. Starting Date: 28/08/2006. https://www.almeezan.qa/LawArticles.aspx?LawArticleID=36311&LawID=2558&language=en

Al Meezan. (2022e). *Article 181. Law No. 22 of 2006 Promulgating 'The Family Law'*. Date:29/06/2006, Official Gazette: Issue:8. Starting Date: 28/08/2006. https://www.almeezan.qa/LawArticles.aspx?LawArticleID=36322&LawId=2558&language=en

Al Shidhani, N. A., Al Kendi, A. A., & Al Kiyumi, M. H. (2020). Prevalence, risk factors and effects of domestic violence before and during pregnancy on birth outcomes: An observational study of literate Omani women. *International Journal of Women's Health, 12*, 911–925. https://doi.org/10.2147/IJWH.S272419

Alaggia, R., Regehr, C., & Jenney, A. (2012). Risky business: An ecological analysis of intimate partner violence disclosure. *Research on Social Work Practice, 22*(3), 301–312. https://doi.org/10.1177/1049731511425503

Alam, M., & Islam, M. (2015). Factors affecting domestic violence against women in Bangladesh. *European Journal of Public Health, 25*(suppl_3). https://doi.org/10.1093/eurpub/ckv175.013

Al-Attiyah, A., & Nasser, R. (2016). Gender and age differences in life satisfaction within a sex-segregated society: Sampling youth in Qatar. *International Journal of Adolescence and Youth, 21*(1), 84–95. https://doi.org/10.1080/02673843.2013.808158

Albrithen, A. A. (2006). *Alcoholism and domestic violence in Saudi society* [Doctoral dissertation, The University of Liverpool]. https://www.cawtarclearinghouse.org/storage/AttachementGender/Alcholisme%20and%20domestic%20violence%20in%20saudi%20socity.pdf

Alejo, K. (2014). Long-term physical and mental health effects of domestic violence. *Themis: Research Journal of Justice Studies and Forensic Science, 2*(1), 5. https://doi.org/10.31979/THEMIS.2014.0205

Al-Ekri, E., Al-Ubaidi, B. A., Husain, H., Bubshait, M., Al-Jamea, L., Al Ubaidi, B. A., Al-Dhubaib, D., Najem, W., & Husain, H. (1994). Prevalence of domestic violence & associated risk factors among adult females attending primary care in the Kingdom of Bahrain. *International Medical Journal, 28*(3), 4413–4425. https://www.researchgate.net/profile/Basem-Al-Ubaidi/publication/350515978_Prevalence_of_Domestic_Violence_Associated_Risk_Factors_among_Adult_Females_attending_Primary_Care_in_the_Kingdom_of_Bahrain/links/60646429a6fdcca78be013e2/Prevalence-of-Domestic-Violence-Associated-Risk-Factors-among-Adult-Females-attending-Primary-Care-in-the-Kingdom-of-Bahrain.pdf

Al-Ghafri, G., Al-Sinawi, H., Al-Muniri, A., Dorvlo, A. S. S., Al-Farsi, Y. M., Armstrong, K., & Al-Adawi, S. (2014). Prevalence of depressive symptoms as elicited by patient health questionnaire (PHQ-9) among medical trainees in Oman. *Asian Journal of Psychiatry, 8*(1), 59–62. https://doi.org/10.1016/j.ajp.2013.10.014

Al-Ghanim, K. (2019). Perceptions of women's roles between traditionalism and modernity in Qatar. *Journal of Arabian Studies, 9*(1), 52–74. https://doi.org/10.1080/21534764.2019.1646502

Al-Ghanim, K. A. (2009). Violence against women in Qatari society. *Journal of Middle East Women's Studies, 5*(1), 80–93. https://doi.org/10.2979/mew.2009.5.1.80

Al-Ghanim, K. A., & Badahdah, A. M. (2017). Gender roles in the Arab world: Development and psychometric properties of the Arab adolescents' gender roles attitude scale. *Sex Roles, 77*(3–4), 169–177. https://doi.org/10.1007/s11199-016-0722-y

Al-Haj, M. (1987). *Social change and family processes.* Westview Press.

Alhojailan, M. I. (2012). Thematic analysis: A critical review of its process and evaluation. *West East Journal of Social Sciences, 1*(1), 39–47. https://faculty.ksu.edu.sa/sites/default/files/ta_thematic_analysis_dr_mohammed_alhojailan.pdf

Ali, A. A., Yassin, K., & Omer, R. (2014). Domestic violence against women in Eastern Sudan. *BMC Public Health, 14*, 1136. https://doi.org/10.1186/1471-2458-14-1136

Alibeli, M. A. (2015). Gender and attitudes toward women in the United Arab Emirates. *Perspectives on Global Development and Technology, 14*(1–2), 109–125. https://doi.org/10.1163/15691497-12341335

Alio, A. P., Nana, P. N., & Salihu, H. M. (2009). Spousal violence and potentially preventable single and recurrent spontaneous fetal loss in an African setting: Cross-sectional study. *The Lancet, 373*(9660), 318–324. https://doi.org/10.1016/S0140-6736(09)60096-9

Al-Krenawi, A., & Graham, J. R. (2000). Culturally sensitive social work practice with Arab clients in mental health settings. *Health & Social Work, 25*(1), 9–22. https://doi.org/10.1093/hsw/25.1.9

Al-Krenawi, A., & Graham, J. R. (2006). A comparison of family functioning, life and marital satisfaction, and mental health of women in polygamous and monogamous marriages. *International Journal of Social Psychiatry, 52*(1), 5–17. https://doi.org/10.1177/0020764006061245

Al-Misnad, S. A. (1984). *The development of modern education in Bahrain, Kuwait and Qatar with special reference to the education of women and their position in modern Gulf society* [Doctoral dissertation, Durham University]. Durham e-Theses. http://etheses.dur.ac.uk/10485/.

Almosaed, N. (2015). Why stay? Saudi Women's adaption's to violence. *International Journal of Humanities and Social Science, 5*(10(1)), 146–162. https://cawtarclearinghouse.org/storage/AttachementGender/Why%20Stay-%20Saudi%20Women%E2%80%99s%20Adaption%E2%80%99s%20to%20Violence.pdf

Almubaddel, A. (2022). Psychometric properties of a Saudi Arabian version of the Positive Mental Health (PMH) scale. *Psicologia: Reflexao e Critica, 35*(1), 29. https://doi.org/10.1186/s41155-022-00232-0

Alquaiz, A. M., Almuneef, M., Kazi, A., & Almeneessier, A. (2021). Social determinants of domestic violence among Saudi married women in Riyadh, Kingdom of Saudi Arabia. *Journal of Interpersonal Violence, 36*(3–4), NP1561–NP1585. https://doi.org/10.1177/0886260517746128

Alsaleh, A. (2022). Violence against Kuwaiti women. *Journal of Interpersonal Violence, 37*(5–6), NP3628–NP3649. https://doi.org/10.1177/0886260520916280

Alsawalqa, R. O. (2020). Economic abuse of women in Amman, Jordan: A quantitative study. *SAGE Open, 10*(4), 1–13. https://doi.org/10.1177/2158244020982616

Alshawi, A. H., & Gardner, A. (2013). Tribalism, identity and citizenship in contemporary Qatar. *Anthropology of the Middle East, 8*(2), 46–59. https://doi.org/10.3167/ame.2013.080204

Anderson, D. K., & Saunders, D. G. (2003). Leaving an abusive partner: An empirical review of predictors, the process of leaving, and psychological Well-being. *Trauma, Violence & Abuse, 4*(2), 163–191. https://doi.org/10.1177/1524838002250769

Anderson, K. L. (2010). Conflict, power, and violence in families. *Journal of Marriage and Family, 72*(3), 726–742. https://doi.org/10.1111/j.1741-3737.2010.00727.x

Anderson, K. L. (2018). Gender, status, and domestic violence: An integration of feminist and family violence approaches. *Domestic Violence, 59*(3), 263–277. https://doi.org/10.4324/9781315264905-20

Anser, L. (2013). Divorce in the Arab gulf countries: A major challenge to family and society. In A. Abela & J. Walker (Eds.), *Contemporary issues in family studies: Global perspectives on partnerships, parenting and support in a changing world* (pp. 59–73). Wiley-Blackwell. https://doi.org/10.1002/9781118320990.ch5

Asli, M. R., & Byouki, M. A. (2016). Forced marriage in Islamic countries: The role of violence in family relationships. In H. Kury, S. Redo, & E. Shea (Eds.), *Women and children as victims and offenders: Background, prevention, reintegration* (pp. 729–753). Springer. https://doi.org/10.1007/978-3-319-08398-8_26

Atiyat, R. B. A. R. (2015). *No redress? Investigating wife abuse through the lens of Feminist Theory and Resource Theory in Jordan* [Doctoral dissertation, University of York]. White Rose eTheses Online. https://etheses.whiterose.ac.uk/10524/

Atkinson, M. P., Greenstein, T. N., & Lang, M. M. (2005). For women, breadwinning can be dangerous: Gendered resource theory and wife abuse. *Journal of Marriage and Family, 67*(5), 1137–1148. https://doi.org/10.1111/j.1741-3737.2005.00206.x

Bacchus, L. J., Ranganathan, M., Watts, C., & Devries, K. (2018). Recent intimate partner violence against women and health: A systematic review and meta-analysis of cohort studies. *BMJ Open, 8*(7), e019995. https://doi.org/10.1136/bmjopen-2017-019995

Bandura, A. (2019). Social learning: Theory. In K. N. Laland & L. Rendell (Eds.), *Encyclopedia of animal behavior* (pp. 380–386). Academic. https://doi.org/10.1016/B978-0-12-813251-7.00057-2

Barakat, H. (1993). *The Arab world: Society, culture and state*. University of California Press.

Bargai, N., Ben-Shakhar, G., & Shalev, A. Y. (2007). Posttraumatic stress disorder and depression in battered women: The mediating role of learned helplessness. *Journal of Family Violence, 22*(5), 267–275. https://doi.org/10.1007/s10896-007-9078-y

Barnawi, F. H. (2017). Prevalence and risk factors of domestic violence against women attending A primary care center in Riyadh, Saudi Arabia. *Journal of Interpersonal Violence, 32*(8), 1171–1186. https://doi.org/10.1177/0886260515587669

Bartolomei, M. R. (2015). Domestic violence and human rights. An anthropological view. *Ex Aequo - Revista Da Associação Portuguesa de Estudos Sobre as Mulheres*, (31), 91–104. https://doi.org/10.22355/exaequo.2015.31.07

Basar, F., Demirci, N., Cicek, S., & Saglam, H. Y. (2019). Attitudes toward violence against women and the factors that affect them in Kutahya, Turkey. *African Journal of Reproductive Health, 23*(1), 16–26. https://doi.org/10.29063/AJRH2019/V23I1.2

Basile, K. C., Jones, K., Smith, S. G., & RAINN Staff. (2021, February 15). *Effects of domestic violence on children*. The Office on Women's Health, National Center for Injury Prevention and Control, Centers for Disease Control and Prevention (CDC). https://www.womenshealth.gov/relationships-and-safety/domestic-violence/effects-domestic-violence-children

Bates, L. M., Schuler, S. R., Islam, F., & Islam, K. (2004). Socioeconomic factors and processes associated with domestic violence in rural Bangladesh. *International Family Planning Perspectives, 30*(4), 190–199. https://doi.org/10.1363/3019004

Bekhet, A. K., & Zauszniewski, J. A. (2012). Methodological triangulation: An approach to understanding data. *Nurse Researcher, 20*(2), 40–43. https://doi.org/10.7748/nr2012.11.20.2.40.c9442

Belfrage, H., & Rying, M. (2004). Characteristics of spousal homicide perpetrators: A study of all cases of spousal homicide in Sweden 1990–1999. *Criminal Behaviour and Mental Health, 14*(2), 121–133. https://doi.org/10.1002/cbm.577

Bell, K. M., & Naugle, A. E. (2008). Intimate partner violence theoretical considerations: Moving towards a contextual framework. *Clinical Psychology Review, 28*(7), 1096–1107. https://doi.org/10.1016/j.cpr.2008.03.003

Bellali, N., Laboudi, F., & Ouanass, A. (2019). Domestic violence and psychopathological impact. *Austin Journal of Psychiatry and Behavioral Sciences, 6*(1), 1070. https://austinpublishinggroup.com/psychiatry-behavioral-sciences/fulltext/ajpbs-v6-id1070.php

Ben-Porat, A., Levy, D., Kattoura, O., Dekel, R., & Itzhaky, H. (2021). Domestic violence in Arab society: A comparison of Arab and Jewish women in shelters in Israel. *Journal of Interpersonal Violence, 36*(1–2), NP26–NP45. https://doi.org/10.1177/0886260517731789

Berrios, D. C., & Grady, D. (1991). Domestic violence: Risk factors and outcomes. *Western Journal of Medicine, 155*(2), 133–135. https://pubmed.ncbi.nlm.nih.gov/1926841/

Bhandari, P. (2020). Pre-marital relationships and violence: Experiences of working middle class women in Delhi. *Gender, Place and Culture, 27*(1), 13–33. https://doi.org/10.1080/0966369X.2019.1618795

Bhona, F. M. C., Gebara, C. F. P., Noto, A. R., Vieira, M. D. T., & Lourenço, L. M. (2019). Socioeconomic factors and intimate partner violence: A household survey. *Trends in Psychology, 27*(1), 205–218. https://doi.org/10.9788/TP2019.1-15

Bird, K. (2007). *The intergenerational transmission of poverty: An overview* (CPRC Working Paper No. 99). SSRN Electronic Journal. https://doi.org/10.2139/ssrn.1629262.

Bohn, D. K., Tebben, J. G., & Campbell, J. C. (2004). Influences of income, education, age, and ethnicity on physical abuse before and during pregnancy. *Journal of Obstetric, Gynecologic & Neonatal Nursing, 33*(5), 561–571. https://doi.org/10.1177/0884217504269009

Bottoms, B. L., Peter-Hagene, L. C., Epstein, M. A., Wiley, T. R. A., Reynolds, C. E., & Rudnicki, A. G. (2016). Abuse characteristics and individual differences related to disclosing childhood sexual, physical, and emotional abuse and witnessed domestic violence. *Journal of Interpersonal Violence, 31*(7), 1308–1339. https://doi.org/10.1177/0886260514564155

Bowen, P. W., Rose, R., & Pilkington, A. (2017). Mixed methods - Theory and practice. Sequential, explanatory approach. *International Journal of Quantitative and Qualitative Research Methods, 5*(2), 10–27. http://www.eajournals.org/wp-content/uploads/Mixed-Methods-Theory-and-Practice.-Sequential-Explanatory-Approach.pdf

Bowlus, A., & Seitz, S. (2000). The economics of abuse. *International Economic Review*, 1–36. http://qed.econ.queensu.ca/pub/faculty/seitz/abuse.pdf

Boy, A., & Kulczycki, A. (2008). What we know about intimate partner violence in the Middle East and North Africa. *Violence Against Women, 14*(1), 53–70. https://doi.org/10.1177/1077801207311860

Braaf, R., & Meyering, I. B. (2013, June 4). *Domestic violence and mental health.* Australian Domestic and Family Violence Clearing House. https://www.nifvs.org.au/wp-content/uploads/2015/01/Domestic-Violence-and-Mental-Health.pdf

Bracewell, K., Jones, C., Haines-Delmont, A., Craig, E., Duxbury, J., & Chantler, K. (2021). Beyond intimate partner relationships: Utilising domestic homicide reviews to prevent adult family domestic homicide. *Journal of Gender-Based Violence, 6*(3), 535–550. https://doi.org/10.1332/239868021x16316184865237

Bramlett, M. D., & Mosher, W. D. (2002). Cohabitation, marriage, divorce, and remarriage in the United States. *Vital and Health Statistics, 23*(22), 1–93. https://pubmed.ncbi.nlm.nih.gov/12183886/

Branigan, E., & Grace, M. (2005). *His money or our money: Financial abuse of women in intimate partner relationships.* 1–22. https://scholar.google.co.uk/scholar?q=his+money+or+our+money+financial+abuse+of+women+in+intimate+partner+relationships&btnG=&hl=en&as_sdt=0%2C5#0%5Cnhttp://csmc.org.au/wp-content/uploads/2014/05/Financial_Abuse.pdf

Braun, V., & Clarke, V. (2006). Using thematic analysis in psychology. *Qualitative Research in Psychology, 3*(2), 77–101. https://doi.org/10.1191/1478088706qp063oa

Breiding, M. J., Basile, K. C., Smith, S. G., Black, M. C., & Mahendra, R. R. (2015). *Intimate partner violence surveillance: Uniform definitions and recommended data elements, Version 2.0.* National Center for Injury Prevention and Control, Centers for Disease Control and Prevention. https://www.cdc.gov/violenceprevention/pdf/ipv/intimatepartnerviolence.pdf

Brignone, L., & Gomez, A. M. (2017). Double jeopardy: Predictors of elevated lethality risk among intimate partner violence victims seen in emergency departments. *Preventive Medicine, 103*, 20–25. https://doi.org/10.1016/j.ypmed.2017.06.035

Bromfield, N. (2014). Interviews with divorced women from the United Arab Emirates: A rare glimpse into lived experiences. *Families, Relationships and Societies, 3*(3), 339–354. https://doi.org/10.1332/204674313X13842674567773

Brownridge, D. A. (2006). Violence against women post-separation. *Aggression and Violent Behavior, 11*(5), 514–530. https://doi.org/10.1016/j.avb.2006.01.009

Bruton, C., & Tyson, D. (2018). Leaving violent men: A study of women's experiences of separation in Victoria, Australia. *Australian & New Zealand Journal of Criminology, 51*(3), 339–354. https://doi.org/10.1177/0004865817746711

Btoush, R., & Haj-Yahia, M. M. (2008). Attitudes of Jordanian society toward wife abuse. *Journal of Interpersonal Violence, 23*(11), 1531–1554. https://doi.org/10.1177/0886260508314313

Bulsara, C. (2015). *Using a mixed methods approach to enhance and validate your research. Brightwater Group Research Centre,* Notre Dame University, 1–82. https://www.academia.edu/23767180/USING_A_MIXED_METHODS_APPROACH_TO_ENHANCE_AND_VALIDATE_YOUR_RESEARCH

Burazeri, G., Roshi, E., Jewkes, R., Jordan, S., Bjegovic, V., & Laaser, U. (2005). Factors associated with spousal physical violence in Albania: Cross sectional study. *British Medical Journal, 331*(7510), 197–201. https://doi.org/10.1136/bmj.331.7510.197

Bureau of Justice Statistics. (2013). *Intimate partner violence: Attributes of victimization, 1993-2011.* https://bjs.ojp.gov/press-release/intimate-partner-violence-attributes-victimization-1993-2011

Burgess, R., & Draper, P. (1989). The explanation of family violence: The role of biological, behavioral, and cultural selection. In L. Ohlin & M. Tonry (Eds.), *Family violence, crime and justice: A review of research* (Vol. II, pp. 59–116). University of Chicago Press. https://www.jstor.org/stable/1147526

Burgos-Muñoz, R. M., Soriano-Moreno, A. N., Bendezu-Quispe, G., Urrunaga-Pastor, D., Toro-Huamanchumo, C. J., & Benites-Zapata, V. A. (2021). Intimate partner violence against reproductive-age women and associated factors in Peru: Evidence from national surveys, 2015–2017. *Heliyon, 7*(7), E07478. https://doi.org/10.1016/j.heliyon.2021.e07478

Caeiro, A. (2018). The politics of family cohesion in the Gulf: Islamic authority, new media, and the logic of the modern rentier state. *Arabian Humanities - International Journal of Archaeology and Social Sciences in the Arabian Peninsula, 10.* https://doi.org/10.4000/cy.3762

Caicedo-Roa, M., Da Veiga Pereira, T., & Carlos Cordeiro, R. (2020). PROTOCOL: Risk factors for femicide. *Campbell Systematic Reviews, 16*(4), e1123, 1–12. https://doi.org/10.1002/cl2.1123

Cameron, P. (2014). *Relationship problems and money: Women talk about financial abuse.* Research Report. WIRE Women's Information. https://apo.org.au/sites/default/files/resource-files/2014-08/apo-nid41025.pdf

Campbell, J. C. (2002). Health consequences of intimate partner violence. *Lancet (London, England), 359*(9314), 1331–1336. https://doi.org/10.1016/S0140-6736(02)08336-8

Campbell, E. (2017). How domestic violence batterers use custody proceedings in family courts to abuse victims, and how courts can put a stop to it. *UCLA Women's Law Journal, 24*(1) https://escholarship.org/uc/item/31z272j1

Campbell, J. C., Webster, D. W., & Glass, N. (2008). The danger assessment. *Journal of Interpersonal Violence, 24*(4), 653–674. https://doi.org/10.1177/0886260508317180

Campbell, J. C., Webster, D., Koziol-McLain, J., Block, C., Campbell, D., Curry, M. A., Gary, F., Glass, N., McFarlane, J., Sachs, C., Sharps, P., Ulrich, Y., Wilt, S. A., Manganello, J., Xu, X., Schollenberger, J., Frye, V., & Laughon, K. (2003). Risk factors for femicide in abusive relationships: Results from a multisite case control study. *American Journal of Public Health, 93*(7), 1089–1097. https://doi.org/10.2105/ajph.93.7.1089

Campbell, J., Torres, S., Ryan, J., King, C., Campbell, D. W., Stallings, R. Y., & Fuchs, S. C. (1999). Physical and nonphysical partner abuse and other risk factors for low birth weight among full term and preterm babies: A multiethnic case-control study. *American Journal of Epidemiology, 150*(7), 714–726. https://doi.org/10.1093/oxfordjournals.aje.a010074

Capaldi, D. M., Knoble, N. B., Shortt, J. W., & Kim, H. K. (2012). A systematic review of risk factors for intimate partner violence. *Partner Abuse, 3*(2), 231–280. https://doi.org/10.1891/1946-6560.3.2.231

Carbone-López, K., Kruttschnitt, C., & Macmillan, R. (2006). Patterns of intimate partner violence and their associations with physical health, psychological distress, and substance use. *Public Health Reports, 121*(4), 382–392. https://doi.org/10.1177/003335490612100406

Cascardi, M., O'Leary, K. D., & Schlee, K. A. (1999). Co-occurrence and correlates of posttraumatic stress disorder and major depression in physically abused women. *Journal of Family Violence, 14*(3), 227–249. https://doi.org/10.1023/A:1022827915757

Castro, H. M., & Ferreira, J. C. (2023). Linear and logistic regression models: When to use and how to interpret them? *Jornal Brasileiro De Pneumologia: publicacao oficial da Sociedade Brasileira de Pneumologia e Tisilogia, 48*(6), e20220439. https://doi.org/10.36416/1806-3756/e20220439

Cavanaugh, C. E., Messing, J. T., Del-Colle, M., O'sullivan, C., & Campbell, J. C. (2011). Prevalence and correlates of suicidal behavior among adult female victims of intimate partner violence. *Suicide and Life-threatening Behavior, 41*(4), 373–383. https://doi.org/10.1111/j.1943-278x.2011.00035.x

CDC. (2020, October 9). *Centers for disease control and prevention.* Intimate Partner Violence, Violence Prevention Injury Center. https://www.cdc.gov/violenceprevention/intimatepartnerviolence/index.html

Chan, Y. H. (2003). Biostatistics 102: Quantitative data - Parametric & non-parametric tests. *Singapore Medical Journal, 44*(8), 391–396. http://www.smj.org.sg/sites/default/files/4408/4408bs1.pdf

Chatterji, S., & Heise, L. (2021). Examining the bi-directional relationship between intimate partner violence and depression: Findings from a longitudinal study among women and men in rural Rwanda. *SSM - Mental Health, 1*(March), 100038. https://doi.org/10.1016/j.ssmmh.2021.100038

Cherlin, A. J. (2017). Introduction to the special collection on separation, divorce, repartnering, and remarriage around the world. *Demographic Research, 37*(1), 1275–1296. https://doi.org/10.4054/DemRes.2017.37.38

Cheung, A. K. L., & Choi, S. Y. P. (2016). Non-traditional wives with traditional husbands: Gender ideology and husband-to-wife physical violence in Chinese society. *Violence Against Women, 22*(14), 1704–1724. https://doi.org/10.1177/1077801216632615

Choudhary, E., Smith, M., & Bossarte, R. M. (2012). Depression, anxiety, and symptom profiles among female and male victims of sexual violence. *American Journal of Men's Health, 6*(1), 28–36. https://doi.org/10.1177/1557988311414045

Christian, M., Safari, O., Ramazani, P., Burnham, G., & Glass, N. (2011). Sexual and gender based violence against men in the Democratic Republic of Congo: Effects on survivors, their families and the community. *Medicine, Conflict and Survival, 27*(4), 227–246. https://doi.org/10.1080/13623699.2011.645144

Clare, C. A., Velasquez, G., Mujica Martorell, G. M., Fernandez, D., Dinh, J., & Montague, A. (2021). Risk factors for male perpetration of intimate partner violence: A review. *Aggression and Violent Behavior, 56*(November 2020), 101532. https://doi.org/10.1016/j.avb.2020.101532

Clark, C. J., Silverman, J. G., Shahrouri, M., Everson-Rose, S., & Groce, N. (2010). The role of the extended family in women's risk of intimate partner violence in Jordan. *Social Science and Medicine, 70*(1), 144–151. https://doi.org/10.1016/j.socscimed.2009.09.024

Clarke, V., & Braun, V. (2013). Teaching thematic analysis: Overcoming challenges and developing strategies for effective learning. *The Psychologist, 26*(2), 120–123. https://uwe-repository.worktribe.com/output/937596

Clements, C. M., Bennett, V. E., Hungerford, A., Clauss, K., & Wait, S. K. (2019). Psychopathology and coping in survivors of intimate partner violence: Associations with race and abuse severity. *Journal of Aggression, Maltreatment & Trauma, 28*(2), 205–221. https://doi.org/10.1080/10926771.2018.1470588

Clements, K. A. V., Sprecher, M., Modica, S., Terrones, M., Gregory, K., & Sullivan, C. M. (2021). The use of children as a tactic of intimate partner violence and its relationship to survivors' mental health. *Journal of Family Violence, 37*, 1049–1055. https://doi.org/10.1007/s10896-021-00330-0

Coker, A. L., Smith, P. H., McKeown, R. E., & King, M. J. (2000). Frequency and correlates of intimate partner violence by type: Physical, sexual, and psychological battering. *American Journal of Public Health, 90*(4), 553–559. https://doi.org/10.2105/AJPH.90.4.553

Coleman, M., Ganong, L., & Fine, M. (2000). Reinvestigating remarriage: Another decade of progress. *Journal of Marriage and Family, 62*(4), 1288–1307. https://doi.org/10.1111/j.1741-3737.2000.01288.x

Collins, C. C., & Dressler, W. W. (2008). Cultural consensus and cultural diversity. *Journal of Mixed Methods Research, 2*(4), 362–387. https://doi.org/10.1177/1558689808322766

Collins, T. W., Grineski, S. E., & Morales, D. X. (2017). Environmental injustice and sexual minority health disparities: A national study of inequitable health risks from air pollution among same-sex partners. *Social Science & Medicine, 191*, 38–47. https://doi.org/10.1016/j.socscimed.2017.08.040

Conroy, A. A. (2014). Gender, power, and intimate partner violence. *Journal of Interpersonal Violence, 29*(5), 866–888. https://doi.org/10.1177/0886260513505907

Conybeare, D., Behar, E., Solomon, A., Newman, M. G., & Borkovec, T. D. (2012). The PTSD Checklist-Civilian Version: Reliability, validity, and factor structure in a nonclinical sample. *Journal of Clinical Psychology, 68*(6), 699–713. https://doi.org/10.1002/jclp.21845

Corradi, C., Marcuello-Servós, C., Boira, S., & Weil, S. (2016). Theories of femicide and their significance for social research. *Current Sociology, 64*(7), 975–995. https://doi.org/10.1177/0011392115622256

CountryReports. (n.d.). *Qatar demographics.* Retrieved March 18, 2023, from https://www.countryreports.org/country/Qatar/population.htm

Creswell, J. W. (2003). Research design: Qualitative, quantitative and mixed methods approach. *Sage Publications.*

Creswell, J. W. (2014). *Research design. Qualitative, quantitative and mixed method approaches* (4th ed.). SAGE.

Creswell, J. W., & Creswell, J. D. (2018). Research design: Qualitative, quantitative, and mixed methods approaches. *Sage Publications.*

Creswell, J. W., & Plano Clark, V. L. (2018). *Designing and conducting mixed methods research* (3rd ed.). SAGE.

Creswell, J. W., Fetters, M. D., & Ivankova, N. V. (2004). Designing a mixed methods study in primary care. *Annals of Family Medicine, 2*(1), 7–12. https://doi.org/10.1370/afm.104

Culross, P. L. (1999). Health care system responses to children exposed to domestic violence. *The Future of Children, 9*(3), 111–121. https://doi.org/10.2307/1602785

Cwikel, J., Lev-Wiesel, R., & Al-Krenawi, A. (2003). The physical and psychosocial health of Bedouin Arab women of the Negev Area of Israel. *Violence Against Women, 9*(2), 240–257. https://doi.org/10.1177/1077801202239008

Dadfar, M., Kalibatseva, Z., & Lester, D. (2018). Reliability and validity of the Farsi version of the patient health questionnaire-9 (PHQ-9) with Iranian psychiatric outpatients. *Trends in Psychiatry and Psychotherapy, 40*(2), 144–151. https://doi.org/10.1590/2237-6089-2017-0116

Dami, C., Karathanos, V., Dimitakopoulou, V. I., Damigos, D., & Gouva, M. (2017). Intimate Partner violence in primary settings and consequences in mental health. *International Journal of Caring Sciences, 10*(1), 17–29. http://www.internationaljournalofcaringsciences.org/docs/3_gouva_original_10_1.pdf

Daoud, N., Berger-Polsky, A., Abu-Kaf, S., & Sagy, S. (2019). Sense of coherence among Bedouin women in polygamous marriages compared to women in monogamous marriages. *Women & Health, 60*(1), 43–59. https://doi.org/10.1080/03630242.2019.1610826

Daoud, N., Sergienko, R., & Shoham-Vardi, I. (2020). Intimate partner violence prevalence, recurrence, types, and risk factors among Arab, and Jewish immigrant and nonimmigrant women of childbearing age in Israel. *Journal of Interpersonal Violence, 35*(15–16), 2869–2896. https://doi.org/10.1177/0886260517705665

Dare, B., Guadagno, R., & Muscanell, N. (2013). Commitment: The key to women staying in abusive relationships. *Journal of Interpersonal Relations, Intergroup Relations and Identity, 6*(January 2013), 58–63. https://www.researchgate.net/publication/236647230

Das, T. K., Bhattacharyya, R., Alam, M. F., & Pervin, A. (2016). Domestic violence in Sylhet, Bangladesh: Analysing the experiences of abused women. *Social Change, 46*(1), 106–123. https://doi.org/10.1177/0049085715618561

Davila, A. L., Johnson, L., & Postmus, J. L. (2021). Examining the relationship between economic abuse and mental health among Latina intimate partner violence survivors in the United States. *Journal of Interpersonal Violence, 36*(1–2), NP287–NP310. https://doi.org/10.1177/0886260517731311

Davis, D. (2010). Who gets the house? Renegotiating property rights in post-socialist urban China. *Modern China, 36*(5), 463–492. https://doi.org/10.1177/0097700410373265

De Bel-Air, F., Safar, J., & Destremau, B. (2018). Marriage and Family in the Gulf Today: Storms over a patriarchal institution? *Chroniques Yéménites, 10*. https://doi.org/10.4000/cy.4399

De Coster, S., & Heimer, K. (2021). Unifying theory and research on intimate partner violence: A feminist perspective. *Feminist Criminology, 16*(3), 286–303. https://doi.org/10.1177/1557085120987615

de Serpa Pimentel, A., Mshana, G., Aloyce, D., Peter, E., Mchome, Z., Malibwa, D., Dwarumpudi, A., Kapiga, S., & Stöckl, H. (2021). Women's understanding of economic abuse in North-Western Tanzania. *Women's Health, 17*, 1–11. https://doi.org/10.1177/17455065211042180

Decima Research Inc. (2002). *National profile of family caregivers in Canada 2002*. Health Canada https://www.canada.ca/content/dam/hc-sc/migration/hc-sc/hcs-sss/alt_formats/hpb-dgps/pdf/pubs/2002-caregiv-interven/2002-caregiv-interven-eng.pdf

Deere, C. D., Contreras, J., & Twyman, J. (2014). Patrimonial violence: A study of women's property rights in Ecuador. *Latin American Perspectives, 41*(1), 143–165. https://doi.org/10.1177/0094582X13492133

DeGregoria, B. (1987). Sex role attitude and perception of psychological abuse. *Sex Roles, 16*(5–6), 227–235. https://doi.org/10.1007/BF00289951

DeKeseredy, W. S. (2021). Bringing feminist sociological analyses of patriarchy back to the forefront of the study of woman abuse. *Violence Against Women, 27*(5), 621–638. https://doi.org/10.1177/1077801220958485

DeKeseredy, W. S., & Dragiewicz, M. (2007). Understanding the complexities of feminist perspectives on woman abuse a commentary on Donald G. Dutton's rethinking domestic violence. *Violence Against Women, 13*(8), 874–884. https://doi.org/10.1177/1077801207304806

Den Otter, R. C. (2015). Three may not be a crowd: The case for a constitutional right to plural marriage. *Emory Law Journal, 64*(6), 1977–2046. https://scholarlycommons.law.emory.edu/elj/vol64/iss6/8

Dery, I. (2021). "Give her a slap or two.. She might change": Negotiating masculinities through intimate partner violence among rural Ghanaian men. *Journal of Interpersonal Violence, 36*(19–20), 9670–9690. https://doi.org/10.1177/0886260519869066

Devers, L. N., & Bacon, S. (2010). Interpreting honor crimes: The institutional disregard towards female victims of family violence in the Middle East. *International Journal of Criminology and Sociological Theory, 3*(1), 359–371. https://ijcst.journals.yorku.ca/index.php/ijcst/article/download/25925/24007

Dhungel, S., Dhungel, P., Dhital, S. R., & Stock, C. (2017). Is economic dependence on the husband a risk factor for intimate partner violence against female factory workers in Nepal? *BMC Women's Health, 17*(1), 1–9. https://doi.org/10.1186/s12905-017-0441-8

Di Napoli, I., Procentese, F., Carnevale, S., Esposito, C., & Arcidiacono, C. (2019). Ending intimate partner violence (IPV) and locating men at stake: An ecological approach. *International Journal of Environmental Research and Public Health, 16*(9), 1652. https://doi.org/10.3390/ijerph16091652

Dichter, M. E., Thomas, K. A., Crits-Christoph, P., Ogden, S. N., & Rhodes, K. V. (2018). Coercive control in intimate partner violence: Relationship with women's experience of violence, use of violence, and danger. *Psychology of Violence, 8*(5), 596–604. https://doi.org/10.1037/vio0000158

Dierickx, S., Coene, G., Jarju, B., & Longman, C. (2019). Women with infertility complying with and resisting polygyny: An explorative qualitative study in urban Gambia. *Reproductive Health, 16*(1), 1–11. https://doi.org/10.1186/s12978-019-0762-1

Dillon, G., Hussain, R., Loxton, D., & Rahman, S. (2013). Mental and physical health and intimate partner violence against women: A review of the literature. *International Journal of Family Medicine, 2013*, 313909. https://doi.org/10.1155/2013/313909

Djamba, Y. K., & Kimuna, S. R. (Eds.). (2015). *Gender-based violence: Perspective from Africa, the Middle East, and India.* Springer. https://doi.org/10.1007/978-3-319-16670-4

Doha International Family Institute (DIFI). (2022). *The state of Qatari Families: Strengths and challenges.* https://doi.org/10.5339/difi_9789927161629

Dokkedahl, S. B., Kirubakaran, R., Bech-Hansen, D., Kristensen, T. R., & Elklit, A. (2022). The psychological subtype of intimate partner violence and its effect on mental health: A systematic review with meta-analyses. *Systematic Reviews, 11*(1), 163. https://doi.org/10.1186/s13643-022-02025-z

Douki, S., Nacef, F., Belhadj, A., Bouasker, A., & Ghachem, R. (2003). Violence against women in Arab and Islamic countries. *Archives of Women's Mental Health, 6*(3), 165–171. https://doi.org/10.1007/s00737-003-0170-x

Dray, J. A. W. (1987). International conflicts in child custody: United States v. Saudi Arabia. *Loyola of Los Angeles International and Comparative Law Review, 9*(2), 413–443. https://digitalcommons.lmu.edu/ilr/vol9/iss2/5

Dutton, M. A., James, L., Langhorne, A., & Kelley, M. (2015). Coordinated public health initiatives to address violence against women and adolescents. *Journal of Women's Health, 24*(1), 80–85. https://doi.org/10.1089/jwh.2014.4884

El Sheikh, M. A. (2019). Post-divorce financial support from the Islamic perspective (Mutʿat al-Ṭalāq). In M. Ayoub (Ed.), *Contemporary approaches to the Quran and Sunnah* (pp. 172–196). International Institute of Islamic Thought. https://doi.org/10.2307/j.ctvk8w26p.14

Eldoseri, H. M., & Sharps, P. (2017). Risk factors for spousal physical violence against women in Saudi Arabia. *Journal of Interpersonal Violence, 35*(5–6), 1269–1293. https://doi.org/10.1177/0886260517696861

Eldoseri, H. M., Tufts, K. A., Zhang, Q., & Fish, J. N. (2014). Adverse health effects of spousal violence among women attending Saudi Arabian primary health-care clinics. *Eastern*

Mediterranean Health Journal, 20(11), 717–725. https://applications.emro.who.int/emhj/v20/11/EMHJ_2014_20_11_717_725.pdf

Elnashar, A. M., El-Dien Ibrahim, M., Eldesoky, M. M., Aly, O. M., & El-Sayd Mohamed Hassan, M. (2007). Sexual abuse experienced by married Egyptian women. *International Journal of Gynecology & Obstetrics, 99*(3), 216–220. https://doi.org/10.1016/j.ijgo.2007.05.049

Enache, R. G., Matei, R. S., & Tuşa, E. (2019). Specialized intervention for protecting victims of domestic violence. *Revista De Asistenta Sociala, 1*, 127–137. https://www.proquest.com/scholarly-journals/specialized-intervention-protecting-victims/docview/2440936908/se-2

Eng, S., Szmodis, W., & Grace, K. (2020). Cambodian remarried women are at risk for domestic violence. *Journal of Interpersonal Violence, 35*(3–4), 828–853. https://doi.org/10.1177/0886260517691520

Ernst, A. F., & Albers, C. J. (2017). Regression assumptions in clinical psychology research practice - A systematic review of common misconceptions. *PeerJ, 2017*(5), 1–16. https://doi.org/10.7717/peerj.3323

Esie, P., Osypuk, T. L., Schuler, S. R., & Bates, L. M. (2019). SSM - population health intimate partner violence and depression in rural Bangladesh: Accounting for violence severity in a high prevalence setting. *SSM – Population Health, 7*(August 2018), 100368. https://doi.org/10.1016/j.ssmph.2019.100368

Etikan, I. (2016). Comparison of snowball sampling and sequential sampling technique. *Biometrics & Biostatistics International Journal, 3*(1), 1–2. https://doi.org/10.15406/bbij.2016.03.00055

Fagan, J. (1988). Contributions of family violence research to criminal justice policy on wife assault: Paradigms of science and social control. *Violence and Victims, 3*(3), 159–186. https://pubmed.ncbi.nlm.nih.gov/3154178/

Fahmy, E., Williamson, E., & Pantazis, C. (2016). *Evidence and policy review: Domestic violence and poverty* (pp. 1–42). Joseph Rowntree Foundation. https://research-information.bristol.ac.uk/files/80376377/JRF_DV_POVERTY_REPORT_FINAL_COPY_.pdf

Falb, K. L., Blackwell, A., Stennes, J., Hussein, M., & Annan, J. (2019). Depressive symptoms among women in Raqqa Governorate, Syria: associations with intimate partner violence, food insecurity, and perceived needs. *Global Mental Health (Cambridge, England), 6*, e22. https://doi.org/10.1017/gmh.2019.20

Ferrari, G., Bonnet, C., & Solaz, A. (2019). "Will the one who keeps the children keep the house?" Residential mobility after divorce by parenthood status and custody arrangements in France. *Demographic Research, 40*(February), 359–394. https://doi.org/10.4054/DEMRES.2019.40.14

Fikree, F. F., Razzak, J. A., & Durocher, J. (2005). Attitudes of Pakistani men to domestic violence: A study from Karachi, Pakistan. *Journal of Men's Health and Gender, 2*(1), 49–58. https://doi.org/10.1016/j.jmhg.2005.01.004

Flynn, A., & Graham, K. (2010). "Why did it happen?" A review and conceptual framework for research on perpetrators' and victims' explanations for intimate partner violence. *Aggression and Violent Behavior, 15*(3), 239–251. https://doi.org/10.1016/j.avb.2010.01.002

Fonseca-Machado, M. d. O., Monteiro, J. C. d. S., Haas, V. J., de Vilhena, A. C. F. A., & Gomes-Sponholz, F. (2015). Intimate partner violence and anxiety disorders in pregnancy: The importance of vocational training of the nursing staff in facing them. *Revista Latino-Americana de Enfermagem, 23*(5), 855–864. https://doi.org/10.1590/0104-1169.0495.2624

Gage, A. N., & Lease, S. H. (2021). An exploration of the link between masculinity and endorsement of IPV myths in American men. *Journal of Interpersonal Violence, 36*(13–14), 6145–6165. https://doi.org/10.1177/0886260518818430

Gangoli, G., Razak, A., & McCarry, M. (2006, June). *Forced marriage and domestic violence among South Asian communities in North East England*. School for Policy Studies, University of Bristol. https://research-information.bris.ac.uk/files/188679401/Final_report.pdf

Gass, J. D., Stein, D. J., Williams, D. R., & Seedat, S. (2011). Gender differences in risk for intimate partner violence among South African adults. *Journal of Interpersonal Violence, 26*(14), 2764–2789. https://doi.org/10.1177/0886260510390960

Gebrewahd, G. T., Gebremeskel, G. G., & Tadesse, D. B. (2020). Intimate partner violence against reproductive age women during COVID-19 pandemic in Northern Ethiopia 2020: A community-based cross-sectional study. *Reproductive Health, 17*(1), 152. https://doi.org/10.1186/s12978-020-01002-w

Ghazi, H. F., & Isa, Z. (2018). Women's attitude and its influence on violence during pregnancy in northern state of peninsular Malaysia: Cross-sectional study. *Journal of Interpersonal Violence, 36*(5–6), 1–25. https://doi.org/10.1177/0886260518759059

Glick, P., & Fiske, S. T. (1997). Hostile and benevolent sexism: Measuring ambivalent sexist attitudes toward women. *Psychology of Women Quarterly, 21*(1), 119–135. https://doi.org/10.1111/j.1471-6402.1997.tb00104.x

Godbout, N., Dutton, D. G., Lussier, Y., & Sabourin, S. (2009). Early exposure to violence, domestic violence, attachment representations, and marital adjustment. *Personal Relationships, 16*(3), 365–384. https://doi.org/10.1111/j.1475-6811.2009.01228.x

Golafshani, N. (2003). Understanding reliability and validity in qualitative research. *The Qualitative Report, 8*(4), 597–607. https://doi.org/10.46743/2160-3715/2003.1870

Gordon, L. (1988). *Heroes of their own lives: The history and politics of family violence.* Viking/Penguin.

Graham, L. M., Macy, R. J., Rizo, C. F., & Martin, S. L. (2022). Explanatory theories of intimate partner homicide perpetration: A systematic review. *Trauma, Violence & Abuse, 23*(2), 408–427. https://doi.org/10.1177/1524838020953800

Gravelin, C. R., Biernat, M., & Bucher, C. E. (2019). Blaming the victim of acquaintance rape: Individual, situational, and sociocultural factors. *Frontiers in Psychology, 9*(JAN), 1–22. https://doi.org/10.3389/fpsyg.2018.02422

Guest, G., & Fleming, P. J. (2015). Mixed methods research. In G. Guest & E. Namey (Eds.), *Public health research methods* (pp. 581–610). Sage. https://doi.org/10.4135/9781483398839.n19

Gultiano, S., Hindin, M., & Upadhyay, U. (2009). Marital status and psychological Well-being of Filipino women. *Philippine Population Review, 8*(1), 16–33. https://www.pssc.org.ph/wp-content/pssc-archives/Philippine%20Population%20Review/2009/05_Martal%20Status%20And%20Psychological%20Well_Being%20Of%20Filipino%20Women.pdf

Haj-Yahia, M. M. (2000). Wife abuse and battering in the sociocultural context of Arab society. *Family Process, 39*(2), 237–255. https://doi.org/10.1111/j.1545-5300.2000.39207.x

Haj-Yahia, M. M. (2002). Attitudes of Arab women toward different patterns of coping with wife abuse. *Journal of Interpersonal Violence, 17*(7), 721–745. https://doi.org/10.1177/08862605020170070

Hamel, J., Desmarais, S. L., Nicholls, T. L., Malley-Morrison, K., & Aaronson, J. (2009). Domestic violence and child custody: Are family court professionals' decisions based on erroneous beliefs? *Journal of Aggression, Conflict and Peace Research, 1*(2), 37–52. https://doi.org/10.1108/17596599200900011

Hammad, A., Kysia, R., Rabah, R., Hassoun, R., & Connelly, M. (1999). *Arab community center for economic and social services guide to Arab culture: Health care delivery to the Arab American community.* ACCESS Community Health Center. https://my.vanderbilt.edu/globalhealth/files/2013/04/Guide-to-Arab-Culture-Health-care-delivery-to-the-Arab-American-Community.pdf

Hanson, W. E., Plano Clark, V. L., Petska, K. S., Creswell, J. W., & Creswell, J. D. (2005). Mixed methods research designs in counseling psychology. *Journal of Counseling Psychology, 52*(2), 224–235. https://doi.org/10.1037/0022-0167.52.2.224

Hardesty, J. L. (2002). Separation assault in the context of postdivorce parenting. *Violence Against Women, 8*(5), 597–625. https://doi.org/10.1177/107780120200800505

Hardesty, J. L., & Ganong, L. H. (2006). How women make custody decisions and manage co-parenting with abusive former husbands. *Journal of Social and Personal Relationships, 23*(4), 543–563. https://doi.org/10.1177/0265407506065983

Harris, R. J., Firestone, J. M., & Vega, W. A. (2005). The interaction of country of origin, acculturation, and gender role ideology on wife abuse. *Social Science Quarterly, 86*(2), 463–483. https://doi.org/10.1111/j.0038-4941.2005.00313.x

Hassouneh-Phillips, D. (2001). American Muslim women's experiences of leaving abusive relationships. *Health Care for Women International, 22*(4), 415–432. https://doi.org/10.1080/07399330119163

Hawcroft, C., Hughes, R., Shaheen, A., Usta, J., Elkadi, H., Dalton, T., Ginwalla, K., & Feder, G. (2019). Prevalence and health outcomes of domestic violence amongst clinical populations in Arab countries: A systematic review and meta-analysis. *BMC Public Health, 19*(1), 315. https://doi.org/10.1186/s12889-019-6619-2

Heise, L. L. (1998). Violence against women: An integrated, ecological framework. *Violence Against Women, 4*(3), 262–290. https://doi.org/10.1177/1077801298004003002

Hetherington, E. M., Bridges, M., & Insabella, G. M. (1992). What matters? What does not? *American Psychologist, 53*(2), 167–184.

Hill, S., & Marshall, T. C. (2018). Beliefs about sexual assault in India and Britain are explained by attitudes toward women and hostile sexism. *Sex Roles, 79*(7–8), 421–430. https://doi.org/10.1007/s11199-017-0880-6

Hindin, M. J., & Adair, L. S. (2002). Who's at risk? Factors associated with intimate partner violence in the Philippines. *Social Science and Medicine, 55*(8), 1385–1399. https://doi.org/10.1016/S0277-9536(01)00273-8

Holmes, S. C., King, K. C., Gonzalez, A., Norton, M. K., Silver, K. E., Sullivan, T. P., & Johnson, D. M. (2023). Associations among intimate partner violence, posttraumatic stress disorder symptoms, and disordered eating among women intimate partner violence survivors residing in shelter. *Journal of Interpersonal Violence, 38*(1–2), NP2135–NP2158. https://doi.org/10.1177/08862605221098968

Hong, J. S., & Espelage, D. L. (2012). A review of research on bullying and peer victimization in school: An ecological system analysis. *Aggression and Violent Behavior, 17*(4), 311–322. https://doi.org/10.1016/j.avb.2012.03.003

Houry, D., Kemball, R. S., Click, L. A., & Kaslow, N. J. (2007). Development of a brief mental health screen for intimate partner violence victims in the emergency department. *Academic Emergency Medicine, 14*(3), 202–209. https://doi.org/10.1197/j.aem.2006.09.056

Hunnicutt, G. (2009). Varieties of patriarchy and violence against women. *Violence Against Women, 15*(5), 553–573. https://doi.org/10.1177/1077801208331246

Ibrahim, H., Ertl, V., Catani, C., Ismail, A. A., & Neuner, F. (2018). The validity of Posttraumatic Stress Disorder Checklist for DSM-5 (PCL-5) as screening instrument with Kurdish and Arab displaced populations living in the Kurdistan region of Iraq. *BMC Psychiatry, 18*(1), 1–8. https://doi.org/10.1186/s12888-018-1839-z

Ibrahim, K., Fahimi, F., Ismail, H., Mamdouh, H., Muhammad, Y., Tawfik, M., El-Sharkawy, O., Sallam, H., (2010, September). *Spousal violence in Egypt.* Population Reference Bureau. https://www.prb.org/wp-content/uploads/2010/09/09282010-spousalviolence-egypt.pdf

IPI Global Observatory. (2021). *Women's political participation in the Arab world.* https://theglobalobservatory.org/2021/01/womens-political-participation-arab-world/

Ivankova, N. V., Creswell, J. W., & Stick, S. L. (2006). Using mixed-methods sequential explanatory design: From theory to practice. *Field Methods, 18*(1), 3–20. https://doi.org/10.1177/1525822X05282260

Izugbara, C. O., Obiyan, M. O., Degfie, T. T., & Bhatti, A. (2020). Correlates of intimate partner violence among urban women in sub-Saharan Africa. *PLoS One, 15*(3), 1–21. https://doi.org/10.1371/journal.pone.0230508

Jacob, S. A., & Furgerson, S. P. (2012). Writing interview protocols and conducting interviews: Tips for students new to the field of qualitative research. *Qualitative Report. ERIC*, 1–10. https://doi.org/10.1016/0168-1702(91)90033-R

Jaffe, P. G., Johnston, J. R., Crooks, C. V., & Bala, N. (2008). Custody disputes involving allegations of domestic violence: Toward a differentiated approach to parenting plans. *Family Court Review, 46*(3), 500–522. https://doi.org/10.1111/j.1744-1617.2008.00216.x

James-Hawkins, L., Qutteina, Y., & Yount, K. M. (2017). The patriarchal bargain in a context of rapid changes to normative gender roles: Young Arab women's role conflict in Qatar. *Sex Roles, 77*(3–4), 155–168. https://doi.org/10.1007/s11199-016-0708-9

Jewkes, R. (2002). Intimate partner violence: Causes and prevention. *The Lancet, 359*(9315), 1423–1429. https://doi.org/10.1016/S0140-6736(02)08357-5

Johnson, R. B., & Onwuegbuzie, A. J. (2004). Mixed methods research: A research paradigm whose time has come. *Educational Researcher, 33*(7), 14–26. https://doi.org/10.3102/0013189X033007014

Jones, J. H., & Ferguson, B. (2009). Demographic and social predictors of intimate partner violence in Colombia: A dyadic power perspective. *Human Nature, 20*(2), 184–203. https://doi.org/10.1007/s12110-009-9064-6

Kalmuss, D., & Seltzer, J. A. (1986). Continuity of marital behavior in remarriage: The case of spouse abuse. *Journal of Marriage and the Family, 48*(1), 113–120. https://doi.org/10.2307/352234

Kalra, N., Hooker, L., Reisenhofer, S., Di Tanna, G. L., & García-Moreno, C. (2021). Training healthcare providers to respond to intimate partner violence against women. *Cochrane Database of Systematic Reviews, 5*(5), CD012423–CD012423. https://doi.org/10.1002/14651858.CD012423.pub2

Karakurt, G., & Cumbie, T. (2012). The relationship between egalitarianism, dominance, and violence in intimate relationships. *Journal of Family Violence, 27*(2), 115–122. https://doi.org/10.1007/s10896-011-9408-y

Karakurt, G., Smith, D., & Whiting, J. (2014). Impact of intimate partner violence on women's mental health. *NIH Public Access Author Manuscript, 29*(7), 693–702. https://doi.org/10.1038/jid.2014.371

Karakurt, G., Whiting, K., Jones, S. E., Lowe, M. J., & Rao, S. M. (2021). Brain injury and mental health among the victims of intimate partner violence: A case-series exploratory study. *Frontiers in Psychology, 12*(October). https://doi.org/10.3389/fpsyg.2021.710602

Kerley, K. R., Xu, X., Sirisunyaluck, B., & Alley, J. M. (2010). Exposure to family violence in childhood and intimate partner perpetration or victimization in adulthood: Exploring intergenerational transmission in urban Thailand. *Journal of Family Violence, 25*(3), 337–347. https://doi.org/10.1007/s10896-009-9295-7

Khadra, C., Wehbe, N., Lachance Fiola, J., Skaff, W., & Nehmé, M. (2015). Symptoms of post-traumatic stress disorder among battered women in Lebanon: An exploratory study. *Journal of Interpersonal Violence, 30*(2), 295–313. https://doi.org/10.1177/0886260514534774

Khalifeh, H., Hargreaves, J., Howard, L. M., & Birdthistle, I. (2013). Intimate partner violence and socioeconomic deprivation in England: Findings from a national cross-sectional survey. *American Journal of Public Health, 103*(3), 462–472. https://doi.org/10.2105/AJPH.2012.300723

Kim, Y. (2011). The pilot study in qualitative inquiry: Identifying issues and learning lessons for culturally competent research. *Qualitative Social Work, 10*(2), 190–206. https://doi.org/10.1177/1473325010362001

King, K., Murray, C. E., Crowe, A., Hunnicutt, G., Lundgren, K., & Olson, L. (2017). The costs of recovery: Intimate partner violence survivors' experiences of financial recovery from abuse. *Family Journal, 25*(3), 230–238. https://doi.org/10.1177/1066480717710656

Koepsell, J. K., Kernic, M. A., & Holt, V. L. (2007). Factors that influence battered women to leave their abusive relationships. *Violence and Victims, 21*(2), 131–147. https://doi.org/10.1891/088667006780644299

Koziol-McLain, J., Webster, D., McFarlane, J., Block, C. R., Ulrich, Y., Glass, N., & Campbell, J. C. (2006). Risk factors for femicide-suicide in abusive relationships: Results from a multisite case control study. *Violence and Victims, 21*(1), 3–21. https://doi.org/10.1891/0886-6708.21.1.3

Krause, E. D., Kaltman, S., Goodman, L., & Dutton, M. A. (2006). Role of distinct PTSD symptoms in intimate partner reabuse: A prospective study. *Journal of Traumatic Stress, 19*(4), 507–516. https://doi.org/10.1002/jts.20136

Krause, K. H., Gordon-Roberts, R., VanderEnde, K., Schuler, S. R., & Yount, K. M. (2016). Why do women justify violence against wives more often than do men in Vietnam? *Journal of Interpersonal Violence, 31*(19), 3150–3173. https://doi.org/10.1177/0886260515584343

Kristiansen, C. M., & Giulietti, R. (1990). Perceptions of wife abuse. *Psychology of Women Quarterly, 14*(2), 177–189. https://doi.org/10.1111/J.1471-6402.1990.TB00013.X

Krueger, R. A., & Casey, M. A. (2009). *Focus groups: A practical guide for applied research*. Sage Publications.

Kucinskas, J. (2010). A research note on Islam and gender egalitarianism: An examination of Egyptian and Saudi Arabian youth attitudes. *Journal for the Scientific Study of Religion, 49*(4), 761–770. https://doi.org/10.1111/j.1468-5906.2010.01545.x

Kurst-Swanger, K., & Petcosky, J. L. (2003). *Violence in the home: Multidisciplinary perspectives*. Oxford Academic. https://doi.org/10.1093/acprof:oso/9780195165180.001.0001

Kutin, J., Russell, R., & Reid, M. (2017). Economic abuse between intimate partners in Australia: Prevalence, health status, disability and financial stress. *Australian and New Zealand Journal of Public Health, 41*(3), 269–274. https://doi.org/10.1111/1753-6405.12651

Kvale, S., & Brinkmann, S. (2009). *Interviews: Learning the craft of qualitative research interviewing* (2nd ed.). Sage Publications.

Kwiatkowski, L. (2019). A "wife's duty" and social suffering: Sexual assault in marital relationships in Vietnam. *Journal of Aggression, Maltreatment and Trauma, 28*(1), 68–84. https://doi.org/10.1080/10926771.2018.1494237

Kyriacou, D. N., Anglin, D., Taliaferro, E., Stone, S., Tubb, T., Linden, J. A., Muelleman, R., Barton, E., & Kraus, J. F. (2018). Risk factors for injury to women from domestic violence. In M. Natarajan (Ed.), *Domestic violence* (pp. 145–151). Routledge. https://doi.org/10.4324/9781315264905-10

Lagdon, S., Armour, C., & Stringer, M. (2014). Adult experience of mental health outcomes as a result of intimate partner violence victimisation: A systematic review. *European Journal of Psychotraumatology, 5*(1), 24794. https://doi.org/10.3402/ejpt.v5.24794

Lakens, D. (2013). Calculating and reporting effect sizes to facilitate cumulative science: A practical primer for t-tests and ANOVAs. *Frontiers in Psychology, 4*, 863. https://doi.org/10.3389/fpsyg.2013.00863

Laland, K. N., & Rendell, L. (2010). Social learning: Theory. In *Encyclopedia of animal behavior* (2nd ed., pp. 380–386). Elsevier Ltd.. https://doi.org/10.1016/B978-0-12-813251-7.00057-2

Lambson, S. H., & Reich, W. A. (2017). *Intimate partner violence as a community problem community perspectives from Bedford-Stuyvesant, Brooklyn*. Center for Court Innovation. http://www.courtinnovation.org/sites/default/files/documents/BedStuy_IPV_Research_Report.pdf

Lamichhane, P., Puri, M., Tamang, J., & Dulal, B. (2011). Women's status and violence against young married women in rural Nepal. *BMC Women's Health, 11*, 19. https://doi.org/10.1186/1472-6874-11-19

Landau, E. M. (2016). Custom or Crime?: Part II of IV: Legal remedies. *American Journal of Family Law, 30*(1), 46–57. https://preventforcedmarriage.org/wp-content/uploads/2016/05/Elizabeth-Landau_Custom-or-Crime-II.pdf

Lari, N. (2022). Toward marriage sustainability: Impacts of delayed marriages in Qatar. *Cogent Social Sciences, 8*(1). https://doi.org/10.1080/23311886.2022.2083480

Lasong, J., Zhang, Y., Muyayalo, K. P., Njiri, O. A., Gebremedhin, S. A., Abaidoo, C. S., Liu, C. Y., Zhang, H., & Zhao, K. (2020). Domestic violence among married women of reproductive age in Zimbabwe: A cross sectional study. *BMC Public Health, 20*(1), 354. https://doi.org/10.1186/s12889-020-8447-9

Lawrence, S. (2002). *Domestic violence and welfare policy research findings that can inform policies on marriage and child well-being*. National Center for Children in Poverty, Columbia University. https://doi.org/10.7916/D87D33S1

Lawson, J. (2012). Sociological theories of intimate partner violence. *Journal of Human Behavior in the Social Environment, 22*(5), 572–590. https://doi.org/10.1080/10911359.2011.598748

Lawton, J., & Schulte, S. J. (2012). The prevalence of mental health symptoms among outpatients in the United Arab Emirates. *Arab Journal of Psychiatry, 23*(2), 138–147. https://platform.almanhal.com/Files/2/17304

Levendosky, A. A., Lannert, B., & Yalch, M. (2012). The effects of intimate partner violence on women and children survivors: An attachment perspective. *Psychodynamic Psychiatry, 40*(3), 397–434. https://doi.org/10.1521/pdps.2012.40.3.397

Li, X., Wong, W., Lamoureux, E. L., & Wong, T. Y. (2012). Are linear regression techniques appropriate for analysis when the dependent (outcome) variable is not normally distributed? *Investigative Ophthalmology & Visual Science, 53*(6), 3082–3083. https://doi.org/10.1167/iovs.12-9967

Loo, R., & Thorpe, K. (1998). Attitudes toward women's roles in society: A replication after 20 years. *Sex Roles, 39*(11–12), 903–912. https://doi.org/10.1023/a:1018832823010

Lotfy, M., Hamdy, M. A., Mansour, A. F. I., Gharib, W. F., Ghoneim, H. M., Abbas, A. M., Ahmed, W. A. S., & Ibrahim, Z. M. (2019). Prevalence and risk factors for domestic violence among infertile Egyptian women: A cross-sectional study. *European Journal of Contraception and Reproductive Health Care, 24*(5), 362–367. https://doi.org/10.1080/13625187.2019.1642467

Lown, E. A., & Vega, W. A. (2001). Prevalence and predictors of physical partner abuse among Mexican American women. *American Journal of Public Health, 91*(3), 441–445. https://doi.org/10.2105/AJPH.91.3.441

Lumley, T., Diehr, P., Emerson, S., & Chen, L. (2002). The importance of the normality assumption in large public health data sets. *Annual Review of Public Health, 23*, 151–169. https://doi.org/10.1146/annurev.publhealth.23.100901.140546

MacMillan, H. L., Wathen, C. N., Jamieson, E., Boyle, M., McNutt, L. A., Worster, A., Lent, B., Webb, M., & McMaster Violence Against Women Research Group. (2006). Approaches to screening for intimate partner violence in health care settings: A randomized trial. *JAMA, 296*(5), 530–536. https://doi.org/10.1001/jama.296.5.530

Madruga, C. S., Viana, M. C., Abdalla, R. R., Caetano, R., & Laranjeira, R. (2017). Pathways from witnessing parental violence during childhood to involvement in intimate partner violence in adult life: The roles of depression and substance use. *Drug and Alcohol Review, 36*(1), 107–114. https://doi.org/10.1111/dar.12514

Maguire, M., & Delahunt, B. (2017). Doing a thematic analysis: A practical, step-by-step guide for learning and teaching scholars. *AISHE-J, 9*, 3351. https://ojs.aishe.org/index.php/aishe-j/article/view/335

Mahapatro, M., Gupta, R. N., & Gupta, V. (2012). The risk factor of domestic violence in India. *Indian Journal of Community Medicine, 37*(3), 153–157. https://doi.org/10.4103/0970-0218.99912

Malik, M., Munir, N., Usman Ghani, M., & Ahmad, N. (2020). Domestic violence and its relationship with depression, anxiety and quality of life: A hidden dilemma of Pakistani women. *Pakistan Journal of Medical Sciences, 37*(1), 1–4. https://doi.org/10.12669/pjms.37.1.2893

Mapayi, B., Makanjuola, R. O. A., Mosaku, S. K., Adewuya, O. A., Afolabi, O., Aloba, O. O., & Akinsulore, A. (2013). Impact of intimate partner violence on anxiety and depression amongst women in Ile-Ife, Nigeria. *Archives of Women's Mental Health, 16*(1), 11–18. https://doi.org/10.1007/s00737-012-0307-x

McIntosh, M. J., & Morse, J. M. (2015). Situating and constructing diversity in semi-structured interviews. *Global Qualitative Nursing Research, 2*. https://doi.org/10.1177/2333393615597674

McLeod, S. (2019). *What does effect size tell you?*. Simply Psychology https://www.simplypsychology.org/effect-size.html

McMullin, C. (2023). Transcription and qualitative methods: Implications for third sector research. *Voluntas, 34*(1), 140–153. https://doi.org/10.1007/s11266-021-00400-3

Melikian, L. H., & Al-Easa, J. S. (1984). Oil and social change in the Gulf. In A. Ghabra (Ed.), *Political behavior in the Arab states* (1st ed., p. 14). Routledge.

Mendoza, J. E., Tolba, M., & Saleh, Y. (2020). Strengthening marriages in Egypt: Impact of divorce on women. *Behavioral Sciences, 10*(1), 1–8. https://doi.org/10.3390/bs10010014

Mercy, J. A., & Saltzman, L. E. (1989). Fatal violence among spouses in the United States, 1976–85. *American Journal of Public Health, 79*(5), 595–599. https://doi.org/10.2105/ajph.79.5.595

Messing, J. T., Campbell, J. C., Brown, S., Patchell, B., Androff, D. K., & Wilson, J. S. (2014). The Association between protective actions and homicide risk: Findings from the Oklahoma lethality assessment study. *Violence and Victims, 29*(4), 543–563. https://doi.org/10.1891/0886-6708.VV-D-13-00013

Miller, S. L., & Manzer, J. L. (2021). Safeguarding children's well-being: Voices from abused mothers navigating their relationships and the civil courts. *Journal of Interpersonal Violence, 36*(9–10), 4545–4569. https://doi.org/10.1177/0886260518791599

Ministry of Development Planning and Statistics (MDPS). (2018). *Marriage & divorce in the State of Qatar, 2017 (Review & analysis)*. https://www.psa.gov.qa/en/statistics/Statistical%20Releases/General/StatisticalAbstract/2017/population-chapters/marriage_divorce_qatar_2017_En.pdf

Ministry of Development Planning and Statistics (MDPS). (2019). *Qatar second national development strategy 2018~2022*. https://www.psa.gov.qa/en/knowledge/Documents/NDS2Final.pdf

Moder, A. (2019). Women, personhood, and the male God: A feminist critique of patriarchal concepts of God in view of domestic abuse. *Feminist Theology, 28*(1), 85–103. https://doi.org/10.1177/0966735019859471

Mojahed, A., Alaidarous, N., Shabta, H., Hegewald, J., & Garthus-Niegel, S. (2020). Intimate partner violence against women in the Arab countries: A systematic review of risk factors. *Trauma, Violence & Abuse, 23*(2), 1–18. https://doi.org/10.1177/1524838020953099

Morland, L. A., Leskin, G. A., Rebecca Block, C., Campbell, J. C., & Friedman, M. J. (2008). Intimate partner violence and miscarriage: Examination of the role of physical and psychological abuse and posttraumatic stress disorder. *Journal of Interpersonal Violence, 23*(5), 652–669. https://doi.org/10.1177/0886260507313533

Moshtagh, M., Amiri, R., Sharafi, S., & Arab-Zozani, M. (2021). Intimate partner violence in the Middle East region: A systematic review and meta-analysis. *Trauma, Violence, and Abuse, 24*(2), 613–631. https://doi.org/10.1177/15248380211036060

Murinkó, L. (2019). Housing consequences of divorce and separation in a "super home ownership" regime: The case of Hungary. *Demographic Research, 40*(June), 975–1014. https://doi.org/10.4054/DemRes.2019.40.34

Mshweshwe, L. (2020). Understanding domestic violence: Masculinity, culture, traditions. *Heliyon, 6*(10), e05334. https://doi.org/10.1016/j.heliyon.2020.e05334

Naseer, S., Farooq, S., & Malik, F. (2021). Causes and consequences of polygamy: An understanding of coping strategies by co-wives in polygamous marriage. *ASEAN Journal of Psychiatry, 22*(9), 1–10. https://doi.org/10.54615/2231-7805.47221

Nelson, M. C. (1988). Reliability, validity, and cross-cultural comparisons for the simplified attitudes toward women scale. *Sex Roles, 18*(5), 289–296. https://doi.org/10.1007/BF00288291

Newman, C. (2010). Expert domestic violence risk assessments in the family courts. *Respect*, 1–19. http://www.fsa.me.uk/uploads/7/6/5/6/7656227/respect_dv_risk_assessment_review_-_c_newman_c_bell.pdf

Obeid, N., Chang, D. F., & Ginges, J. (2010). Beliefs about wife beating: An exploratory study with Lebanese students. *Violence Against Women, 16*(6), 691–712. https://doi.org/10.1177/1077801210370465

Ogbe, E., Harmon, S., van den Bergh, R., & Degomme, O. (2020). A systematic review of intimate partner violence interventions focused on improving social support and/ mental health outcomes of survivors. *PLoS One, 15*(6), 1–27. https://doi.org/10.1371/journal.pone.0235177

Ogden, S. N., Dichter, M. E., & Bazzi, A. R. (2022). Intimate partner violence as a predictor of substance use outcomes among women: A systematic review. *Addictive Behaviors, 127*, 107214. https://doi.org/10.1016/j.addbeh.2021.107214

Oram, S., Khalifeh, H., & Howard, L. M. (2017). Violence against women and mental health. *The Lancet Psychiatry, 4*(2), 159–170. https://doi.org/10.1016/S2215-0366(16)30261-9

Otieno, F. O. (2017). *A Meta-analysis of the association between intimate partner violence and age disparity in sub-Saharan Africa* [Master's thesis, University of Stellenbosch]. SUNScholar. https://scholar.sun.ac.za/server/api/core/bitstreams/6651d00b-23bc-482f-bdb5-c649c649010a/content

Owusu Adjah, E. S., & Agbemafle, I. (2016). Determinants of domestic violence against women in Ghana. *BMC Public Health, 16*, 368. https://doi.org/10.1186/s12889-016-3041-x

Usta, J., Makarem, N. N., & Habib, R. R. (2013). Economic Abuse in Lebanon: Experiences and Perceptions. *Violence Against Women, 19*(3), 356–375. https://doi.org/10.1177/1077801213486313

Papreen, N., Sharma, A., Sabin, K., Begum, L., Ahsan, S. K., & Baqui, A. H. (2000). Living with infertility: Experiences among urban slum populations in Bangladesh. *Reproductive Health Matters, 8*(15), 33–44. https://doi.org/10.1016/S0968-8080(00)90004-1

Paris, W. L., Wang, T., Laumann, E. O., Pan, S., & Luo, Y. (2004). Intimate partner violence in China: National prevalence, risk factors and associated health problems. *International Family Planning Perspectives, 30*(4), 174–181. https://doi.org/10.1363/3017404

Paulino, M. (2016). The different forms of spousal violence. In *Forensic psychology of spousal violence* (pp. 33–43). Elsevier. https://doi.org/10.1016/b978-0-12-803533-7.00003-x

Peltzer, K., Pengpid, S., McFarlane, J., & Banyini, M. (2013). Mental health consequences of intimate partner violence in Vhembe district, South Africa. *General Hospital Psychiatry, 35*(5), 545–550. https://doi.org/10.1016/j.genhosppsych.2013.04.001

Pervin, D. (2014). Post-divorce maintenance for Muslim women : Which path to follow in Bangladesh? *Society & Change, 8*(1), 7–26. https://societyandchange.com/uploads/1509597310.pdf

Peterman, A. (2011). Women's property rights and gendered policies: Implications for women's long-term welfare in rural Tanzania. *Journal of Development Studies, 47*(1), 1–30. https://doi.org/10.1080/00220381003600366

Peterson, J. E. (1990). Change and continuity in Arab Gulf society. In C. Davies (Ed.), *After the War: Iraq, Iran and the Arab Gulf* (pp. 287–312). Carden Publications. http://jepeterson.net/sitebuildercontent/sitebuilderfiles/Peterson_Change_and_Continuity_in_Gulf_Society_1990.pdf

Pinto, I. V., Bernal, R. T. I., Souza, M. d. F. M. d., & Malta, D. C. (2021). Fatores associados ao óbito de mulheres com notificação de violência por parceiro íntimo no Brasil. *Ciência & Saúde Coletiva, 26*(3), 975–985. https://doi.org/10.1590/1413-81232021263.00132021

Postmus, J. L., Plummer, S. B., & Stylianou, A. M. (2016). Measuring economic abuse in the lives of survivors: Revising the scale of economic Abuse. *Violence Against Women, 22*(6), 692–703. https://doi.org/10.1177/1077801215610012

Postmus, J. L., Plummer, S. B., McMahon, S., Murshid, N. S., & Kim, M. S. (2012). Understanding economic abuse in the lives of survivors. *Journal of Interpersonal Violence, 27*(3), 411–430. https://doi.org/10.1177/0886260511421669

Preece, D., & Williams, K. (2017). Transcription: A review of the literature and implications for psychotherapy research. *Psychology and Psychotherapy: Theory, Research and Practice, 90*(3), 406–423. https://doi.org/10.1111/papt.12126

Priestley, S., & Lee, K. A. (2021). Understanding IPV perpetration among young Jamaican men: The role of socialization and attitudinal factors. *Journal of Interpersonal Violence, 36*(17–18), NP9053–NP9077. https://doi.org/10.1177/0886260519854553

Qureshi, K. (2020). Transnational divorce and remarriage between Pakistan and Britain: Intersectionality, harmful immigration rules and internal racism. *Population, Space and Place*, (September), e2396. 1–11. https://doi.org/10.1002/psp.2396

Rabaan, H., Young, A. L., & Dombrowski, L. (2021). Daughters of men: Saudi women's sociotechnical agency practices in addressing domestic abuse. *Proceedings of the ACM on Human-Computer Interaction, 4*(CSCW3), 1–31. https://doi.org/10.1145/3432923

Rahaman, M., Sen, S., Rana, M. J., & Ghosh, S. (2021). Is consanguineous marriage related to spousal violence in India? Evidence from the National Family Health Survey, 2015–16. *Journal of Biosocial Science, 1–16*, 959–974. https://doi.org/10.1017/S0021932021000626

Rahebi, S. M., Rahnavardi, M., Rezaie-Chamani, S., Nazari, M., & Sabetghadam, S. (2019). Relationship between domestic violence and infertility. *Eastern Mediterranean Health Journal, 25*(8), 537–542. https://doi.org/10.26719/emhj.19.001

Rahman, M., Nakamura, K., Seino, K., & Kizuki, M. (2013). Does gender inequity increase the risk of intimate partner violence among women? Evidence from a national Bangladeshi sample. *PLoS One, 8*(12), e82423. https://doi.org/10.1371/journal.pone.0082423

Raj, A., Santana, M. C., La Marche, A., Amaro, H., Cranston, K., & Silverman, J. G. (2006). Perpetration of intimate partner violence associated with sexual risk behaviors among young adult men. *American Journal of Public Health, 96*(10), 1873–1878. https://doi.org/10.2105/AJPH.2005.081554

Rashad, H., Osman, M., & Roudi-Fahimi, F. (2005). Marriage in the Arab World. *Population Reference Bureau*, 2–8. https://citeseerx.ist.psu.edu/viewdoc/download?doi=10.1.1.738.1360&rep=rep1&type=pdf

Rathi, P., Pachauri, J., & Pooja Rathi, C. (2018). Problems faced by divorced women in their pre and post-divorce period: A sociological study with reference to District Meerut. *Journal of Pharmacognosy and Phytochemistry, 7*(1), 207–212. https://www.phytojournal.com/archives/2018/vol7issue1/PartC/6-6-234-823.pdf

Renzetti, C. M., Follingstad, D. R., & Coker, A. L. (Eds.). (2017). *Preventing intimate partner violence: Interdisciplinary perspectives* (1st ed.). Bristol University Press. https://doi.org/10.2307/j.ctt1t89gf6

Rhodes, N. R., & McKenzie, E. B. (1998). Why do battered women stay?: Three decades of research. *Aggression and Violent Behavior, 3*(4), 391–406. https://doi.org/10.1016/S1359-1789(97)00025-6

Riggs, D. S., Caulfield, M. B., & Street, A. E. (2000). Risk for domestic violence: Factors associated with perpetration and victimization. *Journal of Clinical Psychology, 56*(10), 1289–1316. https://doi.org/10.1002/1097-4679(200010)56:10<1289::AID-JCLP4>3.0.CO;2-Z

Rioli, G., Sgarbi, C., Moretti, V., & Sinisi, A. (2017). An update on intimate partner violence and mental health. *Minerva Psichiatrica, 58*(4), 216–233. https://doi.org/10.23736/S0391-1772.17.01943-4

Rizo, C. F., Givens, A., & Lombardi, B. (2017). A systematic review of coping among heterosexual female IPV survivors in the United States with a focus on the conceptualization and measurement of coping. *Aggression and Violent Behavior, 34*, 35–50. https://doi.org/10.1016/j.avb.2017.03.006

Roberts, A. L., Gilman, S. E., Fitzmaurice, G., Decker, M. R., & Koenen, K. C. (2010). Witness of intimate partner violence in childhood and perpetration of intimate partner violence in adulthood. *Epidemiology, 21*(6), 809–818. https://doi.org/10.1097/EDE.0b013e3181f39f03

Rocca, C. H., Rathod, S., Falle, T., Pande, R. P., & Krishnan, S. (2009). Challenging assumptions about women's empowerment: Social and economic resources and domestic violence among young married women in urban South India. *International Journal of Epidemiology, 38*(2), 577–585. https://doi.org/10.1093/ije/dyn226

Ruffin, A. K. (2021). *Family structure and women's experiences of intimate partner violence* [Unpublished doctoral dissertation]. University of Pennsylvania.

Ruiz-Pérez, I., Plazaola-Castaño, J., Álvarez-Kindelán, M., Palomo-Pinto, M., Arnalte-Barrera, M., Bonet-Pla, Á., et al. (2006). Sociodemographic associations of physical, emotional, and sexual intimate partner violence in Spanish women. *Annals of Epidemiology, 16*(5), 357–363. https://doi.org/10.1016/j.annepidem.2005.03.007

Sabri, Y. (2021). Depression and post-traumatic stress disorder in females exposed to intimate partner violence. *Middle East Current Psychiatry, 28*(1). https://doi.org/10.1186/s43045-021-00157-x

Sarkar, K., & Rizzi, E. (2020). Love marriage in India. Document de Travail 14, Centre de recherche en démographie. *Louvain-la-Neuve*, 1–42. https://doi.org/10.13140/RG.2.2.14596.55687

Sato-Dilorenzo, A., & Sharps, P. W. (2007). Dangerous intimate partner relationships and women's mental health and health behaviors. *Issues in Mental Health Nursing, 28*(8), 837–848. https://doi.org/10.1080/01612840701493535

Semahegn, A., & Mengistie, B. (2015). Domestic violence against women and associated factors in Ethiopia: Systematic review. *Reproductive Health, 12*(1), 78. https://doi.org/10.1186/s12978-015-0072-1

Sezgin, A. U., & Punamäki, R. L. (2021). Type of traumatic events, mental health problems, and posttraumatic cognitions among eastern Anatolian women. *Journal of Interpersonal Violence, 36*(17–18), NP9501–NP9525. https://doi.org/10.1177/0886260519858385

Shahid, A. (2013). Post-divorce maintenance for Muslim women in Pakistan and Bangladesh: A comparative perspective. *International Journal of Law, Policy and the Family, 27*(2), 197–215. https://doi.org/10.1093/lawfam/ebt004

Shamu, S., Abrahams, N., Temmerman, M., Musekiwa, A., & Zarowsky, C. (2011). A systematic review of African studies on intimate partner violence against pregnant women: Prevalence and risk factors. *PLoS One, 6*(3), 1–9. https://doi.org/10.1371/journal.pone.0017591

Sharma, A. (2001). Healing the wounds of domestic abuse: Improving the effectiveness of feminist therapeutic interventions with immigrant and racially visible women who have been abused. *Violence Against Women, 7*(12), 1405–1428. https://doi.org/10.1177/10778010122183928

Sharp-Jeffs, N. (2015). *Money matters: Research into the extent and nature of financial abuse within intimate relationships in the UK*. London Metropolitan University. http://repository.londonmet.ac.uk/1481/1/Money-Matters.pdf

Sheikhan, Z., Ozgoli, G., Azar, M., & Alavimajd, H. (2014). Domestic violence in Iranian infertile women. *Medical Journal of the Islamic Republic of Iran, 28*(1), 152. https://pubmed.ncbi.nlm.nih.gov/25695010/

Sheykhi, M. T. (2020). World perspective of divorce in selected countries: A sociological appraisal. *World Family Medicine, 18*(6), 66–70.

Shockley, B. (2018). Competence and electability: Exploring the limitations on female candidates in Qatar. *Journal of Women, Politics & Policy, 39*(4), 467–489. https://doi.org/10.1080/1554477x.2018.1511125

Siegel, S. Y. (2012). Non parimetric tests statistics. *The American Statistician, 11*(3), 13–19. http://www.jstor.org/stable/2685679

Siganporia, M. (1993a). Indian Muslim women: Post divorce problems and social support. *Indian Journal of Social Work, 54*(3), 355–355. TISS – The Indian Journal of Social Work Achieve. https://journals.tiss.edu/archive/index.php/ijswarchive/article/view/3274

Siganporia, M. (1993b). Indian Muslim women: Post divorce problems and social support. *Indian Journal of Social Work, 54*(3), 355–355. https://journals.tiss.edu/archive/index.php/ijswarchive/article/view/3274

Signorelli, M. S., Arcidiacono, E., Musumeci, G., Di Nuovo, S., & Aguglia, E. (2014). Detecting domestic violence: Italian validation of Revised Conflict Tactics Scale (CTS-2). *Journal of Family Violence, 29*(4), 361–369. https://doi.org/10.1007/s10896-014-9594-5

Singer, J. B. (1989). Divorce reform and gender justice. *North Carolina Law Review, 67*(5), 1103–1121. https://scholarship.law.unc.edu/nclr/vol67/iss5/8

Singh, S., & Wassenaar, D. (2016). Contextualising the role of the gatekeeper in social science research. *South African Journal of Bioethics and Law, 9*(1), 42. https://doi.org/10.7196/sajbl.2016.v9i1.465

Smith, M. D. (1990). Sociodemographic risk factors in wife abuse: Results from a survey of Toronto women. *Canadian Journal of Sociology, 15*(1), 39. https://doi.org/10.2307/3341172

Smith-Marek, E. N., Cafferky, B., Dharnidharka, P., Mallory, A. B., Dominguez, M., High, J., Stith, S. M., & Mendez, M. (2015). Effects of childhood experiences of family violence on adult partner violence: A meta-analytic review. *Journal of Family Theory & Review, 7*(4), 498–519. https://doi.org/10.1111/jftr.12113

Solanke, B. L., Bisiriyu, A. L., & Oyedokun, A. (2018). Is the likelihood of spousal violence lower or higher among childless women? Evidence from Nigeria demographic and health surveys. *BMC Women's Health, 18*(1), 1–12. https://doi.org/10.1186/s12905-018-0514-3

Soliman, A., Alyafie, A., & Gomaa, A.-S. (2019). *Factors that influence Qatari family stability: Testing a vulnerability and resiliency model.* Doha International Family Institute (DIFI), 1–27. https://www.difi.org.qa/wp-content/uploads/2022/09/B-h-1.pdf

Song, Y. Y., & Lu, Y. (2015). Decision tree methods: Applications for classification and prediction. *Shanghai Archives of Psychiatry, 27*(2), 130–135. https://doi.org/10.11919/j.issn.1002-0829.215044

Speizer, I. S., & Pearson, E. (2011). Association between early marriage and intimate partner violence in India: A focus on youth from Bihar and Rajasthan. *Journal of Interpersonal Violence, 26*(10), 1963–1981. https://doi.org/10.1177/0886260510372947

Spencer, C., Mallory, A. B., Cafferky, B. M., Kimmes, J. G., Beck, A. R., & Stith, S. M. (2019). Mental health factors and intimate partner violence perpetration and victimization: A meta-analysis. *Psychology of Violence, 9*(1), 1–17. https://doi.org/10.1037/vio0000156

Stein, M. B., & Kennedy, C. (2001). Major depressive and post-traumatic stress disorder comorbidity in female victims of intimate partner violence. *Journal of Affective Disorders, 66*(2–3), 133–138. https://doi.org/10.1016/S0165-0327(00)00301-3

Stepney, E. (2016). *Housing tenure and economic inequality among Qatari citizens.* SESRI Policy Brief, 2016(3), 3–4. The Social and Economic Survey Research Institute, Qatar University. https://qspace.qu.edu.qa/bitstream/handle/10576/5116/Qatari-Renters-Eng-Final.pdf?sequence=2&isAllowed=y

Stöckl, H., Devries, K., Rotstein, A., Abrahams, N., Campbell, J., Watts, C., & Moreno, C. G. (2013). The global prevalence of intimate partner homicide: A systematic review. *The Lancet, 382*(9895), 859–865. https://doi.org/10.1016/S0140-6736(13)61030-2

Straus, H., Cerulli, C., McNutt, L. A., Rhodes, K. V., Conner, K. R., Kemball, R. S., Kaslow, N. J., & Houry, D. (2009). Intimate partner violence and functional health status: Associations with severity, danger, and self-advocacy behaviors. *Journal of Women's Health, 18*(5), 625–631. https://doi.org/10.1089/jwh.2007.0521

Straus, M. A. (2008). Dominance and symmetry in partner violence by male and female university students in 32 nations. *Children and Youth Services Review, 30*(3), 252–275. https://doi.org/10.1016/j.childyouth.2007.10.004

Straus, M. A., Hamby, S. L., Boney-McCoy, S., & Sugarman, D. B. (1996). The Revised Conflict Tactics Scales (CTS2): Development and preliminary psychometric data. *Journal of Family Issues, 17*(3), 283–316. https://doi.org/10.1177/019251396017003001

Stuart, G. L., Moore, T. M., Gordon, K. C., Ramsey, S. E., & Kahler, C. W. (2006). Psychopathology in women arrested for domestic violence. *Journal of Interpersonal Violence, 21*(3), 376–389. https://doi.org/10.1177/0886260505282888

Stylianou, A. M. (2018). Economic abuse experiences and depressive symptoms among victims of intimate partner violence. *Journal of Family Violence, 33*(6), 381–392. https://doi.org/10.1007/s10896-018-9973-4

Sultana, A. (2012). Patriarchy and women's subordination: A theoretical analysis. *Arts Faculty Journal, 4*(2010–2011), 1–18. https://doi.org/10.3329/afj.v4i0.12929

Suntornkanit, N., & Varma, P. (2018). Influence of gender role attitude, quality of alternatives, investment size, and commitment on marital satisfaction between Thai women who married Thai men and Thai women who married foreign men. *Scholar: Human Sciences, 9*(2), 106–119. https://core.ac.uk/download/pdf/233619845.pdf

Sutherland, C. A., Sullivan, C. M., & Bybee, D. I. (2001). Effects of intimate partner violence versus poverty on women's health. *Violence Against Woman, 7*(10), 1122–1143. https://doi.org/10.1177/10778010122183775

Taft, C. T., Resick, P. A., Watkins, L. E., & Panuzio, J. (2009). An investigation of posttraumatic stress disorder and depressive symptomatology among female victims of interpersonal trauma. *Journal of Family Violence, 24*(6), 407–415. https://doi.org/10.1007/s10896-009-9243-6

Tahirih. (2016, October 20). *Arranged marriage*. Tahirih Justice Center. Forced Marriage Initiative. https://preventforcedmarriage.org/understanding-arranged-and-forced-marriage/.

Tanimu, T. S., Yohanna, S., & Omeiza, S. Y. (2021). The pattern and correlates of intimate partner violence among women in Kano, Nigeria. *African Journal of Primary Health Care and Family Medicine, 8*(1), 1–7. https://doi.org/10.4102/phcfm.v8i1.1209

Tashakkori, A., Johnson, R. B., & Teddlie, C. (2020). *Foundations of mixed methods research: Integrating quantitative and qualitative approaches in the social and behavioral sciences* (2nd ed.). Sage Publications.

Tashkandi, A., & Rasheed, F. P. (2009). Wife abuse: a hidden problem. A study among Saudi women attending PHC centres. *Eastern Mediterranean health journal = La revue de sante de la Mediterranee orientale = al-Majallah al-sihhiyah li-sharq al-mutawassit, 15*(5), 1242–1253. http://apps.who.int/iris/bitstream/handle/10665/117755/15_5_2009_1242_1253.pdf?sequence=1&isAllowed=y

Taylor, J. A. (1953). A personality scale of manifest anxiety. *Journal of Abnormal and Social Psychology, 48*(2), 285–290. https://doi.org/10.1037/h0056264

Tehreem, A., Zakar, R., Khan, B. S., Hussain, M. F., & Afza, R. (2021). Factors associated with termination of pregnancy among married adolescent girls in Pakistan: Secondary analysis of data from Pakistan demographic and health survey. *JAMDC, 3*(3), 95–102. https://doi.org/10.51127/JAMDCV3I3OA01

Tekkas Kerman, K., & Betrus, P. (2020). Violence against women in Turkey: A social ecological framework of determinants and prevention strategies. *Trauma, Violence & Abuse, 21*(3), 510–526. https://doi.org/10.1177/1524838018781104

Terrazas-Carrillo, E. C., & McWhirter, P. T. (2015). Employment status and intimate partner violence among Mexican women. *Journal of Interpersonal Violence, 30*(7), 1128–1152. https://doi.org/10.1177/0886260514539848

Thabet, A. A., Tawahina, A. A., El Sarraj, E., & Vostanis, P. (2008). Exposure to war trauma and PTSD among parents and children in the Gaza strip. *European Child and Adolescent Psychiatry, 17*(4), 191–199. https://doi.org/10.1007/s00787-007-0653-9

Thabet, A., Tawahina, A., Victoria, T., & Vostanis, P. (2015). PTSD, depression, and anxiety among Palestinian women victims of domestic violence in the Gaza strip. *British Journal of Education, Society & Behavioural Science, 11*(2), 1–13. https://doi.org/10.9734/bjesbs/2015/18960

The Shura Council. (2018). *History*. https://www.shura.qa/en/Pages/About-Council/History

Thomson, D. R., Bah, A. B., Rubanzana, W. G., & Mutesa, L. (2015). Correlates of intimate partner violence against women during a time of rapid social transition in Rwanda: Analysis of the 2005 and 2010 demographic and health surveys. *BMC Women's Health, 15*(1), 1–13. https://doi.org/10.1186/s12905-015-0257-3

Tiruneh, F. N., Chuang, K. Y., Ntenda, P. A. M., & Chuang, Y. C. (2018). Unwanted pregnancy, pregnancy loss, and other risk factors for intimate partner violence in the Democratic Republic of the Congo. *Women and Health, 58*(9), 983–1000. https://doi.org/10.1080/03630242.2017.1377800

Tiruye, T. Y., Harris, M. L., Chojenta, C., Holliday, E., & Loxton, D. (2020). Intimate partner violence against women in Ethiopia and its association with unintended pregnancy: A national cross-sectional survey. *International Journal of Public Health, 65*(9), 1657–1667. https://doi.org/10.1007/s00038-020-01510-3

Tiwari, A., Chan, K. L., Cheung, D. S. T., Fong, D. Y. T., Yan, E. C. W., & Tang, D. H. M. (2015). The differential effects of intimate terrorism and situational couple violence on mental health outcomes among abused Chinese women: A mixed-method study. *BMC Public Health, 15*(1), 1–12. https://doi.org/10.1186/s12889-015-1649-x

Tokuç, B., Ekuklu, G., & Avcioğlu, S. (2010). Domestic violence against married women in Edirne. *Journal of Interpersonal Violence, 25*(5), 832–847. https://doi.org/10.1177/0886260509336960

Tracy, S. R. (2007). Patriarchy and domestic violence: Challenging common misconceptions. *Journal of the Evangelical Theological Society, 50*(3), 573–594.

Treuthart, M. P., & Rosenbaum, S. A. (2013). Engendering a clinic: Lessons learned from a domestic violence clinical course in Qatar. *International Review of Law, 2013*(4), 1–24. https://doi.org/10.5339/irl.2013.dv.1

Ugwuanyi, B. C., Formella, Z., & Szadejko, K. (2022). *Reporting domestic violence on women. An exploratory research in Igboland of Nigeria* (No.:16). Transdisciplinary Studies on Culture and Education. Scientific Yearbook of the Kuyavian-Pomeranian University in Bydgoszcz. https://www.researchgate.net/publication/358187209_REPORTING_DOMESTIC_VIOLENCE_ON_WOMEN_AN_EXPLORATORY_RESEARCH_IN_IGBOLAND_OF_NIGERIA

Ulloa, E. C., & Hammett, J. F. (2016). The effect of gender and perpetrator–victim role on mental health outcomes and risk behaviors associated with intimate partner violence. *Journal of Interpersonal Violence, 31*(7), 1184–1207. https://doi.org/10.1177/0886260514564163

Umubyeyi, A., Mogren, I., Ntaganira, J., & Krantz, G. (2014). Intimate partner violence and its contribution to mental disorders in men and women in the post genocide Rwanda: Findings from a population based study. *BMC Psychiatry, 14*, Article 315. https://doi.org/10.1186/s12888-014-0315-7

Usta, J., Farver, J. A., & Pashayan, N. (2007). Domestic violence: The Lebanese experience. *Public Health, 121*(3), 208–219. https://doi.org/10.1016/j.puhe.2006.09.014

Uyanık, G. K., & Güler, N. (2013). A study on multiple linear regression analysis. *Procedia - Social and Behavioral Sciences, 106*, 234–240. https://doi.org/10.1016/j.sbspro.2013.12.027

van Teijlingen, E., & Hundley, V. (2002). The importance of pilot studies. *Nursing Standard, 16*(40), 33–36. https://doi.org/10.7748/ns2002.06.16.40.33.c3214

Varma, D., Chandra, P. S., Thomas, T., & Carey, M. P. (2007). Intimate partner violence and sexual coercion among pregnant women in India: Relationship with depression and post-traumatic stress disorder. *Journal of Affective Disorders, 102*(1–3), 227–235. https://doi.org/10.1016/j.jad.2006.09.026

Vassiliou, V., Georgas, J. G., & Vassiliou, G. (1967). Variations in manifest anxiety due to sex, age, and education. *Journal of Personality and Social Psychology, 6*(2), 194–197. https://doi.org/10.1037/h0024572

Volpe, E. M., Hardie, T. L., Cerulli, C., Sommers, M. S., & Morrison-Beedy, D. (2013). What's age got to do with it? Partner age difference, power, intimate partner violence, and sexual risk in urban adolescents. *Journal of Interpersonal Violence, 28*(10), 2068–2087. https://doi.org/10.1177/0886260512471082

Vujadinovi, D., Fröhlich, M., & Giegerich, T. (Eds.). (2023). *Gender-competent legal education*. Springer. https://doi.org/10.1007/978-3-031-14360-1

Walklate, S., Fitz-Gibbon, K., & McCulloch, J. (2018). Is more law the answer? Seeking justice for victims of intimate partner violence through the reform of legal categories. *Criminology and Criminal Justice, 18*(1), 115–131. https://doi.org/10.1177/1748895817728561

Walton-Moss, B. J., Manganello, J., Frye, V., & Campbell, J. C. (2005). Risk factors for intimate partner violence and associated injury among urban women. *Journal of Community Health, 30*(5), 377–389. https://doi.org/10.1007/s10900-005-5518-x

Wang, T., Wong, J. Y. H., & Fong, D. Y. T. (2022). Subjective socioeconomic status: An indicator of intimate partner violence in middle-aged adults in Hong Kong. *Health and Social Care in the Community, 30*(5), 1–8. https://doi.org/10.1111/hsc.13760

Watson, L. B., & Ancis, J. R. (2013). Power and control in the legal system: From marriage/relationship to divorce and custody. *Violence Against Women, 19*(2), 166–186. https://doi.org/10.1177/1077801213478027

Watts, C., & Zimmerman, C. (2002). Violence against women: Global scope and magnitude. *Lancet, 359*(9313), 1232–1237. https://doi.org/10.1016/S0140-6736(02)08221-1

Weiner, S. (2016). Rethinking patriarchy and kinship in the Arab Gulf states. *Women and gender in Middle East politics workshop* (March 11, 2016). Project on Middle East Political Science. https://pomeps.org/rethinking-patriarchy-and-kinship-in-the-arab-gulf-states

Wickrama, K. A. S., Lorenz, F. O., Conger, R. D., Elder, G. H., Abraham, W. T., & Fang, S.-A. (2006). Changes in family financial circumstances and the physical health of married and recently divorced mothers. *Social Science & Medicine, 63*(1), 123–136. https://doi.org/10.1016/j.socscimed.2005.12.003

World Health Organization (WHO). (2012a, November 23). *Understanding and addressing violence against women: Intimate partner violence.* 1–12. https://apps.who.int/iris/bitstream/handle/10665/77432/WHO_RHR_12.36_eng.pdf

World Health Organization (WHO). (2012b, November 23). *Understanding and addressing violence against women: Femicide.* 1–8. https://apps.who.int/iris/bitstream/handle/10665/77421/WHO_RHR_12.38_eng.pdf

World Health Organization (WHO). (2021). *Caring for women subjected to violence: a WHO training curriculum for health care providers (Revised edition).* https://apps.who.int/iris/handle/10665/349539

Wright, E. N., Hanlon, A., Lozano, A., & Teitelman, A. M. (2019). The impact of intimate partner violence, depressive symptoms, alcohol dependence, and perceived stress on 30-year cardiovascular disease risk among young adult women: A multiple mediation analysis. *Preventive Medicine, 121*(August 2018), 47–54. https://doi.org/10.1016/j.ypmed.2019.01.016

Xu, X., Zhu, F., O'Campo, P., Koenig, M. A., Mock, V., & Campbell, J. (2005). Prevalence of and risk factors for intimate partner violence in China. *American Journal of Public Health, 95*(1), 78–85. https://doi.org/10.2105/AJPH.2003.023978

Yadav, A., Kumar, P., & Kumar, J. (2022). Domestic violence: Consequences, causes and preventive measures. *Indian Journal of Psychology and Education, 12*(2), 40–43. https://www.researchgate.net/publication/362760828_Domestic_Violence_Consequences_Causes_and_Preventive_Measures

Yau, J. H. Y., Fong, D. Y. T., & Wong, J. Y. H. (2020). Risk factors for and mental well-being outcomes of economic abuse in Hong Kong Chinese population. *Violence and Victims, 35*(2), 246–265. https://doi.org/10.1891/VV-D-18-00057

Yau, J. H. Y., Wong, J. Y. H., Choi, E. P. H., & Fong, D. Y. T. (2019). Transcultural validation of the 12-item scale of economic abuse in Chinese population. *Violence and Victims, 34*(5), 804–817. https://doi.org/10.1891/0886-6708.VV-D-17-00164

Yoshihama, M., Blazevski, J., & Bybee, D. (2014). Enculturation and attitudes toward intimate partner violence and gender roles in an Asian Indian population: Implications for community-based prevention. *American Journal of Community Psychology, 53*(3–4), 249–260. https://doi.org/10.1007/s10464-014-9627-5

Yount, K. M. (2011). Women's conformity as resistance to intimate partner violence in Assiut, Egypt. *Sex Roles, 64*(1–2), 43–58. https://doi.org/10.1007/s11199-010-9884-1

Yüksel-Kaptanoğlu, I., Türkyilmaz, A. S., & Heise, L. (2012). What puts women at risk of violence from their husbands? Findings from a large, nationally representative survey in Turkey. *Journal of Interpersonal Violence, 27*(14), 2743–2769. https://doi.org/10.1177/0886260512438283

Zahidi, S. (2018). *Fifty million rising: The new generation of working women transforming the Muslim World* (1st ed.). Nation Books.

Zakar, R., Nasrullah, M., Zakar, M. Z., & Ali, H. (2016). The association of intimate partner violence with unintended pregnancy and pregnancy loss in Pakistan. *International Journal of Gynecology & Obstetrics, 133*(1), 26–31. https://doi.org/10.1016/j.ijgo.2015.09.009

Zara, G., & Gino, S. (2018). Intimate partner violence and its escalation into femicide. Frailty thy name is "violence against women". *Frontiers in Psychology, 9*, 1–11. https://doi.org/10.3389/fpsyg.2018.01777

Zeoli, A. M., Rivera, E. A., Sullivan, C. M., & Kubiak, S. (2013). Post-separation abuse of women and their children: Boundary-setting and family court utilization among victimized mothers. *Journal of Family Violence, 28*(6), 547–560. https://doi.org/10.1007/s10896-013-9528-7

Zhang, Y., & Breunig, R. V. (2021). Gender norms and domestic abuse: Evidence from Australia (March 31, 2021). Tax and transfer policy institute - working paper 5/2021. *SSRN Electronic Journal*. https://doi.org/10.2139/ssrn.3824466

Zlotnick, C., Johnson, D. M., & Kohn, R. (2006). Intimate partner violence and long-term psychosocial functioning in a national sample of American women. *Journal of Interpersonal Violence, 21*(2), 262–275. https://doi.org/10.1177/0886260505282564

Zweiri, M., & Al Qawasmi, F. (Eds.). (2020). *Contemporary Qatar - Examining state and society* (4th ed.). Springer. https://doi.org/10.1007/978-981-16-1391-3

MIX
Papier aus verantwortungsvollen Quellen
Paper from responsible sources
FSC® C105338

FSC
www.fsc.org

If you have any concerns about our products,
you can contact us on
ProductSafety@springernature.com

In case Publisher is established outside the EU,
the EU authorized representative is:
Springer Nature Customer Service Center GmbH
Europaplatz 3, 69115 Heidelberg, Germany

Printed by Libri Plureos GmbH
in Hamburg, Germany